WRITING FOR PUBLICATION IN NURSING

SECOND EDITION

Marilyn H. Oermann, PhD, RN, FAAN, ANEF, is a Professor and Chair of Adult and Geriatric Health at the School of Nursing, University of North Carolina at Chapel Hill, Chapel Hill, North Carolina. She is author/co-author of 12 nursing education books and many articles on clinical evaluation, teaching in nursing, and writing for publication. She is the Editor of the *Journal of Nursing Care Quality* and past editor of the *Annual Review of Nursing Education*. Dr. Oermann lectures widely on teaching and evaluation in nursing and on writing for publication.

Judith C. Hays, PhD, RN, is Associate Professor Emerita at the Duke University School of Nursing in Durham, North Carolina. She is author/co-author of a psychiatric epidemiology textbook and more than 70 scientific articles on late-life living arrangements, religiousness, depression, palliative care and bereavement, and nursing history. She is co-Editor of the journal *Public Health Nursing*. Dr. Hays teaches scientific writing to graduate nurses in master's and doctor of nursing practice (DNP) programs.

WRITING FOR PUBLICATION IN NURSING

SECOND EDITION

Marilyn H. Oermann, PhD, RN, FAAN, ANEF

Judith C. Hays, PhD, RN

SPRINGER PUBLISHING COMPANY
NEW YORK

Springer Publishing Company, LLC
11 West 42nd Street
New York, NY 10036
www.springerpub.com

Acquisitions Editor: Margaret Zuccarini
Production Editor: Gayle Lee
Cover Design: Mimi Flow
Composition: Ashita Shah at Newgen Imaging Systems, Ltd.

ISBN: 978–0–8261–1802–8
E-book ISBN: 978–0–8261–1804–2

13 14 15 16 17 18 / 12 11 10 9 8 7 6

The author and the publisher of this Work have made every effort to use sources believed to be reliable to provide information that is accurate and compatible with the standards generally accepted at the time of publication. Because medical science is continually advancing, our knowledge base continues to expand. Therefore, as new information becomes available, changes in procedures become necessary. We recommend that the reader always consult current research and specific institutional policies before performing any clinical procedure. The author and publisher shall not be liable for any special, consequential, or exemplary damages resulting, in whole or in part, from the readers' use of, or reliance on, the information contained in this book. The publisher has no responsibility for the persistence or accuracy of URLs for external or third-party Internet Web sites referred to in this publication and does not guarantee that any content on such Web sites is, or will remain, accurate or appropriate.

Library of Congress Cataloging-in-Publication Data

Oermann, Marilyn H.
    Writing for publication in nursing/Marilyn H. Oermann, Judith C. Hays.
      2nd ed.
        p. ; cm.
    Includes bibliographical references and index.
    ISBN 978-0-8261-1802-8
    1. Nursing—Authorship. 2. Nursing literature—Marketing. 3. Nursing—Periodicals.
I. Hays, Judith C. II. Title.
    [DNLM: 1. Writing—Nurses' Instruction. 2. Periodicals as Topic—Nurses' Instruction.
3. Publishing—Nurses' Instruction. 4. Research—methods—Nurses' Instruction.
WZ 345 O29w 2011]
    RT24.O35 2011
    808'.06661—dc22   2010012536

Printed in the United States of America by Courier Corporation.

To our students and readers,
whose enthusiasm for disseminating
the best of their nursing practice, research, and education
to the broadest possible audience
in the widest variety of formats
inspired the second edition of this book.

CONTENTS

Writing for publication in nursing is essential to disseminate evidence, share initiatives and innovations with others, provide new information to keep nurses up-to-date, communicate the findings of research studies, and develop the science base of the profession. Writing manuscripts is hard work, but the process can be simplified by understanding how to develop a manuscript and submit it for publication. *Writing for Publication in Nursing* was prepared for beginning and experienced authors, for nurses who want to learn how to write for publication, and for graduate students in nursing who need to learn how to write research reports, clinical articles, systematic reviews, and other types of articles.

The book describes the process of writing, beginning with an idea, searching the literature, preparing an outline, writing a draft and revising it, and developing the final paper. How to select a journal and gear the writing to the intended audience, submit a manuscript to a journal, revise a paper and respond to reviewers, and carry out other steps to facilitate publication are discussed in the book. A chapter is devoted to writing research articles to assist nurses in preparing their work for publication; strategies are included for developing manuscripts from theses and dissertations. Other chapters describe principles for preparing articles that disseminate the outcomes of reviews of research evidence, articles on clinical practice topics, case reports, and other types of papers. A new chapter in this edition guides authors in writing chapters and books.

The book serves as reference for students at all levels of nursing education to guide them in writing papers for courses. Many nursing programs expect students to demonstrate competency in writing as an outcome of the program. *Writing for Publication in Nursing* is a good resource for that purpose. Graduate students in particular can use the book to learn how to write for publication, an essential skill for advanced practice nurses, researchers, educators, administrators, and nurses in other roles to disseminate their work and for their career advancement.

Writing for Publication in Nursing can be used in conjunction with the style manual in the nursing program. While style manuals direct students in preparing citations, references, tables, and figures, and guide them on other aspects of style, these manuals do not teach students the process of writing nor how to prepare a paper for publication in nursing.

The book contains many examples and resources for writing in nursing and other healthcare professions. These resources make writing easier for both beginning and experienced authors.

Writing for publication in nursing is essential to disseminate the findings of research and evidence for practice, communicate knowledge and share expertise with other nurses, inform nurses of initiatives and innovations developed for patient populations and settings, and advance the profession. Chapter 1 introduces the steps the author follows in planning, writing, and publishing manuscripts in nursing. The focus is on early writing decisions, such as generating ideas, selecting a topic, and deciding on the type of article to be written. The author evaluates if the ideas to be presented are worth writing about and are important enough to be published.

The next steps are to identify the audience to whom the manuscript will be directed and to select a journal that might be interested in publishing it. The purpose of the manuscript and how it will be developed guide the author in deciding on possible journals. The goal is to match the topic and type of manuscript with an appropriate journal and readers who would be interested in it. Chapter 2 discusses how to evaluate possible journals, select an appropriate one, and write a query letter to gauge the interest of the journals' editors. Valuable resources in this chapter include a description of Web sites of directories of journals, checklists for determining the audience and the "right" journal, and a sample query letter.

Decisions about the focus of the manuscript, audience, and journal are important early in the writing process. Other decisions pertain to authorship; if these are not made before beginning the writing project, they may create problems and conflict among the authors later on. Each individual designated as an author on a manuscript or other type of paper should have contributed sufficiently to it. Chapter 3 addresses authorship and author responsibilities in preparing to write. Because many papers are written in groups, strategies are provided to facilitate this process.

Chapter 4 prepares the author for reviewing the literature and writing a literature review for a manuscript and other types of papers. Although literature reviews for research studies, theses and dissertations, course work, evidence syntheses, and other purposes vary in the types of literature used, their comprehensiveness, and how they are summarized for the reader, the process of reviewing the literature is the same. Chapter 4 describes bibliographic databases useful for literature reviews in nursing, selecting databases to use, search strategies, analyzing and synthesizing the literature, and writing the literature review. This chapter provides many resources to help nurse-authors with their literature reviews. Strategies to avoid plagiarism and information about obtaining permission to reproduce copyrighted material in a manuscript are included in the chapter.

Research projects are not complete until the findings are communicated to others. All too often nurses conduct important research studies but fail to disseminate the results of their work. Some nurses are not prepared for their role as an author and are unsure how to proceed; others may believe that their work does not warrant publication. However, rigorous research is important to communicate to others, regardless of whether the findings were anticipated or not. Research papers present the findings of quantitative and qualitative research based on original data. Chapter 5 begins with a discussion of how to report research using the conventional format of an introduction and literature review; a methods section, including design and sample, measurements, and analytic strategy; a results section; and a discussion. This basic structure of research articles is known as IMRAD, i.e., **I**ntroduction, **M**ethods, **R**esults, and **D**iscussion. Examples are provided of quantitative and qualitative research articles for authors to learn how to write different sections of these manuscripts. Ethical considerations when writing research papers include deciding the appropriate number of articles to write from a single study and avoidance of redundant or duplicate publications. Authors should take care to protect the privacy rights of their subjects and to avoid defamation of other members of the research community. The chapter concludes by describing pitfalls to avoid when reporting research findings and revising academic papers as research manuscripts.

Nurses in all clinical settings require the most current and complete evidence of effective approaches to guide their decision making and practice. The evidence should be based on a critical appraisal of studies that answer a specific clinical question or examine best practices and the synthesis of findings from across these studies. The preferential use of such approaches is known as evidence-based practice (EBP). With EBP, nurses rely on the review and synthesis of evidence from multiple studies rather than the report of one original research study. Methods are now available to nurse-authors for reviewing and integrating individual studies and summarizing the evidence from them to answer a clinical question or explore a topic of interest. These review methods include integrative reviews, systematic reviews, meta-analyses, and metasyntheses. In addition to review papers, nurses also prepare manuscripts on research utilization, which focus on the structures, process, and outcomes of transferring research knowledge and findings into clinical practice. Manuscripts on EBP address the effectiveness of new approaches or changes in practice as well as the resources needed for implementation and the process used by nurses in a clinical setting to engage in EBP. Chapter 6, a new chapter in this edition, presents guidelines for preparing articles that disseminate the outcomes of reviews of research and other types of papers related to EBP in nursing.

Chapter 7 presents strategies for writing articles about clinical practice. There are many opportunities for preparing these manuscripts: nurses can write about their innovations in practice, unit-based initiatives and projects, updates on clinical topics, new directions in patient care, and research studies and quality improvement projects done in the clinical setting. Considering the wealth of clinical journals in nursing, these publications provide a venue for nurses to share their work with others. General guidelines for writing clinical articles are presented in the chapter including writing research reports for clinical journals and preparing papers on quality improvement projects.

Although research and clinical practice articles are primary formats for nurses to present knowledge to readers, other forms of writing are equally important. Some articles address emerging issues that affect nursing practice, education, or research. These articles may include case reports; descriptions of theory development; commentaries on policies, ethics, or legal aspects of nursing; innovative research methods; historical studies; editorials; and letters to the editor. Nurses also write book reviews and articles for consumer and non-professional audiences. These other types of writing differ in the purposes they are trying to achieve, their format, and often their writing style. Yet all are similar because they address non-trivial topics, provide original insight, and have implications for advancing health and well-being. Chapter 8 describes these other types of papers and provides many examples to guide these forms of writing.

Writing a book or book chapter is different from an article because the author has more opportunity to provide background information and discuss related content, with more pages allowed, than in a manuscript for a journal. Whereas articles generally focus on one topic, books address multiple but related content areas and also require a significant time commitment. Chapter 9 provides information for nurse-authors who are interested in writing a book, including contacting a publisher, developing the prospectus, responsibilities of the author and publisher, the process of writing the book, and working with contributors in an edited book. There also is a section on writing a book chapter.

At this point in the process of writing, the author has identified the type of manuscript, the purpose of the paper, potential journals, and the audience to which the paper will be geared. The author has obtained author guidelines from the target journal, has conducted or updated the literature review, has completed other preparations for writing, and is now ready to begin writing the manuscript. Chapter 10 focuses first on preliminary questions to ask before starting to write and on organizing the content into an outline. Next, the chapter describes how to write the first draft of the manuscript. Finally, the chapter describes the steps in revising the content and organization of the paper and then revising the writing structure and style. Some principles are provided for improving how the paper is written.

Most papers written for publication in nursing include references. The references in the manuscript document the literature reviewed by the author who prepared the paper and provide support for the ideas in it. In Chapter 11 the focus is on citing the references in the manuscript and preparing the reference list. Journals have different reference formats, and the author must prepare the references according to the journal guidelines. Examples are provided of how to cite references in the text and on the reference list using different reference styles.

Tables are essential when the author needs to report detailed information and numeric values. It is often clearer and more efficient to develop a table than to present the information in the text. Figures are valuable for demonstrating trends and patterns, and for some manuscripts the author may include an illustration of a new procedure or a photograph of a patient. Not every manuscript, though, needs tables and figures, and whether to include them is a decision made during the drafting phase of writing the paper. Chapter 12 provides guidelines for deciding when to prepare tables and figures and how to develop them. Examples are included of different types of tables, presenting information in a table and as text when text is preferred and when a table is preferred, and developing figures for a manuscript.

When the author has completed the revisions of the content and format of the paper and prepared the references, tables, and figures, the author is ready to submit the paper to the journal. Prior to submission, the author has some final responsibilities to ensure that the manuscript is consistent with the journal requirements and contains all the required parts for submission. The manuscript is then ready to send to the journal for review. Chapter 13 describes the steps in preparing all elements of the final paper to submit to the journal and details associated with this submission. Examples of these elements are provided in the chapter, and a checklist is included for authors to ensure that all items are submitted with the manuscript to avoid delays in its review.

Chapter 14 presents the editorial review process from the point at which the paper is received in the journal office through the final editorial decision. The roles and responsibilities of the editor, editorial board, and peer reviewers are discussed, and examples are provided of criteria used by reviewers when asked to critique a manuscript for publication. Peer review is not without issues, and some of these are examined in the chapter. Manuscripts submitted to a journal may be accepted without revision or accepted provisionally pending revision, may be returned to the author for a major revision and resubmission, or may be rejected. Each of these editorial decisions has implications for the author and how the author responds to the editor: these are presented in the chapter. Resources for readers include sample peer review forms and sample letters to send with revised manuscripts.

When the manuscript is accepted for publication, the paper moves into the publishing phase. The author has some responsibilities here, such as answering queries and correcting page proofs, but most of the work is done by the publisher of the journal or by the group or individual responsible for the publication. Chapter 15 describes the publishing process that begins with the acceptance of the paper through its publication. Publishers have different ways of handling the manuscript editing phase and forms of the manuscript that they return to the author for proofing. The publishing process is described in the chapter, but the author should recognize that it may differ across journals. Copyright also is presented in the chapter.

Many individuals have contributed to the preparation and writing of this book. The authors extend a special acknowledgment to Margaret Zuccarini who recognized the need for this resource for nursing authors and students and encouraged us to prepare this second edition. Her enthusiasm for writing in nursing is contagious.

Marilyn H. Oermann and Judith C. Hays

PREPARING TO WRITE

1

GETTING STARTED

Writing for publication in nursing is essential to disseminate evidence, share initiatives and innovations with others, provide new information to keep nurses up-to-date, communicate the findings of research studies, and develop the science base of the profession. Writing manuscripts is hard work, but the process can be simplified by understanding how to develop a manuscript and submit it for publication.

Chapter 1 introduces the steps the author follows in planning, writing, and publishing manuscripts in nursing. The focus of chapter 1 is on early writing decisions, such as, generating ideas, selecting a topic, and deciding on the type of article to be written. These are important decisions because they guide the author in selecting potential journals, which is addressed in chapter 2.

■ REASONS TO WRITE

Writing for publication is an important skill for nurses to develop. By communicating initiatives and innovations in clinical practice, findings of research studies and evidence-based practice projects, and new ideas, nurses direct the future of their practice and advance the development of the profession. As nursing attempts to build its evidence base, it is increasingly important for nurses to write about studies they are doing in their clinical practice: the findings of these studies provide the evidence for practice. Writing for publication cannot be considered the responsibility of only nurses in academic settings, for clinicians have a major responsibility to describe the effectiveness of their nursing interventions and the innovations they have developed for patient care. Nurse educators, administrators, managers, and researchers have a similar responsibility—to share knowledge and ideas for the benefit of others.

There are five main reasons to write for publication: (1) to share ideas and expertise with other nurses; (2) to disseminate evidence and the findings of nursing research studies; (3) for promotion, tenure, and other personnel decisions; (4) for development of own knowledge and skills; and (5) for personal satisfaction.

3

Share Ideas and Expertise

Writing for publication provides a way of sharing ideas with other nurses. Through publications, nurses can describe best practices; innovations developed for patients, staff, and students; and new techniques they are using in clinical practice, teaching, management, and administration. Publications keep nurses abreast of new developments in nursing. McGaghie and Webster (2009) identified the opportunity to share knowledge with others as an intrinsic motive to write for publication.

Disseminate Evidence and Research Findings

For nurses involved in research studies and evidence-based practice projects, writing for publication is critical: disseminating research findings and the outcomes of projects to evaluate the effectiveness of nursing interventions are essential to build the knowledge base of nursing, provide new evidence for practice, and develop studies that build on one another. Many clinicians are engaged currently in evidence-based practice projects. Some of these projects are to review and synthesize the available evidence to decide on best practices or if a change in practice is warranted. In other settings nurses are studying the effects of nursing interventions, contributing to the evidence base of nursing. However, those contributions are not realized unless nurses disseminate the findings of their studies and projects. Carlson, Masters, and Pfadt (2008) emphasized the need for clinicians to share their research findings not only within the clinical agency but also to a wider audience; that requires publishing in professional journals.

The essence of a discipline is its body of scientific knowledge, the values and ethics that guide practice in the discipline, and its worth to society (American Association of Colleges of Nursing, 2006). In practice disciplines such as nursing, an added responsibility is the use of research findings and other evidence to guide decisions about patient care. Research findings can only be applied to practice if they are published and made available for use by other clinicians and nursing professionals. All too often nurses conduct important research without disseminating the findings of these studies to others.

Meet Promotion, Tenure, and Other Job Requirements

For nursing faculty in colleges and universities, writing for publication is required for promotion, tenure, and other personnel decisions. Not all articles carry the same weight in these decisions. Typically, databased papers, which report the findings of a research study, published in peer-reviewed journals are highly valued and more important in tenure and promotion decisions than other types of publications such as non-databased articles, chapters, and books. McGaghie and Webster (2009) suggested that articles that report original research data (databased) and are published in peer-reviewed journals are the "gold standard" for faculty in academic settings.

Peer-reviewed journals, also called refereed, use peer reviewers to critique the manuscript as a basis for the acceptance decision. Peer reviewers are experts, external to the journal staff, who provide an independent, critical assessment of the quality of the manuscript, including the scientific process (International Committee of Medical Journal Editors, 2009). Although the responsibilities of peer reviewers differ with each journal, in general, they critique the manuscript, identify areas for revision, and give expert opinions on the quality of the paper. With some journals, the peer reviewers also suggest to the editor if the manuscript should be accepted, revised and resubmitted, or rejected. The peer review process is discussed in chapter 14 of the book. Publishing an article in a peer-reviewed journal is important in tenure and promotion decisions because it indicates that the quality of the paper was assessed by experts based on standards. Most nursing and healthcare journals are peer-reviewed although the process and standards vary for their reviews of papers.

The importance given to writing chapters and books varies across institutions. Most chapters are not peer reviewed and thus do not carry the same weight in tenure and promotion decisions as does an article in a peer reviewed journal. Completion of a book requires a significant amount of time, and prior to the tenure decision, that time might be better spent writing papers for journals. Because the standards for tenure and promotion vary widely across schools of nursing, faculty should be well informed about this process in their own institutions.

While nurses in clinical settings are not faced with tenure and promotion decisions, writing for publication is often a requirement for job mobility in that setting and career advancement. Whether or not the article is databased or published in a peer reviewed journal is less important than writing for journals read by nurses who need this new information and perspective to guide their practice.

Expand Personal Knowledge and Skills

Another reason to write for publication is the learning gained in the process of preparing the manuscript. Rarely is the nurse able to write a manuscript without completing a thorough review of the literature. This literature review and the thinking that is done in developing the manuscript contribute to the knowledge base and understanding of the author.

Writing skills are useful in many settings as nurses fulfill both professional and personal roles. Writing about a topic facilitates understanding it and oneself. A good writer, i.e., a well-practiced writer, brings a valuable skill to endeavors that range far beyond writing for publication.

Gain Personal Satisfaction

Writing also gives the nurse a sense of personal satisfaction in sharing expertise with other nurses and contributing to the development of their profession. Most journals do not pay authors for their manuscripts; however, writing for publication is personally fulfilling. Winslow, Mullaly, and Blankenship (2008) suggested that through publications, nurses share with a wider audience their stories about personal and professional challenges they experience in the work setting on a daily basis and their satisfactions.

BARRIERS TO WRITING

Writing is time consuming, and authors may be frustrated as to their progress in preparing the manuscript. Developing a publishable paper requires practice, and the more writing the author does, the easier will be completion of the manuscript. Similar to the development of clinical skills, writing improves with practice. Some of the barriers to writing are a lack of understanding of this process, writer's block, lack of time, and fear of rejection.

Lack of Understanding of How to Write for Publication

Many faculty members have had limited experience in writing for publication and are unsure of the process but need to publish in their academic settings. Similarly, clinicians may be reluctant to assume the role of author because they too are unsure of the process of manuscript development and have never been prepared for this role in their nursing education programs (Carlson, Masters, & Pfadt, 2008).

Before beginning any manuscript, the author needs to first understand the writing and publishing processes. Often, students believe that the A+ paper they completed as a requirement in one of their nursing courses is publishable; this may or may not be true. Papers prepared for a course may be at too low a level for readers of a journal who have specialized knowledge and more advanced understanding of the topic. Or, the course paper may not be in an appropriate writing style for the journal to which submitted: the paper may be too theoretical or the literature review may be too long. Or, the paper may not contain material that is original or represent an added value to readers. An understanding of how to write for publication and a particular journal and its readership helps the author avoid situations such as these.

Rickard et al. (2009) evaluated the effectiveness of a one-week writing for publication course for nursing and other faculty followed by a monthly writers' support group. Submissions of manuscripts to peer reviewed journals increased from 9 to 33 over a two-year period. Participants reported that this preparation and continued support from colleagues increased their confidence in and satisfaction with the process of writing for publication. Regardless of whether nurses take courses in writing for publication or use a book such as this one, learning how to write for publication in professional journals and other venues is critical for success.

Writer's Block

Some authors experience writer's block that keeps them from writing. This may occur from anxiety about the project, uncertainty as to how to proceed, and past unsuccessful experiences with writing. It is important for authors to be clear about the topic and intent of their writing project—recording these on paper before beginning, discussing them with colleagues, and "presenting" ideas to others often help to avoid writer's block. Brainstorming, identifying alternate ways of approaching the topic, and diagramming or outlining ideas are strategies that can be used to overcome writer's block. Another strategy is to draw a concept map of the topics in the manuscript and how they relate to each other, providing a visual representation of the ideas and encouraging thinking about how best to proceed.

If these techniques are not effective, authors can review the literature, prepare the references, and engage in other activities that do not require the same degree of creativity as does writing. Often a short break from writing and use of some of the strategies identified earlier will resolve writer's block, but if not, authors should seek a mentor who can guide them through this process and completion of the paper.

Lack of Time

The extensive time for preparing a manuscript is another barrier to writing. Time is needed for preliminary work such as developing the idea and reviewing the literature, for preparing the draft and rewriting it until suitable for submission, and for subsequent revisions suggested by the editor and reviewers. In a qualitative study of 16 novice researchers, many viewed writing as complex and demanding, particularly when considering their other responsibilities; they identified barriers such as a lack of time, procrastination, and anxiety, among others (Shah, Shah, & Pietrobon, 2009). Time for writing is a problem encountered by both novice and experienced authors.

Fear of Rejection

One other barrier to writing is fear of rejection (Oermann, 1999b, 2010). In submitting a manuscript, the author is open to criticism and possible rejection; for some nurses this is a barrier to writing for publication. Having a manuscript rejected is part of the writing process and may not be related to the quality of the writing. The manuscript may be rejected because a similar one has already been accepted, or the information in the manuscript is not new enough for publication in that particular journal. Rejections for reasons such as these do not mean that the ideas are questionable or poorly presented. Even if the manuscript is rejected because of criticisms of the research design, ideas in the manuscript, or format, the author can use this feedback as a way of learning more about the writing process, for developing writing skills further, and for revising the manuscript for submission elsewhere. Reflective scholars use these rejections and feedback from the critiques to revise and resubmit their work (McGaghie & Webster, 2009).

■ PERSONAL STRATEGIES

Writing manuscripts requires set dates for completion and personal strategies to keep on target, meet deadlines, and use wisely the limited time available. A manuscript can be doomed to failure if the author does not manage the time allotted for writing and completing other aspects of preparing the manuscript for submission to a journal.

Set Due Dates

First, a due date should be set for completion of the manuscript, whether it is a journal article, chapter in a book, research proposal, or other writing project. The due date for completing the final copy should be realistic considering work and personal responsibilities and should not be altered; modifying the due date for completion of a manuscript often becomes a pattern, and the manuscript is never finished or takes too long to complete.

Second, after setting the due date for completion of the final manuscript, the author can divide the content areas into manageable parts and identify dates for completing each of these. In this way smaller content areas are viewed as separate writing assignments with individual due dates. If the author is working from an outline, which will be discussed in a later chapter, dates can be assigned to different sections of the outline. Third, in addition to dividing the manuscript into sections, each with its own due date, the author can assign dates to complete other activities related to the manuscript, for example, preparing the references and registering at the journal's website. It is important not to waiver from these due dates because with busy schedules, delays are difficult to make up later.

Even with firm dates, some writers have difficulty getting started and others have difficulty finishing. Viewing the manuscript in terms of smaller writing assignments and completing a few sections of the content often provide sufficient momentum and reinforcement to continue writing until the manuscript is completed.

Identify Prime Time for Writing

Authors should identify their prime time for writing, when they are most productive and creative, and protect that time (Oermann, 1999a, 2010). For some people, a large block of time is most effective, but for others smaller segments of time are easier to allow for in a busy work schedule. For example, authors might set aside 1 to 2 hours a day for writing plus the weekend or 3 to 4 hours a few days of the week. Heinrich (2008) recommended allowing 15 minutes a day to write and dividing the writing project into segments that could be written in that short time period.

The author should avoid interruptions and distractions during the time allotted for writing. Checking emails and answering the phone, even if they take limited time, affect concentration and distract the author from thinking about the topic and how best to present it to readers. In addition to removing distractions, the author should have a comfortable chair, good computer screen, and writing resources at hand.

▧ STEPS IN WRITING FOR PUBLICATION

Every article written for publication begins with a planning phase; progresses to writing a draft, revising it, and submitting the final copy to the journal; and concludes with its publication. These phases, which provide a framework for the organization of the book, are discussed in more detail in later chapters.

Planning Phase

Prior to writing the manuscript, the author proceeds through a series of steps. These steps are important to assist the author in selecting a topic that is publishable, choosing an appropriate journal with readers who are interested in the topic, and gearing the content and format for the journal. The unpublished document submitted to a journal for review is called the manuscript or paper (American Medical Association, 2007). Once that document is published, it is referred to as an article.

Identify Purpose of Manuscript

The first step in the planning phase is to identify the topic and purpose of the manuscript. In some cases the purpose is to present research findings, describe evidence-based practices, and explain how practice changes were made based on a review of the evidence. The intent of other manuscripts may be to present new nursing interventions and approaches to managing patient problems, describe nursing interventions for patients with particular health problems, analyze trends and issues in practice, and present new directions in nursing education or management.

For some manuscripts, identifying the purpose is easy because the author has a specific goal in mind at the outset such as presenting the findings of a project done in the clinical setting. Other times, though, generating the idea for the manuscript or deciding how to develop it is more involved. Every manuscript needs a primary message that is communicated to readers; this message directs how the manuscript is then developed.

Before proceeding, the author should be able to answer these questions: What is the purpose of writing the manuscript? Why is this information important for readers? What difference will it make in clinical practice, teaching, administration, and research? The author should be able to answer these questions clearly and succinctly.

Once the purpose of the manuscript is clearly thought out, the author should record it somewhere, for example, on an index card or as a document saved in the computer, and keep it in view during the writing phase. This helps to stay on target as the writing proceeds. Often novice writers have enthusiasm about a topic but conceptualize ideas that are too global. A useful strategy in the early planning phase is to write the purpose of the manuscript in one sentence to confirm it is clear and focused.

Decide on Importance of Topic

After deciding on the purpose of the manuscript, the author needs to ask if the ideas to be presented are worth writing about. Will the paper present important information that readers need? The goal in this step in the writing process is to avoid preparing a manuscript that has a limited chance of being accepted for publication. Exhibit 1.1 presents questions the author can ask to evaluate if the manuscript is worth writing and if the content is important enough to warrant publication. The author should answer these questions before spending any more time on the manuscript.

EXHIBIT 1.1

Assessing Importance of Content of Manuscript

Does the manuscript present new ideas?

Is the topic already in the literature? If so, how does the planned manuscript differ from the existing literature?

If the content is not new and articles have already been published on similar content, what is different about the manuscript to be worthy of publication? What new perspective is offered?

If the manuscript is published, how important is the message? Will it make a difference in patient care? Will it change nursing practice, education, administration, management, or research?

Who is the audience, and will readers be interested in the topic?

Is this a manuscript a journal would be interested in publishing?

Search for Related Articles

In generating ideas for a manuscript, the author should keep in mind that journals are interested in publishing new ideas and communicating information to readers that they may not already know. If the topic or idea is not new, then the question is whether it presents a unique perspective or a different way of looking at a well known topic.

To determine this, the author should do a literature review on the topic and related content areas. The literature search may reveal that the topic is indeed new to the nursing literature or at least to the readers for whom the manuscript is intended. An article may have been published for the general nursing audience, but the intended manuscript focuses instead on how the content would be used by nurses in a specialty area. Or, the articles are research-oriented and the intended topic is related to clinical practice or professional issues. If there have been articles published on the same topic, they may have been in other journals than those targeted for the manuscript being planned, or the focus at present will add to what is already known about the topic.

The goal in searching the literature at this point is to scan articles to determine if others have been published on the same topic. Authors should not spend much time with the search in case the decision is made not to write about that topic because it has already been addressed in the literature. If the author finds, though, that the manuscript will present new information, this beginning literature search may be used later as the manuscript is developed. For this reason, the author should record complete information about the articles and other publications reviewed for ease in returning to them at a later time.

The next steps in the process of writing for publication are to identify the audience to whom the manuscript will be directed and select a journal that might be interested in publishing it. These steps are discussed in the next chapter. The goal is to match the purpose and type of manuscript with an appropriate journal and readers who would be interested in it.

Identify Type of Article to be Written

The purpose of the manuscript indicates the type of article to be written. While there are many ways of categorizing articles in the nursing and healthcare literature, one way is: research; evidence-based practice including integrative literature reviews, critical appraisals of research studies with implications for practice, and reports on evidence-based practice projects; clinical practice; and other forms of writing such as case reports and editorials. These types of manuscripts differ in their goals, format, and writing style, and frequently reach different audiences. Often manuscripts are rejected because they do not match the type of articles that the journal publishes. Identifying the type of manuscript, therefore, helps the author make a decision about possible journals for submission. Nurses also prepare manuscripts and other documents for patients and non-professional audiences, which require careful writing to avoid using technical terms and to be at a level that readers without any healthcare background can understand; chapters; and books.

Research Articles Research (databased) articles present the findings of quantitative and qualitative studies. Quantitative research papers typically follow the IMRAD format, **I**ntroduction, **M**ethods, **R**esults **a**nd **D**iscussion, or an adaptation of this depending on the journal and type of research. There is no one style, however, for presenting qualitative research findings because the format necessarily depends on the purpose of the research, methods, and data (Sandelowski, 1998). Blignault and Ritchie (2009) indicated that qualitative research papers may be written in the first person, which differs from the usual style of reporting research.

With some manuscripts, the intent is to present the original research study, with less of a focus on its clinical implications. For example, *Nursing Research* reports quantitative and qualitative studies, the latest research techniques, and methodological strategies. Although articles in that journal may present clinical research studies, the focus is more on the research itself rather than translating the findings for use by clinicians. Many clinical journals also publish papers on research studies in their area of practice, and these generally emphasize the clinical implications of the research findings and are written for clinicians as readers. In a study of 768 articles published in clinical journals, nearly a third of those articles were reports on original research studies (Oermann, et al., 2008). Journals in other areas of nursing, such as nursing education and administration, often publish databased papers but expect authors to emphasize the implications of those studies for teaching, administration, and other areas of practice.

Evidence-Based Practice Articles Many nurses are engaged in projects to critically appraise evidence to answer questions about their practice and to evaluate the effectiveness of using those new approaches in patient care. In an integrative literature review, the author completes a comprehensive review of the literature on a topic, critiques the research, and then draws conclusions about the findings. The review of the literature is guided by a research question or problem to be solved, and the author may generate recommendations for practice based on the review. In evidence-based practice, nurses identify a clinical question or problem for which more information is needed, search for evidence to answer that question, critically appraise studies and assess the quality of the evidence, and make decisions about the use of the evidence for practice. Outcomes of these reviews are potential manuscripts for publication in nursing and other journals. In clinical settings nurses are using evidence to change practice and evaluating the effectiveness of those new approaches. The findings of those projects also can be prepared as manuscripts.

Clinical Articles Another type of manuscript addresses topics in clinical practice. Clinical articles may be written for nurses across specialties or for nurses practicing in a particular clinical area. The goals of the *American Journal of Nursing* (AJN) are to disseminate evidence-based clinical information and original research, discuss relevant and controversial professional issues, and promote nursing perspectives to the healthcare community and public (AJN, 2009). In contrast, articles in journals such as *Cancer Nursing* are more focused on specific patient populations and health problems.

The format for writing clinical articles differs with the journal but usually includes a description of the patient problems and nursing interventions, with an emphasis on the clinical implications of whatever topic is presented. Some journals have different departments each of which has a certain format for its articles.

Other Types of Articles Nurses write many other types of papers for publication. For example, case reports provide new information on nursing practice or care of patients with particular health problems through the presentation of an actual case. These manuscripts often begin with why the case was selected and its importance to nursing practice and continue with a description of the case and related care by nurses and other disciplines. Manuscripts also address topics in nursing education, administration, management, and other non-clinical areas. Articles may describe innovations, new practices, and issues in teaching, administration, and management. Other papers may focus on policy, ethics, legal aspects, historical studies, theory development or testing, issues affecting nurses in an area of clinical practice, and editorials. Nurses may respond to an article in a letter to the editor and complete book reviews for publication in a journal, both of which provide valuable experiences for a novice author.

Writing Phase

The writing phase involves preparing the first and subsequent drafts of the manuscript, completing the final revision, and submitting the manuscript to the journal. The steps in the writing phase include:

- Develop a formal or an informal outline to guide writing.
- Write the first draft focusing on presenting the content rather than on grammar, spelling, punctuation, and writing style.
- Revise the first and later drafts continuing to focus on the content of the manuscript.
- Then revise the manuscript for grammar, spelling, punctuation, and writing style.
- Prepare tables, figures, and the references paying close attention to the journal's format for references.
- Prepare the final version of the manuscript, accompanying materials required by the journal, and the submission or cover letter, and
- Submit the manuscript to the journal.

Publishing Phase

The final phase in writing for publication occurs after the manuscript is submitted to the journal. The manuscript is critiqued by peer reviewers who have expertise in the topic or methodology and can assess its quality. Peer reviewers provide feedback to authors on needed revisions to strengthen the manuscript and to the editor on the suitability of the manuscript for publication in the journal. It is through this process that the best papers are accepted for publication, ensuring quality of the information and meeting ethical standards.

Editors of nursing journals are nurses who have expertise in the content area of the journal. The final decision on acceptance of a manuscript is made by the editor, considering the peer reviews, the editor's own assessment of the quality and suitability of the paper for the journal, and other factors such as how many similar papers have been published or are in the queue to be published and upcoming themes planned for the journal. Different editorial decisions are possible ranging from acceptance of the manuscript without revision or pending revision; a request that the manuscript be revised and resubmitted, in which case the paper will be peer reviewed again; to rejection. If the manuscript is rejected, the author should revise the paper using feedback from the peer review process and submit it to another journal. With the wealth of nursing and other healthcare journals, if authors are willing to revise their papers, it is likely they will find a journal interested in their manuscript. Writing for publication requires perseverance and a willingness to use feedback and guidance from others to craft a paper that is appropriate for a particular journal and audience.

The publishing phase also includes responsibilities of the author once the manuscript is accepted for publication. At this point the author answers queries from the journal or production editor, reads carefully and corrects the page proofs, and returns promptly all materials to the publisher.

SUMMARY

Writing for publication is an important skill for nurses to develop. By disseminating new initiatives and innovations in clinical practice, research findings, and other ideas about nursing, nurses direct the future of their practice and advance the development of the profession. There are barriers to writing, but the nurse can overcome these by setting due dates for completion of writing projects, meeting these deadlines, and using wisely the available time for writing.

Every article written for publication begins with a planning phase; progresses to writing a draft, revising it, and submitting the final copy to the journal; and concludes with its publication. The manuscript or paper is the unpublished document submitted to a journal for review; once published it is referred to as an article. The first step in the planning phase is to identify the topic and purpose of the manuscript. After deciding on the purpose of the manuscript, the author needs to assess if the ideas to be presented are worth writing about. Will the paper present important information that readers need? To determine this, the author should do a literature review on the topic and related content areas. The literature search may reveal that the topic is indeed new to the nursing literature or at least to the readers for whom the manuscript is intended.

The next steps in the process of writing for publication are to identify the audience to whom the manuscript will be directed and select a journal that might be interested in publishing it. The goal is to match the purpose and type of manuscript with an appropriate journal and readers who would be interested in it. While there are many ways of categorizing articles in the nursing and healthcare literature, one way is: research articles, review papers that disseminate the outcomes of a synthesis of individual studies and articles addressing evidence-based practice, clinical practice articles, and other forms of writing such as case reports and editorials.

The writing phase involves preparing the first and subsequent drafts of the manuscript, completing the final revision, and submitting the manuscript to the journal. The final phase in writing for publication occurs after the manuscript is submitted to the journal. The manuscript is critiqued by peer reviewers, who have expertise in the topic or methodology, and can assess its quality. Peer reviewers provide feedback to authors on needed revisions to strengthen the manuscript and to the editor on the suitability of the manuscript for publication in the journal. As the manuscript proceeds through the production process, the author answers queries about the paper and reads carefully the page proofs.

Writing for publication is hard work, but the satisfaction gained from completing a manuscript and making a lasting contribution to the literature outweighs the effort and time. Writing is a skill that can be developed with practice. Once a manuscript is completed, the author should begin planning the next one.

REFERENCES

American Association of Colleges of Nursing. (2006). *Position Statement on Nursing Research*. Retrieved from http://www.aacn.nche.edu/Publications/positions/NsgRes.htm.

American Journal of Nursing. (2009). *About the Journal.* Retrieved from http://journals.lww. com/ajnonline/Pages/AbouttheJournal.aspx.

American Medical Association (AMA). (2007). *AMA manual of style: A guide for authors and editors* (10th ed.). New York: Oxford University Press.

Blignault, I., & Ritchie, J. (2009). Revealing the wood and the trees: Reporting qualitative research. *Health Promotion Journal of Australia, 20*(2), 140–145.

Carlson, D. S., Masters, C., & Pfadt, E. (2008). Guiding the clinical nurse through research publication development. *Journal of Nurses in Staff Development, 24,* 222–225. doi: 10.1097/01.NND.0000320679.73448.bf

Heinrich, K. T. (2008). *A nurse's guide to presenting and publishing: Dare to share.* Boston: Jones and Bartlett Publishers.

International Committee of Medical Journal Editors. (2009). *Ethical Considerations in the Conduct and Reporting of Research: Peer Review.* Retrieved from http://www.icmje.org/ ethical_3peer.html.

McGaghie, W. C., & Webster, A. (2009). Scholarship, publication, and career advancement in health professions education: AMEE Guide No. 43. *Medical Teacher, 31,* 574–590.

Oermann, M. H. (1999a). Extensive writing projects: Tips for completing them on time. *Nurse Author & Editor, 9*(1), 8–10.

Oermann, M. H. (1999b). Writing for publication as an advanced practice nurse. *Nursing Connections, 12*(3), 5–13.

Oermann, M. H., Nordstrom, C., Wilmes, N. A., Denison, D., Webb, S. A., Featherston, D. E., ... Striz, P. (2008). Dissemination of research in clinical nursing journals. *Journal of Clinical Nursing, 17,* 149–156. doi: 10.1111/j.1365–2702.2007.01975.x

Oermann, M. H. (2010). Writing for publication in nursing: What every nurse educator needs to know. In L. Caputi (Ed.), *Teaching nursing: The art and science* (2nd ed., 146–166). Glen Ellyn, IL: College of DuPage.

Rickard, C., McGrail, M., Jones, R., O'Meara, P., Robinson, A., Burley, M., et al. (2009). Supporting academic publication: Evaluation of a writing course combined with writers' support group. *Nurse Education Today, 29,* 516–521. doi: 10.1016/j.nedt.2008.11.005

Sandelowski, M. (1998). Writing a good read: Strategies for re-presenting qualitative data. *Research in Nursing & Health, 21,* 375–382.

Shah, J., Shah, A., & Pietrobon, R. (2009). Scientific writing of novice researchers: What difficulties and encouragements do they encounter? *Academic Medicine, 84,* 511–516. doi: 10.1097/ACM.0b013e31819a8c3c

Winslow, S. A., Mullaly, L. M., & Blankenship, J. S. (2008). You should publish that: Helping staff nurses get published. *Nursing for Women's Health, 12,* 120–126. doi: 10.1111/j.1751–486X.2008.00298.x

2

SELECTING A JOURNAL

The first step in writing for publication is to identify the topic or focus of the manuscript. The next steps are to identify the intended audience for the manuscript and a journal that might be interested in publishing it. Chapter 2 discusses how to evaluate possible journals, select an appropriate one, and write a query letter to gauge the interest of the journals' editors.

■ WHO IS THE AUDIENCE?

The author needs to be clear as to the intended readers of the manuscript. Identifying the audience is an important first step because the manuscript needs to be written for readers who have a keen interest in the topic and a need to know about it. Then, the next step is to identify a journal that publishes manuscripts on that topic for the same audience. Otherwise, the manuscript will be inappropriate for the journal to which it is submitted. A manuscript written for a general nursing audience but then submitted to a specialty journal read predominantly by advanced practice nurses will probably be rejected, and the author will lose valuable time.

The author can begin by asking who will likely read the manuscript and need the content in it. Most articles are read by people who need answers to questions about their practice, teaching, management, or research, or about other aspects of their work. Early decisions about the audience include if the readers are nurses in general practice or in a specialized area of nursing practice; whether they are staff nurses, advanced practice nurses, faculty, managers, or in other roles; whose needs would be met from reading the manuscript; and who would benefit from the content in the manuscript. Exhibit 2.1 provides questions to help the author characterize the audience of the manuscript.

The audience also may be consumers. Many health journals to which nurses contribute are written for the public. Writing for patients and consumers has implications for the depth and complexity of the content, technical words used in the writing, presentation style, and length of the manuscript. Chapter 8 discusses writing for patients and non-professional audiences.

Once the author has described the intended readers of the manuscript, this information should be recorded for use in selecting journals. During the writing process, the author keeps the intended audience in mind when deciding on

EXHIBIT 2.1

Identifying the Audience of Manuscript

- For whom will the article be written?
- Is the manuscript geared to a specialized audience, or is the content intended for nurses in general?
- If specialized, what is the reader's area of clinical nursing practice (e.g., pediatrics)?
- What is the primary role of the reader, such as staff nurse, advanced practice nurse, educator, manager, and others, that would influence how the manuscript is written?
- What is the work setting (e.g., hospital) of the reader?
- What are the needs of the reader that the manuscript will meet?
- Who will benefit from reading the paper?
- How will the information improve the reader's practice, teaching, management, or research, or other aspects of his or her work?
- What should the intended reader already know about the content area, and how will the manuscript build on this understanding?
- What is the educational level of the audience?

the content and how it is presented to the readers, types of examples to use, and writing style.

WHAT ARE THE PURPOSES OF THE PAPER?

Closely related to the audience of the manuscript is its purpose. Because science is a social enterprise and develops within a larger society, it depends upon clear communication among its practitioners and consumers (Penrose & Katz, 2004). The purpose of scientific communication varies widely. Original research, including its critical evaluation and replication, is the backbone of medical and scientific communication (American Medical Association [AMA], 2007). The purpose of such communication is to advance our understanding of health promotion and disease prevention strategies by specifying research questions or hypotheses to be addressed using rigorous protocols. But there are many other crucial reasons to communicate the work of nurses and other scientists and practitioners.

Some authors propose to review and summarize the diffuse or obscure evidence concerning a population at risk, a health problem, a theory or model, an historical event, or a treatment regimen and to recommend next steps in research or practice. Other authors provide a description or set of clinical or managerial observations that are less rigorously formulated than research articles but are nevertheless informative to readers functioning in relevant roles. Some authors represent panels of experts that prepare consensus statements or practice guidelines based on available evidence on a healthcare topic of importance

(AMA, 2007). Opinion pieces, such as editorials and letters to the editor, marshal the most persuasive evidence available to promote a specific point of view. Before the author can select the appropriate journal, one must be clear about the purpose of the article to be submitted.

IDENTIFYING APPROPRIATE JOURNALS

Selecting a journal is an early step in writing for publication. The number of journals related to nursing and health sciences is so large that the choice can feel overwhelming. Journals differ widely in their topics, the types of articles published, and readership. Selecting an appropriate journal is important because the author's goal is to submit the manuscript to a journal whose readers are interested in that subject area and looking for the type of manuscript planned, for example, research reports. The choice of journals for manuscript submission, therefore, should be carefully made; otherwise, it is unlikely that the manuscript will be accepted.

If a paper is submitted to an inappropriate journal, three actions may occur. First, the editor may return the manuscript to the author, having decided not to send it to experts for peer review. The editor may determine that the paper is unsuitable for the journal either due to its topic or its type. Second, the paper may be reviewed by peer experts but then rejected because reviewers reported a lack of fit with the journal's mission and readers. The comments made by reviewers, though, may not facilitate revision because of their lack expertise in the topical area. With these first two possibilities, valuable time is lost. Third, the manuscript may be accepted and subsequently published but in a journal never read by the intended readers who most need the information provided in the manuscript.

Match With Topic

The primary consideration in selecting a journal is whether the journal publishes articles in the subject area of the proposed manuscript. Is the topic appropriate for the journal? Although the author may be familiar with prominent journals in a particular area of nursing, other journals also may publish articles on the topic or in related content areas. Although there is no single core list of nursing journals, two sources for identifying journal titles for further exploration are the Medical Library Association's (MLA) project on Mapping the Literature of Nursing (MLA, 2009a) and Allen's Key and Electronic Nursing Journals Chart© (Allen, 2007). The MLA mapped articles cited by published authors in 53 generalist and specialty nursing journals over a three-year period. The MLA devoted separate articles in 2007 to journals that publish in specific clinical and functional areas (e.g., pediatric, home care, emergency nursing, nursing informatics, and education). The list developed by Allen evaluates 257 nursing journals. Use of these two tools is described more fully below.

The author should review all possible journals in nursing and other health fields that might be interested in the manuscript and should keep a list of them with related materials such as Author Guidelines. If an editor is not interested in reviewing the proposed manuscript, or the manuscript is rejected, then the author has other possible journals to consider for submission.

Match With Type of Article

The second consideration in choosing a journal is whether it publishes the type of article being planned. Different types of articles were identified in Chapters 5–8, including research, clinical practice, issue, theoretical, review articles, case reports, and manuscripts focused on policy, history, education, methods, and ethics. The journals appropriate for the topic may not publish the type of manuscript being considered. For instance, the goal of the proposed manuscript may be to present research on teaching effectiveness. While *Nurse Educator* publishes articles on teaching and the role of the teacher, it typically does not publish research reports. The *Journal of Nursing Education*, which publishes research, would be more appropriate. If the intended manuscript will provide a critical review of the literature in a particular area of nursing practice, then the author needs to identify a journal that publishes comprehensive reviews rather than short descriptions of innovations in clinical practice.

The review of journals also guides the author in planning the manuscript. From this review, the author develops ideas how to write the manuscript to fit with other articles in the journal as well as about alternative strategies for publishing. For instance, a nurse reporting on a complex patient care improvement project on her unit might write one manuscript for a journal that regularly publishes results of program evaluation studies and a second manuscript for a journal that publishes case studies of individual patients who were benefited from excellent nursing practice.

Match With Intended Audience

Is the audience that the author wants to reach the same audience that will read the target journal? Every journal has its own readers and style of presentation that meets their needs. There is a primary audience, readers for whom the journal is targeted, and a secondary audience, people outside of the journal's target audience who read an article to meet a particular need. The goal, however, is to learn as much as possible about the primary or target audience of the journal. The primary audience may be highly specialized and narrow in focus, or the journal may be geared to a general readership. The primary audience for the *Journal of Intravenous Nursing*, for instance, is nurses involved in the administration of intravenous therapy to patients, a specialized area of nursing practice, in comparison with the *American Journal of Nursing*, for which the primary audience is nurses in general. The targeted audience guides the choice of journals for manuscript submission (Albarran & Scholes, 2005).

The author can develop an understanding of a journal's target audience in several ways. First, the journal's mission or aims and scope may specify the kind of readers whom the editors and publishers intend to serve. For example, the *Journal of Nursing Education* published articles "for nurse educators in various types and levels of nursing programs" (Journal of Nursing Education, 2009), whereas the *Journal of Cardiovascular Nursing* targets "advanced practice nurses in cardiovascular care, providing thorough coverage of timely topics and information…for daily, on-the-job use" (Journal of Cardiovascular Nursing, 2009). Second, sample articles throughout the journal reflect the range of issues and problems relevant to its readers in specific roles and circumstances as well as what format and writing style are appropriate to those readers. Finally, the author may use personal experience as a guide; the journals read most often by the author can be a good starting point when developing a list of journals that may be targets for the planned submission.

In the same way that reviewing journals informs what types of manuscripts are most appropriate, reviewing journals can suggest different audiences and expand the possible journals for submission. For example, the author may have planned to develop a manuscript for critical care nurses but realized from the review of journals that nurses working in non-critical care settings are facing challenges of a similar nature and would benefit as much or more from the information, also expanding the choice of publications.

Open Access Literature

Over the past decade open access literature sites have emerged as alternatives to traditional subscription-based journals as repositories for scientific literature. *Open access* sites provide published papers that are "digital, online, and free of charge, regardless of the timing of availability" (Matsubayashi et al., 2009, p. 5). The rationale for this emerging trend has been the demand for increased worldwide accessibility to information (and particularly biomedical information), as exemplified by the National Institutes of Health's (NIH) public access policy requiring their funded researchers to upload accepted articles to PubMed Central within 12 months of publication (NIH, 2009).

In lieu of subscriptions, open access literature sites depend on six types of sponsorship support: individuals, universities and research institutes on behalf of affiliated members, academic guilds, governments and public institutions, "journals" that charge authors for making their articles freely available, and third-party sponsors affiliated with multiple publishers (Matsubayashi et al., 2009). To establish a baseline description of this emerging phenomenon, Matsubayashi and colleagues studied a random sample of 4,667 articles published in the nine months prior to implementation of the NIH policy. They found approximately one in four articles was freely accessible to the public as a downloadable file; 70% of these were available from journal Web sites, most frequently from journals owned by scholarly associations.

The Directory of Open Access Journals (Lund University Libraries, 2009) lists 28 nursing journals in 2009, including the *Online Journal of Issues in Nursing*, the *Online Journal of Nursing Informatics*, and the *Online Journal of Rural Nursing and Health Care*. Nursing journals owned by some publishers, such as Wiley-Blackwell's *Journal of Advanced Nursing* (JAN), offer their authors a pay-to-publish service: manuscripts accepted for publication may be viewed and downloaded freely from the publisher's website for a one-time fee of $3,000 "to be met by or on behalf of the Author in advance of publication" (JAN, 2009).

This trend towards open access publishing has been controversial because many open access sites do not incorporate an expert peer review procedure prior to publication, thus calling into question the rigor of the published science. Commercial publishers also question the sustainability of a publication business model that is not dependent on subscriptions (Matsubayashi et al., 2009). Nevertheless, as these and other new opportunities and decisions confront nurse authors, the underlying reasons to write and strategies for selecting publishers, as described in this text, remain the most relevant guideposts for selecting a publication venue.

Internet Resources for Identifying Journals

To choose the "right" journal for the manuscript, the author needs to review available journals in nursing and other health fields. There are a number of different ways to identify possible journals.

Key and Electronic Nursing Journals Chart©

A valuable resource for reviewing nursing journals is the Key and Electronic Nursing Journals chart© (Allen, 2007). The chart is available as a .pdf file at http://www.utexas.edu/nursing/norr/docs/keyjournals07.pdf.

The chart describes characteristics of nursing journals including:

- if they are peer-reviewed;
- the number and percentage of articles based on primary research, evidence-based nursing (EBN), and continuing education units (CEU) published in each journal, derived from Cumulative Index to Nursing and Allied Health Literature® (CINAHL®) database searches;
- indexes in which they are listed; and
- limited information on where to obtain full-text articles on-line if available.

The chart is helpful in identifying journals that are peer-reviewed and that publish research. Most of the journals in nursing are peer-reviewed, even though the review process may differ widely across the journals. The information in the chart is particularly useful if planning on writing a research manuscript or presenting information that will be useful in developing the evidence base for nursing practice. For instance, the *Journal of Nursing Scholarship* is peer-reviewed and published 124 (75%) research articles in a three-year period. In contrast, in *AORN Journal* (Association of periOperative Registered Nurses), which is also peer-reviewed, only 41 or 7% of the articles were research reports in the same time period (Allen, 2007).

The chart also may be used to identify journals that might be interested in a research report in a specific clinical area. If the manuscript is on research in critical care nursing, for example, the chart may be used to select journals that publish these studies. The *American Journal of Critical Care* had 162 (63%) research articles in a three-year period, similar to *Heart & Lung* (96 articles or 60%). *Critical Care Nurse*, in contrast, published only 7 (3%) research articles in the same time period (Allen, 2007). An article that describes a critical care research project would be more suited for submission to *American Journal of Critical Care* or *Heart & Lung* than to *Critical Care Nurse*. The author can then go to the web sites of the prospective journals to review the table of contents of recent issues to confirm their appropriateness. For instance, the web-based Information for Authors of the *American Journal of Critical Care* (2009) describes many areas of interest to the journal's editors.

The Key and Electronic Nursing Journals chart© (Allen, 2007) also reports a summary rating score that combines an assessment of content (research, evidence-based nursing [EBN], continuing education units [CEU]), reputation, and citations into a scale of quality from 0–10. Authors may easily compare and contrast the overall scores of possible target journals and what are their relative strengths during 2003–2005.

CINAHL® Database

The *Cumulative Index to Nursing and Allied Health Literature* (CINAHL®–EBSCO Publishing Company, 2009) database is a comprehensive guide to nursing and allied health literature from 1982 to the present. There are more than 2000 journals currently indexed in CINAHL®, including 546 nursing journals, 434 allied health journals, 87 biomedical journals, 91 consumer health journals, and others (*EBSCO Publishing Company*). The complete list of journals is available to the public on-line at http://www.cinahl.com/library/jourlist.pdf.

Authors may have access to a medical, academic, government, corporate or public library that subscribes to EBSCO*host*, the research platform of the CINAHL databases. These databases can be used to review the journals that published articles about the topic of the manuscript and in related content areas. The author can find this information by doing a subject search. This often assists the author in identifying journals that might be interested in the manuscript and in determining if the idea is new or is already in the literature. By reviewing the abstracts of the articles, the author can learn more about the focus of the journal and types of papers published in it.

Databases are also searchable to retrieve material specific to clinical specialties. These databases can be set to retrieve articles according to "special interest", such as advanced practice nursing, critical care, emergency care, and hospice/palliative care, which the author can use to identify possible target journals.

Directories of Journals

There are Web sites that provide directories of journals in nursing and other health fields (Exhibit 2.2). These web sites contain an alphabetical listing of hundreds of journal titles. Many of the sites have links to the information for authors page of the journal as well as email addresses of editors for querying them about the proposed manuscript. They do not describe characteristics of the journals, though, as does the Key Nursing Journals chart©, but they provide easy access to editors for the author to query about manuscript ideas.

EXHIBIT 2.2

Web Sites of Directories of Journals

Public Access Resources

http://www.utexas.edu/nursing/norr/docs/keyjournals07.pdf
Allen's Key and Electronic Nursing Journals: Characteristics and Database Coverage compares 257 journals according to review protocol; percentage of primary research, evidence-based nursing (EBN), and continuing education units (CEU) published; database coverage; and full-text availability. The journals are also ranked on research content, representation on core lists of journals, and frequency of citation in other journals.

http://www.ncbi.nlm.nih.gov/journals
PubMed is an indexing tool of 19+ million citations for biomedical articles from MEDLINE and life science journals, sponsored by the National Library of Medicine at NIH. Journals can be identified via search by topic, journal title or abbreviation, ISSN, or subject terms.

http://www.nurseauthor.com/library.asp
This site provides an alphabetical list of nursing journals with email connections to editors and author information pages.

Elsevier: *http://www.elsevier.com/wps/find/journal_browse.cws_home*

Lippincott: *http://www.nursingcenter.com/*

Wiley Interscience: *http://www3.interscience.wiley.com/browse/?type=JOURNAL*

Publishing company Web sites provide lists of their journals, access to some current and past issues, information about the journal, author guidelines, some full-text articles and/or web-only Supplements. The examples above include Elsevier (79 nursing journal titles), Lippincott's NursingCenter.com (61 journals and 21 journal Supplements), and Wiley Interscience (38 nursing journals). Additional publishers of nursing materials are available at: *http://www.lights.ca/publisher/db/topics/Nursing.html*

http://nahrs.mlanet.org/activity/mapping/nursing/refs.html
The nursing literature mapping project of the Medical Library Association identified 54 major journals in 17 generalist and specialty nursing areas (general nursing, home health, maternal-child/gynecological, medical-surgical, nephrology, midwifery, administration, informatics, case management, emergency, nurse practitioner, education, pediatrics, rehabilitation, transcultural, international, and public/community health.) Journals were characterized by the source and age of their citations, how frequently specific titles were cited, and coverage of highly cited journals in 12 databases.

Subscription-based Resources (accessible to affiliated users via library Web sites)

Web of Science is a citation database covering 23,000 journals, 87 nursing journals in the Expanded Science Edition Index and 85 nursing journals in the Social Science Edition Index.

- For journal Impact Factors: at the IS Web of Knowledge portal, click on tab for Select a Database/Journal Citation Reports. Under Select an Option, choose Search for a Specific Journal and click Submit. Type in the journal name, and click submit.
- For Most Frequently Cited Articles in a journal: at the ISI Web of Knowledge portal, click on tab for Web of Science/Cited Reference. Cut and paste the journal abbreviation from the provided list; type in the year desired; hit Search.

http://www.cinahl.com/cgi-bin/jlookup?cdbysset.dat+Nursing
CINAHL®, the Cumulative Index to Nursing and Allied Health Literature, is the most comprehensive resource for nursing and allied health literature, recently expanded to offer four databases including two full-text versions. CINAHL enables authors to search 546 nursing journals.

http://www.ulrichsweb.com/ulrichsweb/
Ulrich's is a global resource for periodicals information, including 1595 titles under the keyword 'nursing.'

Libraries also provide Tools for Authors with links to multiple databases, lists of e-journals, and more, e.g., Duke University Medical Center Library/ Tool Sets/Nursing

OBTAINING AUTHOR GUIDELINES

After identifying possible journals, the author should read each journal's information for authors page, also referred to as Author Guidelines and Instructions for Contributors. The information for authors page usually describes the:

- Topics the journal is interested in publishing
- Types of articles published, e.g., research, clinical practice, case studies, commentaries, theory, and others
- Manuscript preparation including the title page, abstract, text, references, figures and tables, photographs, permission to reprint, and copyright transfer
- Editorial process, peer review, and related information
- Length of manuscripts
- Other guidelines for writing the manuscript and submitting it.

The information for authors page may be found in each issue of the journal or in a specific issue such as the first one of a volume (i.e., January). Typically, this page also is available at the web site of the journal and therefore may be easily obtained once the potential journals have been selected.

For most journals, the author guidelines are consistent with the *Uniform Requirements for Manuscripts Submitted to Biomedical Journals* (International Committee of Medical Journal Editors, 2008). Sometimes referred to as the "Vancouver Style", the Uniform Requirements are instructions to authors on how to prepare manuscripts.

After reviewing the Author Guidelines and narrowing the list of possible journals, the author might read a few articles in each journal to get a better perspective on the types of papers published, their format and length, the writing style, and other characteristics. Authors might also read a few recent journal editorials to gauge what topics the editors find compelling. It is helpful to keep a file of author guidelines and sample articles from the most promising journals for use with the current and later writing projects.

OBTAINING OTHER RELEVANT INFORMATION ABOUT THE JOURNAL

Circulation of Journal

While quality of the journal is certainly important, the circulation of the journal also may be considered. Manuscripts are time-consuming to prepare, and authors want to reach as many nurses as possible who will be interested in the topic and can use the new information in their practice. The circulation, though, is typically not a major consideration in deciding on journals for submission. In addition, circulation may not equate with quality of the publication.

Journal circulation data are proprietary and belong to publishers. Circulation data include the number of individual and library subscriptions to print copies as well as digital subscriptions to groups of journals on related topics. These bundled subscriptions are more cost effective for libraries than would be individual subscriptions. If available to the public, circulation data will usually appear on the publisher's journal website. Open access journals, as described above, are free of charge to the public, which renders circulation considerations moot.

Frequency of Publication, Response Time, and Acceptance Rates

Some final considerations are the frequency with which the journal is published, the average length of time for review and editorial decisions and between acceptance and publication, and what proportion of submitted articles are accepted. The time from acceptance to publication of a manuscript is usually shorter for journals that are published more often. For journals that publish the acceptance date of the manuscript, the author can easily determine the length of time between acceptance and publication. Keep in mind that many journals, whether monthly, bimonthly or quarterly, have backlogs; the projected time between acceptance and publication may be a factor in the consideration of journals. To address this delay, some journals post accepted articles on their Web sites as soon as they are accepted, with subsequent print issues drawing exclusively from the posted manuscripts.

It is sometimes worthwhile to ask colleagues about their experiences in publishing in a journal, and some editors will estimate for prospective authors the probable wait-time for publication of accepted manuscripts. The length of time from submission through publication also depends on how promptly reviewers respond with comments and authors resubmit their revised manuscripts.

Editors and publishers routinely calculate the acceptance and rejection rates of their journals. This information is not often published on Web sites. However, editors may respond to individual queries about this statistic.

Impact Factors and Other Measures of Quality

There is no gold standard system for ranking the quality of nursing journals. The author may make an informed judgment of the quality and prestige of the journals by identifying the ones that present new and important information for readers and whose articles are clearly written.

Another way of assessing the quality of the journal is by reviewing the number of times articles in one journal are cited in other publications. The *Journal Citation Reports®* counts the number of articles published in each journal and the number of times each article has been cited by other scholarly publications, and then calculates an Impact Factor. The Impact Factor is the number of current citations to articles published in a specific journal in a two year period, divided by the total number of articles published in the same journal over the same two year period (Institute for Scientific Information [ISI], 2009). The *Journal Citation Reports®* Science Edition provides citation data on more than 5,700 leading science journals; the Social Sciences Edition provides citation data on approximately 1,700 leading social sciences journals (ISI, 2000). The *Journal Citation Reports®* is useful if intending to publish in medical or social science journals. There are limited nursing journals in each of these citation databases, and some nursing journals such as *Public Health Nursing* are listed in both. *Journal Citation Reports®* is accessible only through subscriber organizations, such as university libraries.

An alternative rating system was developed by Allen (2007) in 1977 and currently ranks 257 nursing journals on a scale of 0–10, based on research content, representation on core lists of journals, and frequency of citation in other journals. Future updates to the most recent Allen Rating System will be conducted by the Nursing and Allied Health Section of the MLA and available, with other essential resources for nurse-authors, at their website (Medical Library Association, 2009b).

▧ CONTACTING EDITORS AND QUERY LETTERS

Journal editors are committed to mentoring and coaching new authors (Kearney & Freda, 2006) and are generally very approachable. Knowing that an editor is interested in the topic can be an important motivating factor for submitting first to that journal. On the other hand, the editor may not be interested in reviewing the manuscript because the journal does not publish that topic or type of manuscript, the journal has recently published too many articles on related topics, or a similar one has already been accepted. Therefore, a query letter can be emailed to the editors of the prospective journals asking about their interest in reviewing the manuscript. The author does not need to send a query letter, though, prior to submitting a manuscript, but it often saves time in the long run.

Query letters may be sent to more than one editor simultaneously. The manuscript, however, may be sent to only one journal at a time. After deciding on the journal to submit the manuscript, the author should notify the other interested editors of the decision not to send the manuscript for review.

The query letter should be no longer than one or two paragraphs. It should indicate the type of manuscript, e.g., description of clinical practice innovation, research report, case review, and so forth, and should explain in a few sentences what the manuscript is about. In the email, the author should include a tentative title of the manuscript, a brief statement of his or her position and expertise to write the manuscript, the anticipated completion date, and contact information. The abstract for the manuscript may be included, if available. Penrose and Katz (2004) cautioned authors to avoid trying to "sell" the editor on the topic but rather to present their material with an awareness of its limits. A sample query email is in Exhibit 2.3.

EXHIBIT 2.3

Sample Query Email

[Date]

Dr. Ann Brown
Editor, *Nursing Journal*
1234 Main Street
Anytown, AnyState 56789
abrown@herjournalemail.com

Dear Dr. Brown:

I am interested in submitting a manuscript to the *Nursing Journal*. The manuscript describes an evaluation we conducted of a new teaching program for patients with congestive heart failure. For our evaluation, we collected information about the learning needs of patients when they were first admitted to the hospital and assessed the effectiveness of our teaching program at two points in time, at discharge and one month after discharge. I have extensive experience caring for patients with cardiac problems and chaired the group that developed and evaluated the teaching program.

Thank you for your consideration.

Sincerely,
Mary Smith
Mary Smith, MSN, RN
Clinical Nurse II

The query letter should be addressed to the email address of the editor or journal administrator. This information is available in the Author Guidelines but also may be found at the web page of the journal, at the publisher's web site, or in the masthead of a current issue of the journal. Querying editors is done easily by email, using the addresses or links available in the directories of journals, such as those in Exhibit 2.2, or at the journal's Web page. In rare cases, the author also may send a letter to the editor. In the latter case, a self-addressed and stamped envelope should be enclosed or an email address for the response.

▉ MAKING THE DECISION

Exhibit 2.4 provides a checklist to help the author decide on the "right" journal. In making this decision, the author considers the appropriateness of the journal for the topic, type of manuscript, and intended audience; the quality of the journal; and other information about the publication that the author has collected. The journals identified for submission, though, may not be the ones with the most important papers nor ones cited more frequently by other authors. The journals chosen for the manuscript should be ones read by nurses or others who are interested in the topic and need the information. Thus, with many manuscripts, the decision as to which journals are appropriate weighs heavily on who reads the journal, who "cares about" the content in the manuscript, and who will use it for improved practice.

EXHIBIT 2.4

Identifying the "Right" Journal

- Does the journal publish articles in the general subject area of the manuscript?
- Is the topic of the manuscript consistent with the goals and mission of the journal?
- Has the topic of the manuscript been published already in the journal? If so, will the manuscript be different enough to warrant publication?
- Does the journal publish the type of manuscript proposed, e.g., research, clinical practice, issue, theoretical, review articles, case reports, and others?
- Who are the readers of the journal, and are they the same as the intended audience of the manuscript?
- What is the quality of the journal, and are there important articles published in it?
- What is the circulation of the journal?
- How frequently is the journal published (e.g., monthly, bimonthly, quarterly)?
- What is the projected time between acceptance and publication?
- Is the journal peer-reviewed?
- Is the journal editor interested in reviewing the manuscript?

One other consideration is the risk of rejection. Prestigious journals also receive more manuscripts for review and have higher rates of rejection. With rejections, the author loses the time it took for the manuscript to be processed and reviewed. Authors may send an email query to the journal editor or administrative office to inquire about rejection rates, although this information may not be available. Novice authors should seek advice from experienced authors in the same field about target journals that provide a higher probability of acceptance and whose editors understand their role to include the mentoring of new authors.

PRIORITIZING JOURNALS FOR SUBMISSION

From the review of journals, the author should select three to five journals for submission of the manuscript and should prioritize them. If the editor of the journal of first choice is not interested in reviewing the manuscript, or it is rejected, then the author can send the manuscript to the next one on the list, without having to review the journals again.

The author also can prepare a secondary list of journals that publish related topics or may be appropriate if the manuscript is adapted for their audience. This list is valuable if the primary journals are not interested in reviewing the manuscript, the author decides not to submit it to one of them, or the manuscript is rejected. Often, the manuscript can be adapted to another journal without much effort. For instance, if the manuscript is on nursing interventions for dyspnea, and the primary journals are not interested in reviewing it, the author might reframe the discussion around caring for the dyspneic patient in the home. Then, the choice of journals extends to those that focus on home care. For rejected manuscripts, the author might refer to this secondary list of publications for ideas how to rewrite the manuscript to fit the different aims and scope of those journals. For example, a research report that has been rejected because of a small sample size may be rewritten as a clinical project or case study with greater emphasis placed on the implications of the study.

SUMMARY

The first step in writing for publication is to identify the topic or focus of the manuscript. From that point, the author decides on the intended readers. The manuscript needs to be written for defined readers and then submitted to a journal that publishes articles on that topic for the same audience.

Considerations in selecting a journal include whether the journal publishes articles in the subject area of the proposed manuscript; whether it publishes the type of article being planned, e.g., research, clinical practice, issue, theoretical, review article, case report, and others; whether the readers of the journal are the same as the intended audience of the manuscript; the quality of the journal; its circulation; how frequently it is published; whether it provides open access; and at what cost.

There are a number of different ways to identify possible journals. These include the Key and Electronic Nursing Journals chart© (Allen, 2007), the CINAHL® database, and web sites that provide directories of nursing and allied health journals. Many of the web sites have links to the information for authors page of the journal and to the editors for querying them about the proposed manuscript.

The author selects three to five journals for submission of the manuscript and prioritizes them. A query letter can be sent to the editors of the prospective journals asking about their interest in reviewing the manuscript. Other decisions made prior to writing the manuscript are discussed in Chapter 3.

▓ REFERENCES

Albarran, J. W., & Scholes, J. (2005). How to get published: Seven easy steps. *Nursing in Critical Care, 10*(2), 72–77. doi: 10.1111/j.1362–1017.2005.00105.x

Allen, M. (2007). *Key and electronic nursing journals: Characteristics and database coverage.* Retrieved from the University of Texas at Austin Nursing Online Resources and Research website: http://www.utexas.edu/nursing/norr/docs/keyjournals07.pdf

American Medical Association. (2007). *AMA manual of style: A guide for authors and editors* (10th ed.). New York: Oxford University Press.

EBSCO Publishing. (2009). *Journal coverage in the CINAHL database.* Retrieved from http://www.cinahl.com/library/journals.htm

Institute for Scientific Information. (2009). *Journal Citation Reports®.* Retrieved from http://admin-apps.isiknowledge.com/JCR/JCR?PointOfEntry=Home&SID=1Bllnb45EmKegcJf3Nj.

International Committee of Medical Journal Editors. (2008). *Uniform requirements for manuscripts submitted to biomedical journals: Writing and editing for biomedical publication.* Retrieved from http://www.icmje.org/urm_main.html

Journal of Advanced Nursing. (2009). *General author guidelines.* Retrieved from http://www.journalofadvancednursing.com/jps.asp?page=authors

Journal of Cardiovascular Nursing. (2009). *About the journal.* Retrieved from http://journals.lww.com/jcnjournal/pages/aboutthejournal.aspx

Journal of Nursing Education. (2009). *About the journal: Profile.* Retrieved from http://www.journalofnursingeducation.com/about.asp

Kearney, M. H., & Freda, M. C. (2006). "Voice of the profession": Nurse editors as leaders. *Nursing Outlook, 54*, 263–267. doi:10.1016/j.outlook.2006.04.002

Lund University Libraries. (2009). Subjects: Health sciences: Nursing. *Directory of Open Access Journals.* Retrieved from http://www.doaj.org/doaj?func=subject&cpid=23.

Matsubayashi, J., Kurata, K., Sakai, Y., Morioka, T., Kato, S., Mine, S. & Ueda, S. (2009). Status of open access in the biomedical field in 2005. *Journal of the Medical Library Association 97*(1), 3–11. doi: 10.3163/1536–5050.97.1.002

Medical Library Association. (2009a). *Mapping the literature of nursing: Publications.* Retrieved from http://nahrs.mlanet.org/activity/mapping/nursing/refs.html

Medical Library Association. (2009b). *Nursing and allied health resources section.* Retrieved from http://nahrs.mlanet.org/

National Institutes of Health. (2009). *PubMed Central: A free archive of life sciences journals.* Retrieved from http://www.ncbi.nlm.nih.gov/pmc/

Penrose, A. M., & Katz, S. B. (2004). *Writing in the sciences: Exploring conventions of scientific discourse* (2nd ed.). New York: Pearson Longman

3

AUTHORSHIP AND PREPARING TO WRITE

Decisions about the focus of the manuscript, audience, and journal are important early in the writing process. Other decisions pertain to authorship; if these are not made before beginning the writing project, they may create problems and conflict among the authors later on. Chapter 3 addresses authorship and author responsibilities in preparing to write.

AUTHORSHIP

The word "author" comes from the Latin word meaning "to produce." Authorship implies production, creation, and origination of new material. In the field of scientific writing, each individual designated as an author on a manuscript or other type of paper should have contributed something substantial to it. Authorship confers professional and personal rewards but involves considerable responsibility (American Medical Association [AMA], 2007). Authors bear responsibility for the truthfulness and trustworthiness of their work, in turn for which fairness dictates that they receive public credit (McKneally, 2006).

Uniform Requirements for Manuscripts Submitted to Biomedical Journals

Who should receive credit as an author of a published manuscript? The *Uniform Requirements for Manuscripts Submitted to Biomedical Journals* specify that authorship credit should be given only when the author made substantial contributions to the:

1. Conception and design of the study, or acquisition of data, or analysis and interpretation of the data;
2. Drafting the manuscript or revising it critically for important intellectual content; and
3. Approval of the version of the manuscript to be published (International Committee of Medical Journal Editors [ICMJE], 2008).

These criteria must be met for a person to be designated as an author on a manuscript.

These criteria have important implications for authors. First, each author listed in the by-line must have participated in designing the project or acquiring, analyzing, or interpreting the data. Their participation may have involved identifying the questions for the study and designing it, identifying the need for a clinical project and planning its development, or critiquing and synthesizing the literature. Individuals who make important contributions to the analysis and interpretation of the data—even though they may not have been involved in the conception and design of the study—qualify for authorship if they meet the other criteria (ICMJE, 2008).

Next, authors must participate in writing the paper, critiquing it as a basis for subsequent revisions, or substantively revising the paper. Many journals require disclosure of evidence in support of authorship (Marusic, 2006). Therefore, authors should be able to document their participation in a group writing activity, such as through logs, data entry sheets, records of meetings held, and drafts of manuscripts. This record keeping may also be important after the paper is published if there are questions about its content or methods.

Last, coauthors must take responsibility for the content of the manuscript. Regardless of the number of drafts that circulate among groups of authors, all authors of a manuscript need to approve the final version, not only by signing the copyright transfer form, but also by approving the content.

Scientific publication requires the assistance of many individuals who do not meet the criteria for authorship. These include those who made suggestions for research questions; acquired funding for the study; recruited subjects or collected the data; provided statistical or technical writing support, editorial assistance, or review; contributed scientific expertise; or provided general supervision for the group, such as a department chair or Dean (AMA, 2007; American Psychological Association [APA], 2009; ICMJE, 2008). For clinical projects involving patients, physicians and nurses who care for patients enrolled in a study do not qualify for authorship unless the above three criteria are met. We discuss below some alternatives available to authors for acknowledging the important contributions of persons who do not meet the three criteria for authorship.

In addition to these three criteria included in the *Uniform Requirements for Manuscripts Submitted to Biomedical Journals*, there are additional responsibilities required of all authors. These include preparing the manuscript for submission; maintenance of the integrity of the copyright; and compliance with ethical, legal, and policy requirements of the journal. The latter includes disclosure of any conflicts of interest or sponsorships that could be interpreted as having been influential over their work and confirmation that they had access to all available data relevant to their research questions (APA, 2009). Conflicts of interest and data access are discussed below as potential abuses of authorship responsibility. Manuscript preparation and copyright requirements are discussed in Chapters 13 and 15.

Information for Authors

Policies related to authorship, if available for a journal, can be found in the Information for Authors or Author Guidelines, as discussed in Chapter 2.

Unfortunately, the information provided to authors may not be sufficient. Wager (2007) examined a random sample of biomedical journals (n = 234) from the World Association of Medical Editors and MEDLINE. Of these, 41% gave no guidance about authorship, 29% used the ICMJE criteria described above, 14% used only the third ICMJE criterion that all authors approve the submitted draft, 14% proposed alternative criteria; and 3% only set limits on the number of authors who could be listed.

Journal editors are responsible for making the authors' responsibilities explicit and concrete; for being honest, fair, collegial, and open in their dealings with authors; and for codifying these values in their information for authors (Penrose & Katz, 2006). Where such policies are not made explicit, authors should clarify with the editor of the target journal what are the expectations and requirements of authorship.

ABUSES OF AUTHORSHIP

Authorship establishes both credit and responsibility for work in nursing, other health fields, and science in general. Misuse of authorship undermines this recognition and responsibility. During the process of writing for publication, authors make many decisions that have important ethical and legal implications (Saver, 2006). The publication of good science has many stakeholders: patients and their families, the media, general readers, publishers, students, faculty, and peer reviewers. But it is ultimately the responsibility of authors and editors to disseminate scientific work in a manner that maintains scholarly integrity within a profession (ICMJE, 2008; Baggs, 2008). Below we address two ethical issues that affect authors: unjustified authorship and conflicts of interest.

Guest Authors and Ghost Authors

Ethical issues related to authorship center around the question of who is entitled to be listed as the author of a scientific publication. There is a trend of increasing numbers of articles with multiple authors published in all scientific fields, including healthcare (Price et al., 2000). While multiple authorship can reflect the increasing complexity of a field, the listing of many author names on a short paper or project description suggests that some individuals listed may be undeserving of authorship credit. The criteria established by the ICMJE provide a framework for determining who should be included as an author of a manuscript and who does not deserve authorship, but authors may not be aware of criteria or may disagree with their extent and rigor (Price et al., 2000). Nursing students and authors should be apprised of these standards for authorship qualifications, and awareness of them should be reinforced.

One type of inappropriate authorship is that of an honorary or guest author. Guest authors are often persons in authority over the actual author but who are listed as authors without having met all appropriate criteria. Guest authorship is a prevalent breach of publication ethics. Mowatt (2002) found that one in three Cochrane reviews included guest authors.

Authorship cannot be conferred upon someone as a gift or seized by someone in a position of power; it is a status that can only be assumed voluntarily by an individual who accepts all the responsibilities inherent in it (AMA, 2007). It is intellectually dishonest to list as a courtesy the name of someone who does not meet all criteria for authorship author. It is unlikely that such individuals would be willing or able to take public responsibility for the accuracy of a paper's content if it were challenged. Inclusion of those not meeting a high standard of contribution also dilutes the meaning of authorship (AMA, 2007).

Some journals have formalized their efforts to reduce the potential for guest authorship by requiring disclosure by authors of the nature of all contributions made by each. Authors must document their specific contributions to conception and design, acquisition of data, and so forth (AMA, 2007). One reliability study of such contribution checklists suggests however that the actual contributions by authors may differ substantially from what authors report on these disclosure forms (Ilakovac et al., 2007). Another study found a substantial number of faculty members resistant to providing such information (Price et al., 2000). As more journals explicitly adopt the Uniform Requirements as criteria for publication and provide authors with instructional guidelines for determining authorship, the attitudes and behavior of authors will likely change (Marusic, 2006).

A related ethical issue is that of "ghost" authorship. Ghost authors may have met all of the criteria for authorship but are not listed as such in the author by-line (AMA, 2007). Mowatt (2002) found evidence of ghost authors in almost 20% of Cochrane reviews.

In some fields, it is a common practice for a medical writer to be hired to write the manuscript, but this "ghost author" does not receive authorship credit. Instead, the name of a prominent scientist in that field is attached before the manuscript is submitted. In such cases, neither the person whose name is listed as author nor the ghost writer qualifies for authorship credit, the former because he or she understands the science but is not accountable for the writing, and the latter because she or he can defend the writing but not the science. Ghost authors may be the actual writers, such as authors' editors and researchers at facilities who write the article but cite others as the authors. Companies have offered to pay ghost writers to write articles that nurse scientists would then submit as the actual author (Baggs, 2008). This is unethical.

Ghost authorship may be appropriate in some circumstances. Ghost authors may be freelance writers who are bound by contract not to receive authorship credit, corporate or governmental agency public relations officers, or authors' editors hired to draft or substantially revise a manuscript. Although they do not qualify as authors, ghost writers should be identified to journal editors and their contributions explained to readers in an acknowledgment.

Conflicts of Interest

To facilitate readers' determining the accuracy and value of published works, authors must disclose any financial or other competing interest that might cast doubt upon their impartiality. Relevant disclosures of potential conflicts include receipt of salaries, consulting fees, personal stock or research grants in products or services relevant to one's publication, or participation in a speakers' bureau for a product relevant to the study (APA, 2009). Does the author or his or her institution or business stand to gain financially from the mention of a commercial product in a publication? If so, questions may arise about whether this financial interest has affected the study results (APA, 2009). If the writer holds stock in a company whose products are promoted in the publication, the writer has an obligation to disclose this association to the editor, who then has a duty to inform readers. Similarly, if a researcher received grant support for a study, he or she should report the source of the funding in any published research report so that readers may determine if the content of the research report relates to the potential vested interest of the funding agency. Other examples of relevant disclosure include copyright holdings or receipts of royalties on an assessment tool used on the study (APA, 2009).

Authors disclose potential conflicts of interest in a variety of ways depending on the journal. Authors may add a statement in the acknowledgement sections, describe the circumstances in the cover letter to the editor, or include the information on the disclosure form, if one is provided by the journal.

WRITING IN A GROUP

Nurses often coauthor scientific manuscripts in a team setting. Writing in a group can produce frustrations and stumbling blocks that are avoidable with pre-planning. The group involved in writing the manuscript should meet with all members present to discuss these areas: (1) who meets the criteria for authorship and who should be acknowledged instead, (2) the types of manuscripts that might be prepared, (3) the roles and responsibilities of each group member and order of names, and (4) the time frame for completion of the manuscript. As in any group effort, the more coauthors involved in planning and writing the manuscript, the more difficult it is to coordinate the writing efforts and keep track of the group's progress. Small working groups focused on an individual writing project may be more manageable. One person in each group working on a manuscript should coordinate their work, track progress, and keep the group on schedule.

Responsibilities and Roles of Group Members

The first responsibility of the group is to review the criteria for authorship and decide who meets them. Other contributors would then be recognized in the acknowledgment section of the manuscript. Discussions of the group and decisions reached should be recorded by one of the group members and kept securely in case questions and issues arise later.

The second responsibility of the group is to determine how many and what types of manuscripts will be prepared, including the audiences to be reached and potential journals. If the project involves research, the authors need to decide how the study findings will be disseminated and whether multiple papers may result and for which types of audiences and journals. If multiple manuscripts may emerge from the work completed by the group, this should be decided in the beginning so the roles and responsibilities associated with preparing the manuscripts may be rotated among the group.

The first priority for dissemination of the work is professional journals, but manuscripts also may be prepared for consumer audiences and other non-professional groups. The discussions also might include presentations to be made at conferences, including oral presentations and posters, so these activities are reflected when the work is divided among the group.

Once the decisions are made about the types and number of manuscripts, the third function of the group is to determine the roles and specific responsibilities of group members for writing the manuscript (APA, 2009; ICMJE, 2008). Research teams may adopt a number of different strategies to complete the writing process. One member may write a first draft and then circulate it to other members for review and refinement (Penrose & Katz, 2006). With some teams there is a natural distribution of labor related to content expertise, which may lend itself to dividing the writing among group members. For example, one member may write the description of the conceptual basis of the study, and another the methodology of the study. Some teams write the manuscript "from the inside out," i.e., first assigning the task of tabling all of the data to one member, followed by other members drafting the results, methods, introduction, and discussion sequentially. Writing groups should divide the work according to the skills, habits, and preferences of its individual members (Penrose & Katz).

A procedure should be established for dating the drafts of the paper and, when writing as a group, labeling sections written and revised by different authors. This is important to keep track of contributions and know who to contact if there is a question about the substantive content or why a particular revision was made. Some word processing programs have an option to include automatically the date with each draft. Another feature that is helpful with group writing is line numbering in which each line of the manuscript is given a number automatically. This makes it easier to revise the manuscript and respond to comments about its content. The annotations feature of word processing software helps coauthors communicate comments about specific parts of the manuscript. Exhibit 3.1 is a tracking form for use in group writing projects.

Depending on the decisions made by members of the writing group, individual members will be assigned specific roles. These include the roles of first author, corresponding author, coauthors, and acknowledged contributors to the manuscript. These roles may shift as the writing project progresses, and with this shift may come a change in the order of author names. But discussion of assigned roles early in the process is important for accountability and productivity in the writing group.

First Author

Typically the first or lead author contributes the most to the project and manuscript (APA, 2009). The first author is often the person who initiated and developed the clinical project, or in the case of research is the primary investigator, and is responsible for moving the group toward completion of a manuscript to describe its work. The assignment of first and subsequent authors should reflect relative contributions to the manuscript rather than organizational status (APA, 2009).

The first author has more responsibilities associated with writing the paper than do the other authors and may be the most experienced in writing for

EXHIBIT 3.1

Tracking Form for Group Writing Projects

Name of research study, clinical project, manuscript:

_____

_____

Authors (list in order):

_____

_____

_____

Acknowledgments (list in order):

_____

_____

Manuscript Responsibilities (list and describe)	Author Assigned	Due Date	Submit to	Date Completed

publication. The first author coordinates preparation of the manuscript. While the group should determine the roles and responsibilities of each author, some common activities completed by the first author are presented in Exhibit 3.2.

EXHIBIT 3.2

Responsibilities of First Author

- Leads the discussion about authorship; the manuscripts to be prepared, their content, and how to organize each one; the order of author names; who will assume responsibility for different parts of the manuscript and for multiple papers if more than one will be prepared; and the time frame
- Obtains author guidelines and assures that they are met
- Arranges for word processing of manuscript
- Completes own writing assignment
- Edits drafts and suggests revisions to coauthors

Continued

Exhibit 3.2 *Continued*

- Maintains copies of all drafts, with dates, and notes about revisions
- Edits a final version of the manuscript for a consistent writing style throughout
- Reads and corrects the final typed manuscript
- Facilitates approval of the final manuscript by coauthors, has each author date and initial the final copy indicating their approval of it, and files these
- Keeps copies of references used in preparing the manuscript and for background work
- Sets up group meetings and keeps records of the discussions
- Assures that coauthors adhere to the time frame and takes the actions established by the group when coauthors do not
- Obtains permissions if needed
- Makes sure that the correct number of copies of the manuscript and other required materials are submitted with it
- May assume responsibilities of corresponding author
- Coordinates subsequent revisions of the manuscript following peer review
- Coordinates signing of the copyright agreement by coauthors
- Reviews page proofs, the typeset manuscript pages that are reviewed for errors before publication, and returns them promptly to the publisher

---

Corresponding Author

The corresponding author communicates with the editor, beginning with the query letter, and is designated as such on the title page of the manuscript or in the cover letter. While the first author usually serves as the corresponding author, the group may decide for another person to assume this role.

The corresponding author is the contact between the authors and the editor, discussing revisions to be made, working with the editor to assure that these are adequately made, and returning the revisions and related materials on time. The corresponding author also receives notification of page proof availability and is responsible for their review and answering all queries in the time frame requested. The contact between the corresponding author and editor helps to establish the credibility of the group and its dependability. Positive working relationships between authors and editors are important in terms of future publications. Once the paper is published, the corresponding author communicates with readers by distributing reprints of the article and answering questions.

Coauthors

Coauthorship of articles has become the norm, especially given the increasing specialization of healthcare, multidisciplinary collaborations, and multi-site research projects (AMA, 2007; Borry, 2006). There is no absolute limit imposed on the number of coauthors permitted on scientific manuscripts (AMA, 2007; APA, 2009; Penrose & Katz, 2006). Coauthors assume responsibility not only for their sections of the manuscript but also for the intellectual content of the paper as a whole. Remember that each author should be able to defend the manuscript publicly.

Writing groups should review the order of author names early and often in order to avoid conflict and problems later on (Baggs, 2008; Price, 2000). Principles to be considered by writing groups for determining the ordering of authors include:

- No contributor should be considered unless the individual has met the three criteria for authorship discussed above.
- Authors should be listed according to level of contribution, from most to least.
- Decisions about order should be discussed early in the project and reviewed regularly as the project progresses and the manuscript emerges.
- Decisions about order are the prerogative of the authors not the journal editor.
- Authors should be provided space to explain the order of authorship if deemed necessary.
- Editors may require disclosure of author contributions.
- Changes made to the author order following submission should be approved by all authors and communicated to the editor. This includes changes related to an author's death or incapacitation (AMA, 2007; ICMJE, 2008).

With the growing number of authors listed with publications, it is more and more difficult to determine the contributions of each person to the project based on the order of author names. In a recent study, only 9% of journals published researchers' contributions to the manuscript (Wager, 2007). If disclosure of the contributions made to the research and to the manuscript were more widespread, the contributors could accept credit and responsibility with more transparency. An example of a contributor list using this system is found in Exhibit 3.3.

EXHIBIT 3.3

Example of Contributor List

Article Citation:
Oermann, M. H., Blair, D., Kowalewski, K., Wilmes, N. A., & Nordstrom, C. K. (2007). Citation analysis of the maternal/child nursing literature. *Pediatric Nursing, 33*, 387–391.

Names on Byline:
Marilyn H. Oermann, Darlene A. Blair, Kathleen Kowalewski, Nancy A. Wilmes, and Cheryl K. Nordstrom

Contributor List:
Study design: MHO; data collection: DAB, KK, NAW; data analysis: MHO, CN; and manuscript preparation: MHO, DAB, KK, NAW, CKN. Jane Long, Christina Morris, Susan Linings, and Clare Davis reviewed the articles and found the original sources. (Note that they are not listed in the article citation).

Group Authors

Group or collaborative authorship may occur when a research project involves multiple academic centers or when organizations or working groups produce a publishable manuscript. In these cases, the manuscript may legitimately be considered as having been authored by the group rather than by individual authors. Authorship of a group-generated document should be determined based on two considerations: appropriate credit for individual contributors and user-friendly indexing of citations for online search and retrieval. When a group authors a manuscript, authorship may legitimately be assigned in several ways (AMA, 2008; ICMJE, 2008):

- One or more authors who meet the standard criteria described above may take responsibility for writing the paper on behalf of or for the specified group and be listed as authors in the by-line; participants who did not meet all of the criteria are listed in the acknowledgements.
- The group name may appear in the byline as the sole collaborative author-group, with all contributing members of the group listed in the acknowledgements or other space in the article.
- Authorship may be attributed to the group as a whole, without identification of group members. In this case, every member of the group must meet criteria for authorship, and one member should be identified as the corresponding author for the group.

Acknowledged Contributors

Acknowledgments are generally used to recognize people who contributed to the research, project, or preparation of the manuscript but do not qualify for authorship. In the acknowledgment section of a manuscript, the author can give credit to people who assisted with the work, such as individuals who:

- critically reviewed the research proposal, design, or methods;
- gave advice on the project;
- collected the data;
- analyzed the data;
- provided statistical support;
- provided technical support;
- assisted in writing and preparing the manuscript; or
- critically reviewed the manuscript.

Acknowledgments also should specify the financial and material support provided for the project (ICMJE, 2008). An example of an acknowledgment for grant support is: "Supported by Heart and Stroke Foundation of Ontario Grant B-2361" (O'Farrell, Murray, & Hotz, 2000, p.97).

Persons mentioned in the acknowledgment section of a manuscript must grant permission to include their names. The inclusion of names in the acknowledgment may suggest endorsement of the content of the manuscript, and for this reason acknowledged contributors should have the opportunity to read the manuscript and consent to be acknowledged.

The acknowledgement section may also contain statements that the authors had full access to datasets. Such disclosure is important under two conditions: where a study was funded by a commercial entity with financial interest in the outcome and where studies are based on data from public archives or repositories. In the latter case, a link to the dataset should be provided, along with any information about independent reliability checks of the analyses by non-compensated scientists (AMA, 2007).

The fourth responsibility of the writing group involves establishing a time frame for completion of each phase in the writing project and manuscript as a whole. The time frame should include the expectations of each group member with accompanying due dates and when the group will meet. The discussion of the time frame also should include the actions to be taken if coauthors do not complete their responsibilities by the due date. This is an important area of discussion because if due dates are not established and adhered to, the writing project may never get completed. The actions to be taken when coauthors do not complete their responsibilities on time might include being dropped entirely from the writing group and listed as a contributor in the acknowledgments or involve a change in responsibilities and reordering of author names. The group should specify its decisions at this point in the discussions, not when required because of noncompliance.

Students Writing With Faculty

Writing groups that include both faculty members and students require special considerations. The relative contributions of each person, professor and student, often are perplexing when the student earns academic credit for his or her work on a project and the professor is being compensated for teaching the student.

Manuscripts coauthored by faculty and students may demonstrate elements of either guest or ghost authorship or both (Price et al., 2000). Unfortunately, under pressure to publish in order to meet criteria for tenure and promotion, some faculty members request or demand authorship credit on any manuscript related to student work guided by faculty. However, unless professors meet all three criteria for authorship specified by the Uniform Requirements (ICMJE, 2008), they should not be listed as authors (guest authorship). If a student and a faculty member jointly plan and carry out a project, and both contribute to drafting and revising the manuscript, both should be listed as authors. It is unethical for a professor to ask a student to draft a manuscript and not give the student authorship credit, or worse, to assign a paper as a course requirement and then to submit the student's work for publication without listing the student as an author (ghost authorship).

The best approach is to negotiate clear expectations for the roles of student and professor with regard to course work and writing for publication. If the student is expected to complete a project for course credit, the teacher should evaluate the work for a grade first, and then discuss the work necessary to author a manuscript for publication. It is at that time that the relative contributions of each person to the manuscript can be negotiated and authorship credit can be assigned fairly. As a general rule, a student is listed as first author on any multiple-authored manuscript that is substantially based on the student's thesis or dissertation (APA, 2009).

▒ SUMMARY

Each individual designated as an author on a manuscript or other type of paper should have contributed sufficiently to it. The *Uniform Requirements for Manuscripts Submitted to Biomedical Journals* specifies that authorship credit should be given only when the author made substantial contributions to: (1) the conception and design of the study, or to the analysis and interpretation of the data, and to (2) drafting the manuscript or revising it for important content, and to (3) the approval of the final version of the manuscript (ICMJE, 1997).

Acknowledgments are generally used to recognize people who contributed to the research, project, or preparation of the manuscript but do not qualify for authorship. People mentioned in the acknowledgment section of a manuscript must grant permission to include their names.

When writing with multiple authors, the first step is to decide on authorship and who qualifies. The second step is to determine the order of author names. Typically the first author contributes the most to the project and manuscript. The order of coauthors' names should be determined by their relative contributions to the work. Coauthors assume responsibility not only for their sections of the manuscript but for the intellectual content of the paper as a whole.

Authors complete other preparations before beginning to write. These preparations allow authors to focus on their writing once they begin.

▒ REFERENCES

American Medical Association. (2007). *AMA manual of style: A guide for authors and editors* (10th ed.). New York: Oxford University Press.

American Psychological Association. (2009). *Publication manual of the American Psychological Association* (6th ed.). Washington, DC: Author

Baggs, J. G. (2008). Issues and rules for authos concerning authorship versus acknowledgements, dual publication, self-plagiarism, and salami publishing. [Editorial.] *Research in Nursing and Health, 31*: 295–297. doi: 10.1002/nur.20280.

Borry, P., Schotsmans, P., & Dierickx, K. (2006). Author, contributor or just a signer? A quantitative analysis of authorship trends in the field of bioethics. *Bioethics, 20*(4), 213–220.

Ilakovac, V., Fister, K., Marusic, M., & Marusic, A. (2007). Reliability of disclosure forms of authors' contributions. *Canadian Medical Association Journal, 176*(1), 41–46. doi: 10.1503/cmaj.060687

International Committee of Medical Journal Editors. (2008). *Uniform requirements for manuscripts submitted to biomedical journals: Writing and editing for biomedical publication.* Retrieved from http://www.icmje.org/urm_main.html

Marusic, A., Bates, T., Anic, A., & Marusic, M. (2006). How the structure of contribution disclosure statements affects validity of authorship: A randomized study in a general medical journal. *Current Medical Research & Opinion, 22*(6), 1035–1044.

McKneally, M. (2006). Put my name on that paper: Reflections on the ethics of authorship. *Journal of Thoracic and Cardiovascular Surgery, 131*(3), 517–519. doi: 10.1016/j.jtcvs.2005.09.060

Mowatt, G., Shirran, L., Grimshaw, J. M., Rennie, D., Flanagin, A., Yank, V.,...Bero, L. A. (2002). Prevalence of honorary and ghost authorship in Cochrane reviews. *Journal of the American Medical Association, 287*(21), 2769–2771.

O'Farrell, P., Murray, J., & Hotz, S.B. (2000). Psychologic distress among spouses of patients undergoing cardiac rehabilitation. *Heart & Lung, 29*(2), 97–104.

Penrose, A. M. & Katz, S. B. (2004). *Writing in the sciences: Exploring conventions of scientific discourse* (2nd ed.). New York: Pearson Longman.

Price, J. H., Dake, J. A., & Oden, L. (2000). Authorship of health education articles: Guests, ghosts, and trends. *American Journal of Health Behavior 24*(4). Retrieved from: http://search.ebscohost.com/login.aspx?direct=true&db=rzh&AN=2000060050&site=ehost-live&scope=site

Saver, C. (2006). Legal and ethical aspects of publishing. *Association of periOperative Registered Nurses Journal, 84*(4), 571–576. doi:10.1016/S0001-2092(06)63936-7

Wager, E. (2007). Do medical journals provide clear and consistent guidelines for authorship? *MedGenMed: Medscape General Medicine, 9*(3), 16.

4

REVIEWING THE LITERATURE

Conducting a literature review is a skill the author needs to develop to be an effective writer. Often, prior to writing the manuscript, the author has reviewed, critiqued, and synthesized the literature as a basis for a research study, an innovation, or a project to be described in the paper. In this situation, the literature may need to be updated, or if the focus of the manuscript is on the implications of the study for clinical practice, another review of the literature from this perspective may be helpful. Other times, though, the author begins with a topic to be considered for a manuscript but has not yet searched the literature. The review enables the author to decide if the manuscript is worth writing in the first place and to gain an understanding of material that has already been published on the topic. Either way, the author cannot begin writing without completing a review of the literature.

Chapter 4 prepares the author for conducting and writing a literature review for a manuscript. Although literature reviews for research studies, theses and dissertations, course work, evidence-based practice, and other purposes vary in the types of literature used, their comprehensiveness, and how they are summarized for the reader, the process of reviewing the literature is the same. Chapter 4 describes bibliographic databases useful for literature reviews in nursing, selecting databases to use, search strategies, analyzing and synthesizing the literature, and writing the literature review for a manuscript and other types of papers. The outcome of this chapter is to develop skill in conducting literature reviews for writing papers in nursing.

PURPOSES OF LITERATURE REVIEW

A literature review is a critique and synthesis of current knowledge about a topic, for research and for use in clinical practice, teaching, administration, and other areas of nursing. There are three main purposes of reviewing the literature. The first purpose is to describe what is known already about a topic. The literature review provides the background for designing a research study, answering questions about clinical practice, developing new projects, and making other decisions in nursing. It reveals existing knowledge about a topic and related areas.

The literature search also lets the author decide whether or not to write the paper. The author may have an idea to share with readers but find from the review of the literature that the topic has already been adequately covered and another article is unnecessary. The opposite also might be true with the proposed paper contributing new ideas and a different perspective to the topic. The review provides the background readings for the manuscript and may help the author decide how to present the content to best meet the needs of particular readers.

The second purpose is to identify gaps in knowledge and where questions still remain. Research studies and other types of projects should build on prior work and fill those gaps. When reviewing the literature to guide practice decisions, nurses can assess the available evidence and identify where further study is needed to build the evidence base of an intervention or a practice.

The third purpose is to determine how the proposed study or project will contribute new knowledge to nursing. How does the work contribute to the literature and answer existing questions? How does it reinforce what is already known? Answering questions such as these is important later in the writing process when the author describes the research or project in the manuscript because readers are interested in how the work expanded what was known about the topic.

TYPES OF LITERATURE REVIEWS

Chapter 4 presents guidelines for conducting literature reviews when writing a manuscript, but these same principles apply when reviewing the literature for papers for courses; a thesis or dissertation; and grants, projects, and other initiatives in which the nurse may be involved.

Literature Reviews for Papers for Courses

When writing the literature review for a term paper and other papers for courses, the author begins with identifying a topic (or the one assigned by the teacher), locates research and other types of articles on that topic using bibliographic databases, critiques and synthesizes the literature, and then writes the review. The keys to this process are understanding the purpose of the paper and pacing oneself to have adequate time to complete the review and write the necessary number of drafts of the paper.

Literature Reviews for Theses and Dissertations

For a thesis, which is a master's level research project, and a dissertation, which is a more extensive and original research study completed at the doctoral level, the same process is used for completing the literature review. The student begins with a topic, approved by the faculty advisor and committee, and then locates, critiques, and synthesizes prior research, identifying how the study contributes new knowledge to nursing or confirms what is already known about the topic.

The literature review for a thesis and dissertation is comprehensive, revealing prior studies on the problem and related areas, and provides the rationale for conducting the research. The student needs to be thorough in identifying the relevant literature, use preset criteria for analyzing studies, and synthesize findings to reveal what is known about the problem and what needs to be examined further. Students defend the research proposal and completed thesis and dissertation, under the scrutiny of the student's committee and other faculty, depending on the procedures established by the college and university. The literature review is a major part of this process, providing the background and rationale for conducting the study and demonstrating how the completed research adds new knowledge to nursing.

Literature Reviews for Grants, Projects, and Other Initiatives

Nurses review and critique the literature as background for developing grants, evidence-based practice and clinical projects, quality improvement studies, and other initiatives. The literature review provides the rationale for these, indicating how they fulfill important needs. Depending on their purposes, the types of literature reviewed may include original research reports, descriptive articles, anecdotal reports, monographs, books, and published case reports. The process of conducting and writing the literature review is similar to other types of papers.

Literature Reviews for Manuscripts

The literature review completed for a course assignment, a thesis or dissertation, and grants, projects, and other initiatives may lead to the preparation of a manuscript and serve as the basis for writing its introduction and literature review section, depending on the format of the manuscript. For other manuscripts, though, the author begins with an idea and then searches the literature to learn what has already been published on the topic and to develop the background for the paper. Regardless of the beginning point for the literature review, the same process is used for identifying, critiquing, and synthesizing the literature.

There are differences, though, in how the literature is presented in a manuscript compared with these earlier papers. In a manuscript there are restrictions in the number of pages, and the author needs to limit the summary of the literature to allow adequate pages for other sections of the paper. As such, the literature reviews in most manuscripts are short and focused, providing the background of the topic and rationale for the research or project described in the manuscript.

Format to Use

Each journal has its own format for how the literature is reported. In many journals, the literature is integrated in the introduction. With this format, the introduction presents the topic of the paper, purpose of the research or project, and why the topic is important, and uses the literature to present the background and rationale for the research or project. Vintzileos and Ananth (2009) suggested that the introduction be two paragraphs: the first one summarizes the background information, rationale, and need for the study and identifies how the new information in the manuscript meets that need. The second paragraph states the purpose of the study. Papers submitted to medical journals often follow this format, and the *AMA Manual of Style* suggests that the introduction should not exceed two or three paragraphs (American Medical Association [AMA], 2007).

In other journals there is a section devoted to the literature review. With these papers, the topic and its importance are discussed in the introduction, often using research and other types of articles as support. The literature is then presented in the next section of the paper. Because ways of presenting the literature review differ across journals, it is important for authors to read the guidelines for the journal and examine a few sample articles published by it.

Extent of Literature and Style of Presentation

The extent of literature presented and writing style used also differ across journals. For research manuscripts the literature review is extensive and includes an analysis of prior studies and synthesis of the findings. A comprehensive review of the literature is important to reveal the gaps in knowledge, which led to the study being presented.

What about other journals? The research paper may be submitted to a clinical journal that publishes reports of research. When writing for a journal that focuses more on clinical practice, the literature review will be less extensive. In many journals the presentation of the literature emphasizes the practice implications of prior studies, and the author needs this information prior to writing the literature review.

It should be apparent why the earlier review of the journals, their goals, and their writing styles is important. That review gives the author a sense of the extent of literature to be presented in a particular journal and how that literature should be reported. In some journals a more formal and academic style of writing is used to present the literature, while in other journals an informal style is used. An example of each style is presented in Exhibit 4.1.

EXHIBIT 4.1

Writing Styles for Literature Reviews

Formal, Academic Style

Studies on patient views of the quality of their healthcare have focused mainly on patient satisfaction with hospital care and the care provided by nursing staff during that hospitalization (Bauleim & Jones, 2009; Heimleich, Dwyer, & Aleive, 2010; Smith, 2007; Zoe, et al., 2010). Patient satisfaction is influenced by the expectations of patients, their prior experiences with the healthcare setting, and their perceptions of quality care (Lazarus, 2008; McMillen, Jones, Smith, & Brown, 2009).

Informal Style

Many studies have been done in nursing on how satisfied patients are with their nursing care in hospitals and other settings (Bauleim & Jones, 2009; Smith, 2007). We know from these studies that patients expect a certain level of nursing care, and these expectations influence their satisfaction with care. Nurses do not always know what aspects of nursing care are important to patients—we need to learn more about this from our patients (McMillen, Jones, Smith, & Brown, 2009).

Current Literature Reported Accurately

Manuscripts submitted to peer reviewed journals are critiqued as a basis for the decision whether to publish them and if published are read critically by others. The literature cited in the paper should present the current state of the research and evidence on the topic and should be accurate. For a research paper, the author may have completed the literature review a year or more prior to beginning the manuscript; in these cases the literature review will probably need to be updated. The author should cite the latest work published on the topic.

Accuracy is essential in interpreting and synthesizing the literature as well as in citing the references. Errors in citing references in the text of papers and on the reference lists must be avoided. Reference accuracy is important for readers to retrieve cited documents and also for authors of those papers to get credit for their work (Oermann, Mason, & Wilmes, 2002). An early study by Taylor (1998) analyzed the references of three nursing research journals and found that 38.3% of the articles had major errors in references, which could impede locating them; the errors were generally mistakes in author names. Oermann and colleagues found errors in references of clinical and general readership nursing journals, suggesting the need for authors to take time in preparing the references and verify their accuracy before submitting the manuscript and in the page proofs (Oermann, Cummings, & Wilmes, 2001; Oermann, Mason, & Wilmes, 2002; Oermann & Ziolkowski, 2002). Use of reference management software such as EndNote® can help prevent many of these citation errors.

Of particular importance is for authors to check the availability of Web references, not only prior to submission of the manuscript but also when revising the paper and checking the page proofs. Web sites and addresses can change frequently. Of 573 web citations in nursing articles randomly selected for analysis, 159 (27.7%) were no longer available and could not be found in an Internet search (Oermann, Nordstrom, Ineson, & Wilmes, 2008).

TYPES OF LITERATURE FOR INCLUSION IN REVIEW

There are different ways of classifying the literature that might be reviewed for manuscripts in nursing. One way of categorizing the literature is by empirical, theoretical, descriptive, anecdotal reports, and reviews. The literature also includes primary and secondary sources.

Empirical

The empirical literature includes reports of research published in journals as well as unpublished studies such as master's theses and doctoral dissertations. These are the original reports of the research study, including its aims, methods, results, discussion of the findings, and implications. In writing research papers, the author focuses predominantly on empirical literature. Because the author has reviewed this literature as a basis for developing the research proposal and conducting the study, frequently only newly published articles need to be examined prior to beginning the manuscript.

Theoretical

Theoretical literature describes concepts, models, and theories in nursing and related fields. Articles, books, and other documents describing theoretical perspectives are useful for developing a conceptual framework for a research study and presenting in a manuscript the concepts and theories that guided the study or project. For example, the literature review for a manuscript on loneliness among older adults may include theoretical articles on loneliness, social isolation, social support, and aging, among others.

Descriptive

Many articles in nursing journals do not describe research or theory but instead report on practices important to nurses regardless of their role. Articles on patient care, new clinical practices and initiatives, educational innovations, nursing management, trends in nursing, issues, and other topics are in this category of literature. These are important to provide the background information for a manuscript and allow the author to assess what others have written about the topic.

Anecdotal

Anecdotal reports are articles that present personal experiences and views of individuals rather than a systematic evaluation or study of the topic. An article about the benefits of preceptors to new graduates based on comments by the graduates, preceptors' evaluations, and observations by others in the clinical setting is an example of an anecdotal report; the effects of using preceptors were not measured through research. Anecdotal reports may be interesting to read and present innovative ideas for consideration, but because they are not based on any type of study with controls or comparison groups, they should be used sparingly in a literature review (Galvan, 2009). For some manuscripts, however, anecdotal reports are useful in presenting the need for study in an area and for getting the reader's interest in the paper.

Reviews

Some journals publish articles that are reviews of the literature. Traditional literature reviews summarize what is known about a particular topic. Integrative reviews critique the research and synthesize the findings, using a well defined and rigorous approach, to answer specific clinical and other types of questions (Cronin, Ryan, & Coughlan, 2008; Torraco, 2005). Journals that publish review articles usually have high standards for accepting these papers (Galvan, 2009). Reviews are valuable to authors in writing for publication because they synthesize the current state of the literature, indicating what is already known and gaps in knowledge. Review articles, though, are secondary sources, and for many papers authors will need to access the original documents.

Primary and Secondary Sources

Primary sources are original sources of information written by the person who developed the ideas. They are original because they are the first published accounts of the research study, theory, innovation, and idea. For research reports, the primary source is the paper written by the researcher who conducted the study. In primary sources the reader finds detailed information about the research problem, methodology, results, and discussion, described by the researchers themselves.

In the theoretical literature the primary source is the theorist who developed the model, theory, or framework. For other types of literature, the primary source is the originator of the innovation or idea.

In secondary sources the information is summarized and reported by someone other than the originator. Summaries of research, literature reviews, descriptions of clinical projects, and discussions of models and theories reported in articles, books, and other references by an author other than the original are secondary sources. The problem with using secondary sources is that the author has interpreted and summarized the writings of someone else. With secondary sources on research, sometimes only limited information is provided about the methodology and findings, or the discussion may highlight only some of the important outcomes.

For secondary theoretical literature, the author may have misinterpreted the model, theory, or framework, or allowed own views to influence the discussion. For other literature authors of secondary sources may omit vital details that would influence use of the innovation or idea in practice and may be biased in the information reported and how it is presented in the paper. In searching the literature in preparation for writing manuscripts and other papers, only primary sources should be used unless those sources cannot be found.

Most literature reviews include predominantly articles published in peer-reviewed journals, which have been critiqued by experts as a basis for their acceptance. These articles can be accessed by searching bibliographic databases, such as MEDLINE® (Medical Literature, Analysis, and Retrieval System Online) and CINAHL® (Cumulative Index to Nursing and Allied Health Literature), which index thousands of journals. By searching these databases, the author can develop a comprehensive review of the literature. Searching the literature is discussed later in this chapter. Some manuscripts also may include in the literature review chapters, books, Web sites, and other gray literature. Gray literature includes reports from government and professional organizations, theses and dissertations, newsletters, and other unpublished documents (Turner, Liddy, Bradley, & Wheatley, 2005). Gray literature is generally accessed by searching the web because most of these documents are not indexed in the bibliographic databases used for a literature review. Information obtained from Web sites and other unpublished documents is typically not peer reviewed and may not available for readers to access in later years. For most manuscripts and papers, authors should rely on journals articles as sources of information for their literature reviews. An exception is surveillance data located in government documents and tables provided to the public on Web sites ending in *.gov*.

DIFFERENCES IN LITERATURE REVIEWS FOR RESEARCH AND USE IN PRACTICE

Literature reviews for developing a research proposal and writing a research paper differ from those conducted when the goal is to locate background information about patient care, an issue in practice, a project being considered, and other topics not related to planning or reporting research.

Reviews for Research Purposes

Literature reviews for research purposes examine studies already completed on the research question and related topics to better understand the problem, identify gaps in knowledge, and provide a basis for conducting the study. These literature reviews are mainly of empirical literature. The goals of a literature review for research reports are to provide readers with a summary of the existing evidence and develop an argument that supports the need for the current study (Polit & Beck, 2008, p. 106). While the study is being conducted, the researcher continues to periodically review the literature to keep current with other relevant studies. When the findings of the study are ready for dissemination, a follow-up literature review may or may not be needed, depending on how consistently the literature was reviewed up to this point.

The literature review for a research report presents prior studies on the topic, not descriptions of practice or anecdotal reports. These other types of articles, as well as chapters and books, provide sources of information for the author to use in writing the introduction and discussion section of the paper. They contribute to establishing the background of the problem and making a case why the study was indicated.

The other type of literature typically reviewed for research proposals and papers relates to theoretical literature, which describes concepts and theories to guide the research. A review of theoretical articles and books provides the background for developing the conceptual framework for the research study and for understanding the research results. Theories often enable the researcher to organize the literature around concepts in the theory and link together pieces of information and evidence from a study.

Quantitative Research

In quantitative studies the literature review directs the development and implementation of the study (Burns & Grove, 2005). The literature is examined prior to beginning the study to identify the work already done on the topic and where further study is indicated. The background and significance of the study are developed from this review of the literature, and theoretical literature is used to construct the conceptual framework for the research. The methodology, including the design, sample, measurement, treatment, and data collection procedure, is based on previous research (Burns & Grove, 2005). The literature review also is used in analyzing the data and reporting the findings so the current study builds on earlier ones. Thus, in quantitative studies, the literature review is used in each phase of the research. Relevant literature may be cited throughout the research paper except for the results section: generally, references to the literature are not included in the results section of the manuscript.

Qualitative Research

In qualitative research, however, the literature review will vary according to the type of study. Burns and Grove (2005) indicated that in phenomenological research, the literature is reviewed after the data are collected and analyzed to avoid influencing the thinking of the researcher and to help the researcher remain objective. For grounded theory studies, while some literature may be examined before the data are collected, to gain a perspective of prior work in the area, the literature is used predominantly to explain and extend the theory generated from the research (p. 96).

Sandelowski (1998) suggested that there is no one style for presenting qualitative research; researchers choose the "story" they will tell in the manuscript and how to tell it (p. 376). For qualitative manuscripts, the style and format of the paper and how the literature is presented depend on the purposes of the research, methods used, and data.

Reviews for Use in Practice

Literature reviews also are done to gain an understanding of best practices and new approaches to patient care, teaching, management, and other areas, and to provide the background for developing and implementing projects that are not related to research studies. To answer questions about practice problems, the nurse begins with a search of the literature to determine how others have approached these same problems and to identify effective strategies. Varied types of literature may be examined including descriptive articles, anecdotal reports, case reports, chapters, books, and empirical studies, among others.

Similar to research reports, if the author reviewed the literature as a basis for developing a project, an innovation, or another initiative, when ready to write the manuscript, the author may need to update and expand the literature review. One literature review as a basis for developing new standards of practice, for instance, may not sufficient for writing later about those standards and how they were used and evaluated in the clinical setting.

BEGINNING THE SEARCH

The author begins the literature review by identifying the topic of the paper. Whether the review is for a course, a thesis or dissertation, a research study, a project, or an idea to be developed into a manuscript, the author starts with a general topic and then narrows it down to one that can searched easily in a bibliographic database. For example, the author may plan to write a manuscript on a project to improve the satisfaction of patients with their care in the clinic. The topic "patient satisfaction" is too broad for reviewing the literature; there are nearly 48,000 publications indexed in the MEDLINE database alone on this topic. Narrowing the topic to patient satisfaction with nursing care in ambulatory settings produces a more manageable literature review, with about 25 citations.

The author then searches the literature. In earlier years this was done by looking up references in the card catalog and in the annual indexes of the periodical literature, which were only in print format. This information is now compiled in electronic databases, which can be accessed via the Internet or may be provided on a local area network or in the library. These databases are searched electronically, making them fast and easy to use. Each publication in the database is reviewed, a record is produced that describes the publication and its characteristics, and then the content is indexed. This allows the user to search the database for specific content areas and other information.

Bibliographic Databases for Nursing Literature

There are varied bibliographic databases for conducting literature searches in nursing. The two databases that are most useful are MEDLINE and CINAHL. When the paper extends beyond nursing practice, there are other bibliographic databases, such as PsycINFO® for psychological literature or Education Resources Information Center (ERIC) for education literature, that also can be searched. In addition, many authors will use the library catalog to locate books and other types of resources. Selecting the database to search is discussed later in the chapter.

Electronic databases provide easy access to the nursing literature when the author is ready to complete a literature review or needs to update the review. With Internet access, some of the databases can be searched from home for no charge, such as MEDLINE, or by subscription.

MEDLINE

The National Library of Medicine (NLM) provides a wide variety of resources related to the biomedical and health sciences. The NLM's premier bibliographic database is MEDLINE, which contains more than 18 million journal citations from 1949 to the present (NLM, 2008a). The citations in MEDLINE are from more than 5,000 biomedical journals worldwide, including nursing journals. MEDLINE is searched through PubMed® available at http://www.ncbi.nlm.nih.gov/pubmed/.

Articles are indexed using Medical Subject Headings (MeSH®), which is the NLM's system to index articles and catalog books. MEDLINE can be searched using MeSH or by key concepts, author last name followed by initials, journal title, publication date, and any combination of these (National Center for Biotechnology Information [NCBI], 2009). A search produces a list of citations to journal articles each with information about the article and an abstract if available; there are often links to the full-text document. Some of those full-text articles might be free, while others might include a link to the web site of the publisher or other full-text provider (NCBI, 2009). Figure 4.1 provides an example of a citation with multiple links to the full-text document.

FIGURE 4.1

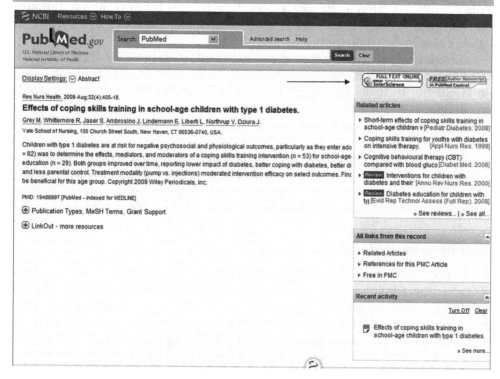

Example of a Citation With Links to Full-Text Document

Sayers, E. W., Barrett, T., Benson, D. A., Bolton, E., Bryant, S. H., et al. (2010). Database resources of the National Center for Biotechnology Information. *Nucleic Acids Research, 38* (Database issue). D5–16. Epub 2009 Nov 12.

The NLM also maintains PubMed Central®, a web-based repository of biomedical journal literature with free and unrestricted access to more than 1.5 million full-text articles; provides access to molecular biology and genomic information; offers extensive healthcare information resources for the public through MedlinePlus®; and maintains the ClinicalTrials.gov database to provide the public with information about all types of clinical research studies, among other resources (NLM, 2009). Links to the many resources of the NLM can be found at http://www.nlm.nih.gov/. The Library's catalog of books, journals, and audiovisuals can be searched through LOCATOR*plus*.

CINAHL

CINAHL is a comprehensive database of nursing and allied health literature. The first edition of CINAHL was published in 1961, indexing the literature from 1956 to 1960, from 16 journals. Currently CINAHL indexes nearly 3,000 journals in nursing and allied health including 71 that are full-text (EBSCO, 2009a). The database also includes access to books and book chapters, nursing dissertations, selected conference proceedings, standards of practice, educational software, and audiovisual media. In addition to the full-text journals, other documents that are available as full text are legal cases, clinical innovations, critical pathways, drug records, research instruments, and clinical trials (EBSCO, 2009a). Initially, CINAHL was a single bibliographic database but has expanded to include four databases with two that are full-text versions.

Material is indexed according to the CINAHL subject headings specifically designed for nursing and allied health literature. The structure is based on MeSH but includes terms and phrases that are tailored to meet the needs of nursing and allied health professionals. There are 12,714 CINAHL subject headings for searching the database and retrieving citations on a specific topic (EBSCO, 2009b).

The CINAHL database is available at medical libraries and libraries with health information, providing access for students and employees for no charge. With this access authors can search the database and often obtain full-text articles. Personal subscriptions to CINAHL are available through varied vendors for a fee.

Other Bibliographic Databases

For many manuscripts, the author will want to review the literature in areas other than nursing. It is worth the time prior to beginning the paper to conduct a thorough search of the literature using multiple databases if appropriate. This provides the author with a broad view of what has already been published on the topic, not only the work done in nursing. Selecting other databases to review depends on the topic of the manuscript. A brief description of selected other databases is found in Table 4.1. This list is not exhaustive but provides an example of the wealth of databases that might be used for reviewing the literature.

Database Structure

Each publication in a bibliographic database has a single *record* with *fields* that contain specific information describing the publication. For instance, the record for a book would include the author's name, title of the book, edition, publisher, and date. There also are fields in the record to indicate the main subject or subjects covered in the book.

Each article in a bibliographic database is indexed similarly. It has a single record with specific information about that article: the author's name, title of the article, journal in which published, publication date and information, and terms or phrases that describe the content of the article. These terms or phrases are important in searching the literature, although sometimes the nurse may begin by searching for particular authors who have done similar work.

Terms for Indexing

MeSH, which stands for Medical Subject Headings, is the NLM's controlled vocabulary thesaurus. A thesaurus is a carefully constructed set of terms in a structure that permits searching at different levels of specificity (NLM, 2008b). The MeSH terms describe the content of an article; thus, authors can search using those

TABLE 4.1

Selected Bibliographic Databases

Database	Subject Area
BIOSIS	Research databases on life sciences information, including biodiversity, biotechnology, drug discovery, gene therapy, and other topics
CINAHL	Nursing and allied health literature
Cochrane Library	High-quality, independent evidence for practice and healthcare decision-making; includes evidence from Cochrane and other systematic reviews, clinical trials, and other evidence reports
Dissertation Abstracts	Abstracts of dissertations in all subjects accepted at US institutions; access to abstracts online through Dissertation Abstracts Online
ERIC	Abstracts of journal articles, books, research syntheses, conference papers, and technical reports in education (including research and practice), and other education-related materials
Education Full Text	Education journals and selected books and annuals
Family and Society Studies Worldwide	Three databases that cover journal and other literature in area of family studies and related topics
Health Source: Nursing/Academic Edition	Nursing and other biomedical fields; includes scholarly full text journals
ISI Citation Indexes	Multiple databases with information from journals, books, book series, reports, conferences, and others. Includes Science Citation Index Expanded™ (SCI™ Expanded), Social Sciences Citation Index® (SSCI®), Arts & Humanities Citation Index® (A&HCI®), and Conference Proceedings Citation Indexes, among others. Covers medicine, nursing (although limited), sciences, social sciences, and humanities. ISI Web of Knowledge also includes Journal Citation Reports® database (impact factors of journals)
MEDLINE/PubMed	Journal articles in life sciences with a concentration on biomedicine and health; includes nursing literature
PsycINFO	Psychological literature
Social Work Abstracts	Social work and related journals on topics such as homelessness, AIDS, child and family welfare, aging, substance abuse, and others
Sociological Abstracts	Sociology and related disciplines, both theoretical and applied

same terms to locate articles on a topic about which they are writing. In addition to its use for indexing articles from the thousands of journals in the MEDLINE/PubMed database, MeSH is also used for the NLM's database on books, documents, and audiovisual materials.

MeSH consists of a set of terms or subject headings that are arranged in both an alphabetical and a hierarchical structure (NLM, 2008b). It uses a tree structure whereby terms are grouped under broad headings, which then have more specific subject headings under them. For example, the heading "education" is at the most general level of the hierarchical structure and at more narrow levels are specific headings such as "baccalaureate nursing education." Exhibit 4.2 provides an example of the MeSH subject headings and levels for the topic "baccalaureate nursing education."

EXHIBIT 4.2

Example of MeSH Subject Headings

Anthropology, Education, Sociology, and Social Phenomena Category
   Education
      Education, Professional
         Education, Nursing
            Education, Nursing, Associate
            Education, Nursing, Baccalaureate
            Education, Nursing, Continuing
            Education, Nursing, Diploma Programs
            Education, Nursing, Graduate
            Nursing Education Research

An advantage of using CINAHL is that the subject headings follow MeSH structure but are specific to the terms used by nurses and allied health professionals, making it easy to search for articles on a topic. For example, if the author is preparing a paper describing a nursing model, there is a major heading "nursing models, theoretical", with many different models and theories listed by both the author's last name and formal name of the model or theory. The search in MEDLINE would be less precise because the headings are more general, such as, "nursing theory" and "models, nursing."

As another example, if the author is writing a paper on a new staffing pattern for maternity nursing, there is a subject heading in CINAHL for obstetric nursing and other headings such as hospital units, alternative birth centers, nursing care, and primary nursing. There are many subheadings for obstetric nursing that might be searched depending on the focus of the paper, for example, administration, economics, manpower, organizations, and trends. Table 4.2 compares the major terms for an article indexed in MEDLINE and the same article in CINAHL.

Keywords

When articles are indexed in a database, an indexer decides what terms or phrases best represent the content in the article, using the MeSH terms or subject

TABLE 4.2

Sample Comparison of Subject Indexing in MEDLINE and CINAHL

Authors: Paton B, Thompson-Isherwood R, Thirsk L
Title: Preceptors matter: An evolving framework
Source: *Journal of Nursing Education* 2009 48(4): 213–216

MEDLINE Terms	CINAHL Major Subject Headings
Alberta[1]	Intuition
*Education, Nursing	Learning Methods
Humans	Nursing Role
Models, Educational	Preceptorship
*Preceptorship	Professional Competence
*Professional	Teaching Methods

[1]Authors from Faculty of Nursing, University of Calgary, Calgary, Alberta, Canada

headings in CINAHL. This ensures that all articles on a particular subject are indexed in the same way, essential when searching for that information. The most specific terms are assigned when possible; for example, an article on pneumonia would be indexed as "pneumonia" rather than "lung diseases" (Lawrence, 2007, p. 780).

The indexed terms are often called keywords in the author guidelines for journals. Many times the guidelines ask authors to submit a short list of keywords with the manuscript when it is submitted. These words are then used for indexing the paper if accepted. To identify keywords for this purpose, the author should go to the thesaurus of the database in which the journal is indexed and select keywords that best describe the content. The indexes are usually listed in the journal on the masthead or table of contents page. If unsure of where the journal is indexed, then author should use MeSH terms or CINAHL subject headings.

Selecting the Database

After choosing the topic and narrowing it down, the next step is to select the most appropriate database for the search. For most clinical topics in nursing, the author should use both CINAHL and MEDLINE and also may search the library catalog. Multiple databases should be included for comprehensive searches of nursing topics (Allen, Jacobs, & Levy, 2006). In a search for articles on problem-based learning in nursing, Oermann (2007) found limited overlap in results between CINAHL and PubMed with the same search strategy, and recommended using more than one database. Searches on nonclinical topics often will extend beyond these into other relevant databases such as those listed in Table 4.1. If unsure of the databases to use, the author should consult with a librarian or should review potential databases and types of articles indexed in them.

Identifying the databases to search is an important decision for the author because otherwise critical articles may be missed. Even though electronic resources are easy to access and convenient to use, a comprehensive search also may involve a review of books and other sources of information.

SEARCH STRATEGIES

Once the databases are selected, it is wise to become familiar with how they are organized. The author should read through some records of articles indexed in them to gain of perspective of the fields and information provided. Many of the databases offer differ views of each record. For instance, one view may include the citation and abstract only while another view adds the terms (e.g., MeSH terms or CINAHL subject headings) and other indexing information.

Before beginning the search, the author should:

- Become familiar with the database and the literature indexed in it
- Learn how the database is organized and how to use it for a search
- Review sample records and different views of each record
- Locate the thesaurus and look up the terms that might be used for the search
- Review search strategies and tips included with information about the database
- Learn how to broaden the search (e.g., by using *or*), narrow the search (e.g., by using *and*), exclude terms in a search (e.g., by using *not*), and other ways of making the search more precise
- Learn how to save searches while in progress and at their completion
- Determine how to order documents if available.

Selecting Search Terms

After selecting an appropriate database, the author should do a quick search to determine how much literature has been published on the topic. A good way of beginning is to look up in the thesaurus of the database the terms to use. This preliminary search allows the author to restate the terms if needed before beginning the actual search. The initial search may reveal that the terms chosen are too broad and need to be more specific to produce more manageable results. If the author is planning on writing a manuscript on using videotapes for teaching patients with asthma, searching in PubMed by using "patient education" yields approximately 63,000 citations. The term "asthma" results in 112,000 citations.

The author needs to choose more specific terms from the thesaurus to best describe the topic and retrieve relevant articles, or modify the search using other techniques. At the other extreme, the terms initially selected for the search may be too specific, thereby excluding some of the relevant literature.

Combining Search Terms

Searches can be modified by choosing other terms to search; by manipulating the fields such as limiting publication dates, looking for selected authors, or restricting the search to certain journals; and by using the Boolean connectors *and, or,* and *not.* These connectors indicate how the computer should combine the search terms and treat them in relation to one another. *And* retrieves results that include all the search terms; *or* means that the results must contain at least one of the search terms; and *not* excludes citations with the selected term (NCBI, 2009).

In the example on a search of the literature on videotapes for teaching patients with asthma, by including *and* between "patient education" *and* "asthma", the list is reduced to nearly 2500 references, but this is still too many to be manageable. Limiting the search to humans and English language produces 2010 citations. Even restricting those to the last five years yields nearly 540 citations. Depending on the purpose of the paper and literature review, the author might decide to review the citations for the most current year to identify relevant ones. This literature would provide background information on educating patients with asthma though not necessarily by using videotapes as the instructional method.

The author may decide to add "videotape" to the search; a look in the MeSH database reveals that "videotape recording" is the term for searching, not videotape. This revision in the search for articles yields 11 citations, which are too few for the complete search but represent citations the author should review.

Searching for "asthma" *and* "videotape recording," and limiting the search to humans and English language, results in 34 citations, all of which should be reviewed. Some of the references, though, pertain to use of videotape for non-instructional purposes, and the author can exclude these quickly by reading the abstract of the article.

Modifying the search to "patient education" *and* "videotape recording" results in 420 citations. Limiting the publication date to the last five years, though, produces 110 citations, a more manageable number. While these articles do not focus on videotapes for teaching patients with asthma, they provide background information on how videotapes have been used for educating patients with other health problems and in varied settings. For example, there are articles on the use of an educational video about prostate cancer screening; effectiveness of informational videotapes for patients in primary care, dialysis units, the emergency department waiting room, and other settings; and studies that compared video instruction to other teaching methods. This literature would contribute to a better understanding of what is known about educating patients by videotape instruction and as such should be reviewed by the author.

This is a good example of how different terms might be combined to retrieve the best citations for the paper and a manageable number without omitting important publications. The same process is used when searching the CINAHL database. Similar to setting limits in PubMed, such as English language only or by publication date, in CINAHL the author refines the search by including limits such as publication date and age limit. Selecting different "filters" in CINAHL eliminates those documents from the search. The author should allow time to experiment with terms and phrases until the search produces the type of literature needed for preparing the paper.

Searching Relevant Databases

With the search strategy planned, the author is ready to begin the search in all relevant databases. The search of the database used to refine the search terms should be done first, then the author should move to other databases if appropriate. When the author finds a relevant citation, some databases allow for searching Related Articles. This feature produces a list of citations to articles that are indexed with the same terms or similar ones.

Reviewing the Literature: How Far Back?

The literature should be reviewed starting with the most recent references and working backwards. When restricting the publication dates to the most recent, which is usually done, the author should be alert to landmark or classic studies that might have been published earlier. Determining how far back to review the literature depends on the topic. Reviewing literature published in the last five years is usually sufficient for most papers. If there are limited publications in this time frame, then the author can continue to work backwards, asking why there are few publications in recent years. It may be a problem with the search terms or may suggest trends in nursing that should be considered in the manuscript. Some areas of nursing practice such as technology are changing so rapidly, articles published a few years earlier are outdated.

Reviewing References Lists

As the citations of articles are retrieved, the author may decide to extend the search using alternate terms or even searching different databases. One other technique is to review the reference lists of relevant articles, chapters, and books to identify other citations that might have been missed. Sometimes the classic references are found there. The author also may find citations to journals not in the databases used for the original search or may identify other subject headings that might extend the search.

A word of caution: there comes a point at which the author must decide to complete the search and begin writing the manuscript. Otherwise the author may delay writing and use valuable time to locate a few more references not even needed for preparation of the paper.

Saving Searches

When searching the literature, it is important to save the results of each search and resulting citations for use in preparing the manuscript and to avoid reviewing a citation more than once. Electronic databases allow authors to save the results of searches and individual citations. Searches in PubMed can be saved temporarily on the Clipboard and permanently as a text file, using My NCBI Collections, as RSS (Really Simple Syndication) feeds, by creating a URL to bookmark the search, or by exporting the citations into a reference management program such as EndNote. The citations also can be emailed or printed. Citations from CINAHL searches can be saved by clicking the "add folder" icon, which automatically places them in a temporary session folder; the searches can be saved permanently in My EBSCOhost. The citations also can be emailed or printed.

The following guidelines provide strategies for authors to manage the searches in addition to saving the results of each search:

- Keep a record of (1) each database searched, (2) terms used for the search, (3) years searched, (4) other limitations placed on the search such as English language only, and (5) resulting citations. Mark the date the search was completed. This record should be kept for writing the current paper and for subsequent searches on the same topic.
- Save the search terms in an electronic file, including terms originally chosen and modified after reviewing the thesaurus of the database. Include any synonyms for the original terms.
- Record how search terms were combined with sample citations produced from each combination; this is helpful in later searches about the same topic.
- Note the dates of any changes in search terms so there is a running record of the progression of the search.
- If Related Records were searched, make a note of how these were accessed and resulting citations.
- Note citations identified from reference lists of articles, chapters, and books, including the original work.
- Record articles, chapters, books, and other materials that will *not* be used for the paper. If another search is done, this will avoid rechecking the same publication.
- Save a copy of publications that will be used in preparing the paper; full-text documents may be accessed during the search. This enables the author to have the material on hand when beginning to write.
- Record all citation information because reference styles differ across journals. This avoids having to recheck a reference when a manuscript is submitted to another journal than originally planned that uses a different style. The author should never rely on memory when it comes to citations.

MANAGING CITATIONS

Considering the large number of citations retrieved in a search, authors need efficient ways of managing and retrieving them for research, writing, and other projects. Frequently a literature search done for one purpose may be expanded for subsequent papers and projects. Along the same line, a review completed for a research study provides the basis for manuscripts written later. It is important to have a system for keeping track of citations for the current project and for use in the future.

Developing a Personalized System

For limited searches of the literature, the author can copy and paste the bibliographic information and abstract into a word document for use later in writing the manuscript or can copy and paste the citation into the paper. However, this is not an efficient way to keep track of citations for a comprehensive literature review. Saving citation information in a reference management program is more efficient and promotes easy access to the citations at a later time.

Reference Management Software

Reference management software, also referred to as citation or bibliographic management software, allows authors to save citations found in a search and access them later. This software sorts citations, retrieves them, and formats references based on the style required by the journal (Steele, 2008). Reference management software such as EndNote, Reference Manager, and ProCite® are proprietary and can be purchased by authors. These software programs allow authors to search online bibliographic databases, store thousands of records, organize citations, create reference lists, and collaborate with others (Thomson Reuters, 2009). They also enable authors to format manuscripts, complete with in-text citations and references based on the journal's style. If the author decides later to submit the manuscript to another publication, which uses a different reference style, the software reformats the in-text citations and reference list, thus avoiding having to retype them. Prior to purchasing reference management software, the author should choose a program that is versatile and easy-to-use, and should first try out the demo version. There also are some free software programs for citation management, and the school or institution library may have free software for use by students and employees.

ANALYSIS OF THE LITERATURE

The author has searched the literature and is now ready to read and analyze the materials. In this phase of the literature review, the author organizes the publications into content areas, develops a format for recording comments, and then analyzes each publication.

Organizing Publications

Initially the author should scan the materials to gain an overview of each publication and its content. This pre-reading enables the author to develop a perspective of the literature as a whole prior to reading separate and sometimes narrow reports (Galvan, 2009).

Then the author should group the articles and other materials by topics or content areas that fit together. While the publications are usually organized by topics, they also might be grouped chronologically or by research design and findings. The decision about how to organize them depends on the purpose of the paper and content area. Organizing them into categories facilitates the literature review because then all the articles and other materials about one topic are read at a time. This helps the author gain an understanding of the content and what has already been published about it and to manage an extensive literature review. Reading the materials in categories also is valuable when writing the draft because the documents are grouped as they might be in the paper.

As the articles and other documents are grouped into topics, the author should attempt to identify more specific content areas, subtopics, which in turn will help organize the literature within each topic. For instance, in a literature review on hospice care in nursing homes, the authors grouped the literature into these topics: (1) background and trends; (2) clinical and quality impact of using hospice in nursing homes; (3) government spending, payment, and efficiency; (4) cost, payment, and profit for nursing homes; (5) barriers to growth and challenges for public policy; and (6) data needs and areas for future research. The literature associated with the first topic, background and trends, was then grouped into subtopics: benefits of hospice, payment for hospice, growth and the changing nature of hospice use, and provision of nursing home hospice (Stevenson & Bramson, 2009).

Hard copies of articles can be placed in file folders or portable document formats (PDFs) of the articles can saved in electronic folders of specific content areas with accompanying notes stored with them. Notes can be added to the folders with important comments about the publications that are critical to the literature review or might be cited in the paper, to keep track of different research methods and subjects, to identify trends in findings of studies or the development of ideas, and to highlight other points.

For searches of Web sites, a similar system should be set up for keeping track of them. This system should include documenting how the web search was conducted and recording information about the material accessed at the Web site including the author's name, title of the document, name of the Web site and its URL, publication date, and date accessed. This information is needed for the reference list of the paper should the site be included in it.

Format for Recording Comments

Before reading the publications and other resources, the author should decide how comments about them will be recorded. This facilitates writing the manuscript and saves the author time later. When reading research articles, consistency in note taking is important in examining patterns across studies and later in synthesizing findings. Care should be taken when recording quotations so they are accurate and the page number noted; this will avoid having to return to the reference at the writing stage.

Exhibit 4.3 and Tables 4.3, 4.4, and 4.5 provide sample formats for recording comments about different types of literature reviewed. Regardless of the format, the key is to develop a consistent method of documenting comments so they are useful later when writing the manuscript.

Guidelines for Analyzing Literature

For some papers the author's intent in reviewing the literature is to learn what has already been on the published on the topic to decide whether to proceed with the manuscript. Once this is determined, then authors need to critically examine each publication before using it as a basis for their own research and writing. Not

EXHIBIT 4.3

Format for Notes About Non-Databased[1] Publications

Reference Information[2]

Article:
Authors' last and first names[3], middle initial(s) _____
Title of article _____
Journal name and publication date _____
Volume, issue, and page numbers_____
DOI_____

Book:
Chapter authors' last and first names, middle initial(s)_____
Title of chapter and page numbers_____
Book authors'/editors' last and first names, initial(s)_____
Title of book and subtitle if any_____
Volume number and title if more than 1 volume; edition number
(other than 1st edition)_____
Place of publication, name of publisher, date of
publication_____

Electronic materials:
Authors' last and first names[3], middle initial(s)_____
Title of document_____
Name of Web site_____
URL_____
Date accessed_____

Notes
1. What is the main point of this publication?
2. What are the major content areas included in it?
3. What background information will it contribute to the paper?
4. How might the publication be used for writing the paper?
5. What are strengths of the publication? Weaknesses?
6. Other comments: _____

[1] Publications that do not report an original research study.
[2] Record complete citation. If using reference management software or have copy of document, record enough information to match notes with reference.
[3] Some reference formats require first name of lead author.

---

every document retrieved from a literature review may be used for preparing a manuscript. Some papers are not used because of poor quality; other times the content is not relevant to the purpose of the paper.

The questions in Exhibit 4.4 are useful for analyzing nursing literature. These are general questions to guide the critique of articles and other documents

TABLE 4.3

Format for Notes About Databased Publications: Quantitative Studies

Reference Information[1]

Article:

Authors' last and first names[2], middle initial(s) _____

Title of article _____

Journal name and publication date _____

Volume, issue, and page numbers _____

DOI _____

Purpose/ Research Questions	Design	Sample (and size)	Instruments (validity and reliability)	Findings	Comments

[1] Record complete citation. If using reference management software or have copy of document, record enough information to match notes with reference.

[2] Some reference formats require first name of lead author.

TABLE 4.4

Format for Notes About Databased Publications: Qualitative Studies

Reference Information[1]

Article:

Authors' last and first names[2], middle initial(s) _____

Title of article _____

Journal name and publication date _____

Volume, issue, and page numbers _____

DOI _____

Type of Qualitative Study	Purpose	Methods	Sample	Findings	Comments

[1] Record complete citation. If using reference management software or have copy of document, record enough information to match notes with reference.

[2] Some reference formats require first name of lead author.

TABLE 4.5

Format for Summarizing Purpose, Methods, and Results of Databased Articles for Literature Review

Author(s)/ Year	Purpose/ Research Questions	Design	Sample (and size)	Instruments (validity and reliability)	Findings	Comments

Note: Add column for treatment/intervention if relevant.

for deciding whether or not to include them in a literature review, assessing their strengths and weaknesses, and planning how they might be incorporated as background for a paper.

Research reports need to be critically appraised to determine the quality of the study and its applicability to answer the research or clinical questions. Studies have strengths and flaws that should be recognized by the author. Problems may exist in how the study was conceptualized and its rationale. There may be issues with the design—its methods, how variables were measured, the instruments used, procedures, and data analysis. The study might have been well designed, but a small sample size limits generalizing the findings to other groups and settings. There may problems with the statistical analysis or how themes were identified and labeled in qualitative studies. Exhibit 4.5 provides a guide for critiquing the research literature in nursing.

Synthesizing the Literature

From this critique of individual articles and other documents, the author develops a view of the literature as a whole and an understanding of what is known about the topic and what still needs to be learned. Synthesis gives the author

EXHIBIT 4.4

Guide for Analyzing Nursing Literature

- What is the purpose of the article, or other type of document, and is it consistent with the author's goals for writing the paper?

- What topics and subtopics are addressed in the article, and are these similar to the content planned for the author's own paper?

- Does the introduction state the problem, issue, need, and so forth, and its significance? Can similarities be drawn between these and the author's own work to be discussed in the paper? If not, how will the article be used in the preparation of the paper?

- Is there a clear and coherent rationale for why the article was written? Why it is important?

- If the article describes nursing practice, a project, an innovation, and so forth, is it comprehensive, providing the reader with information essential to using the content in own setting?

- If the article suggests a change in practice, is there evidence provided for this change?

- Is the literature review in the article accurate and up-to-date? Are primary sources used?

- Does the literature support the discussion and establish the background?

- Does the article make it clear how it fills gaps in the literature? Is this accurate?

- Does the article make significant contributions to the nursing field? Why or why not? What is the relationship between these contributions and the author's goals for writing own paper?

- What concepts, models, and theories are described in the article, and are they relevant to the author's paper? How can these be used to develop the paper?

- Are key terms defined similarly?

- Does the article provide solutions to the problem, issue, need, and so forth, identified in the introduction? Are these solutions applicable to the author's own work?

- If the article evaluated the effectiveness of an intervention, was the methodology sound? Was it described sufficiently to be replicated?

- What is unique about the problem, issue, need, intervention, subjects, setting, and resources described in the article? Are these relevant to the author's own situation? Why or why not?

- What are strengths and weaknesses of the article? How can they be used in preparing the author's own paper?

EXHIBIT 4.5

Guide for Analyzing Research Literature in Nursing

Title
Does it describe the study? Is it informative?

Abstract
Does it emphasize the study's purpose, method, major findings, and
  conclusions?
Is this a quantitative or qualitative study?

Introduction
Does it state the problem and its significance to nursing?
Does the introduction provide the background and rationale for the study?
What is the purpose of the study, and is it clear?
If a conceptual framework is presented, does it relate to the purpose and
  describe the concepts underlying the study and their relationships?

Literature Review
Is the literature critically reviewed?
Are strengths and weaknesses of earlier studies presented?
Does the review support the rationale for conducting the study as reported
  in the article?
Is the literature review up-to-date?
Are important studies included in it?
Are primary sources used?

Research Questions or Hypotheses
Are the research questions or hypotheses clear, specific, and stated
  appropriately?
Are variables defined if appropriate?

Design
Is the design consistent with the problem?
What type of design is used?
What are strengths and weaknesses of the design?

Sample
Is the sampling procedure described?
What criteria were used to select the sample?
Is the sample size adequate?
Is the sample representative, and how will this affect generalizing the
  findings?

Instruments
Are the instruments and other measures described, and are they
  appropriate?
Are they valid and reliable?

Data Collection Procedure

Is the procedure clearly described?

Are methods for collecting qualitative data appropriate for the type of study?

Findings

Are the findings interpreted correctly including any statistical analyses?

Are the statistics appropriate for analyzing the data?

Are the findings presented clearly and in relation to the study questions or hypotheses?

Are the findings presented logically?

Are any tables and figures easy to read, and do they support the text?

Discussion

Are the conclusions based on the study results?

Is the discussion related to the literature, and does it include how the study builds on earlier research?

Are the limitations identified, and could they have been resolved?

Can the findings be generalized and if so, to what populations?

Are there implications for practice, teaching, administration, and others, and are they relevant?

Strengths and Weaknesses

Overall, what are the study's major strengths and weaknesses?

a sense of how studies and other types of projects relate to one another and a perspective of how own topic relates to prior work. Synthesizing the research literature is critical because it allows the author to identify relationships among studies, gaps in the research, and where further study is needed before using the findings in practice.

In developing evidence-based practice, the synthesis of related research provides the evidence to support a change in practice or indicates if further study is needed. As part of this process, nurses critique the literature and weigh the evidence; synthesize the best evidence; and assess feasibility, benefits, and risks (Larrabee, Sions, Fanning, Withrow, & Ferretti, 2007). If the synthesis provides sufficient evidence to support a change in practice, which is feasible, then nurses have a basis for considering a change in practice.

When the publications have been reviewed and analyzed, the author's task is to integrate them and present a summary in the manuscript. First, the author returns to the original purpose of completing the literature review. Was the goal to develop the background for a research study, answer questions about clinical practice, use evidence in practice, develop new projects, or make other decisions? Was the literature review conducted for a paper in a course, thesis, dissertation, grant, or project in which the nurse may be involved? Was the purpose of the literature review to decide whether to write the manuscript, and if so how it should be developed to fill gaps in the literature? The synthesis should meet these original goals for reviewing the literature.

Second, for each topic and subtopic, the author should identify similarities and common points of view in the publications. For research reports, the author should indicate when findings are consistent across studies and when different, propose explanations for those differences (Galvan, 2009). For instance, were the studies done at varied points in time? Were there differences in methodologies and subjects that might account for the discrepancies in findings? Were different instruments used, or were there variations in statistical analyses that might account for the lack of consistency in the results?

Third, the author should recognize gaps in the literature. In writing the paper, the author makes a case how the paper fills these gaps and contributes new knowledge to nursing.

WRITING THE LITERATURE REVIEW

The first step in writing the literature review is to consider the audience of the journal to which the manuscript will be submitted. If writing the literature review for a research journal, it should be comprehensive, each research study should be critiqued as described earlier, and research findings should be synthesized, noting where further study is indicated. In the review authors should justify their study by pointing out how it:

1. closes a gap in the literature,
2. tests an important aspect of current theory,
3. replicates an important study,
4. extends earlier work using a different sample or new methods, and
5. resolves conflicts in the literature (Galvan, 2009, p. 89).

For other journals, the literature review will not have the same depth nor will readers expect this same level of critique as in a research journal. Often, the literature is used to present the topic and why it is important for readers. The literature may be integrated throughout the paper rather than discussed in a separate section. Once again, the importance of identifying possible journals prior to writing the paper is apparent when deciding on how the present the literature review.

Introductory Statement

The literature review should begin an introductory statement about what literature will be presented and why it is important to the problem or purpose of the paper. This introductory statement should not be too broad.

In the example that follows, the first introductory statement to the literature review is too broad; it does not tell the reader what types of literature will be discussed. The methods for assessing critical thinking could be standardized tests, strategies used in classroom instruction, or methods for evaluating cognitive skills in clinical practice. The revised statement indicates more specifically that the literature reviewed is on methods for assessing the critical thinking of nursing students in clinical practice.

Too Broad: Critical thinking is an important competency for nursing students to develop. Varied methods can be used for assessing critical thinking.

Specific and focused: Five methods of assessing nursing students' critical thinking skills within the context of clinical practice are: (1) observation of students in practice, (2) higher-level questions, (3) post clinical conferences, (4) case method, and (5) written assignments. The literature is reviewed on each of these methods.

Important Studies

In writing the literature review, the author should highlight important studies and describe why they are significant. Classic studies should be noted and some discussion provided as to how they contributed to development of the topic. These papers are frequently pivotal works and can be used in the review to show the progression of research in an area. Other than these classic works, however, the literature review should describe current publications, within the last five years.

Lack of Publications on Topic

At times the author may not locate any relevant literature about a topic. Galvan (2009) cautioned against writing "no studies were found" in a manuscript and recommended instead that authors justify these gaps in the literature by explaining how they arrived at this conclusion. For example, the author can indicate the databases that were searched, the years searched, and other limits applied in the search. Details on the search strategy provide support for the statement about no studies found in the literature review.

Grouping Publications

In the synthesis of the literature, authors should group studies, identify similarities and differences across them, and describe how individual studies relate to one another rather than listing and discussing each publication separately. The following example demonstrates this principle:

The demand for registered nurses (RNs) continues to exceed the supply, and this problem will worsen as more nurses retire in upcoming years (Buerhaus, Auerbach, & Staiger, 2009; Chapman, et al., 2009; Palumbo, McIntosh, Rambur, Naud, 2009). This is a particular problem in hospitals, where most new graduates work (Duchscher, 2008; Kovner et al., 2007; Zhao et al., 2009). Many factors affect the demand for RNs, including the aging population, acuity of patients in hospitals, shortened hospital length of stay, and new technologies for care.

There are six different articles cited in this paragraph of the literature review, but rather than discussing each one separately, they are integrated in the review.

When findings are inconsistent, however, the author should report studies separately so the discrepancies are clear to readers. For instance, in the first example below it is not clear which studies had a low return rate of 25% and which had the higher rate of return (65%) after sending reminder postcards.

Original: Previous studies have shown a return rate of surveys ranging from 25% to 65% after clinic staff sent postcards reminding patients to send back their surveys (Adams, 2008; Gabow, 2009; Smith & Jones, 2007).

Revised: Previous studies have shown that sending reminder postcards from clinic staff to patients results in survey return rates ranging from 25% (Adams, 2008; Smith & Jones, 2007) to 65% (Gabow, 2009).

Accuracy of References

As mentioned earlier in the chapter, studies have documented errors in citations in journal articles in nursing (Oermann, Mason, & Wilmes, 2002; Oermann, Nordstrom, Ineson, & Wilmes, 2008; Oermann & Ziolkowski, 2002) similar to other biomedical journals. The citations in a manuscript reflect the quality and thoroughness of the author's work and allow others to retrieve documents cited in the paper. Errors in the authors' names, article title, journal name, page numbers, and publication date may inhibit retrieval of the publication. It is important to be accurate with citations in the literature review, in which many publications are often cited, and on the reference list. Each reference should be checked carefully for errors.

Reference management software does not guarantee accuracy of citations. There may be errors because of data entry mistakes made by the author, limitations of the software such as with citing electronic references, and discrepancies between the software and author guidelines of a journal (Brahmi & Gall, 2006; Kessler & Van Ullen, 2005; Steele, 2008).

▪ PERMISSIONS

Copyright is a form of legal protection to authors of their original works that prevents others from copying them. The copyright is held initially by the author, or coauthors, of a manuscript, but the copyright typically transfers to the publisher either at the time the manuscript is submitted or when it is accepted. Publishers usually require assignment of the copyright to them so they in turn may publish the article and distribute it in different forms. When authors are reviewing the literature and deciding on text, tables, figures, and other illustrations to include in their papers, they need permission from the copyright holder, for example, the publisher of the journal or book, to adapt or reproduce the copyrighted materials in their manuscript. Copyright is described in more detail in chapter 15.

Permission should be obtained for quotes that extend for a few paragraphs. The length quoted should not diminish the "value of the original work" (AMA, 2007, p. 198). Entire tables, figures, and illustrations may not be reproduced without permission. This includes use of a table, figure, or other type of graphic in a paper prepared for a course. Using one or two sentences from a table is acceptable if the original source is referenced, but reprinting the entire table is not.

The request for this permission should be done early in the writing process to avoid delays in the submission and publication of the manuscript. While permission to reprint is required before the article is published, some journal editors may request letters indicating permission has been received when the manuscript is submitted for review.

For journal articles, which are usually copyrighted by the publisher of the journal, the author requests permission from the publisher to reproduce the selection of text, table, figure, or other illustration in the manuscript. Information on how to obtain this permission is included in the masthead of the journal, which lists the editor, staff, and other journal details, or information for the author page. This information also is found at the journal's Web site, and many journals have links to the Copyright Clearance Center to facilitate obtaining permission to adapt and reprint materials. For a book the copyright holder is specified on the page following the title page. When the authors of the original works hold the copyrights, they would grant permission to reprint their material and would be contacted directly.

The Copyright Clearance Center (http://www.copyright.com/) manages the rights for many copyrighted works, for publishers, and for authors. At the Web site authors can purchase permission to adapt, reproduce, and distribute published materials, and post them to a Web site (Copyright Clearance Center, 2009).

As part of the permission to adapt and use copyrighted materials, copyright holders will often specify how the credit line should be written and also may require certain conditions when granting permission to use the material. Examples of credit lines are in Exhibit 4.6. In all situations, authors need to include a credit line with copyrighted materials and the copyright notice if applicable (AMA, 2007).

EXHIBIT 4.6

Sample Permission Credit Lines

Journal:
From "SQUIRE Guidelines for Reporting Improvement Studies in Healthcare: Implications for Nursing Publications," by M. H. Oermann, 2009, *Journal of Nursing Care Quality, 24*, p. 93. Copyright 2009 by Wolters Kluwer Health. Reprinted with permission.

Book:
From *Evaluation and Testing in Nursing Education* (p. 24), by M. H. Oermann and K. B. Gaberson, 2009, New York: Springer. Copyright 2009 by Springer. Adapted with permission.

Permissions Letter

An example of a letter requesting permission to reprint copyrighted materials is in Exhibit 4.7 and a form for this same purpose is in Exhibit 4.8. However, in most instances, requests for permission to reprint from journals can be done online. An electronic form may be available from the publisher, through a service such as Rightslink that is linked to the Web site of the journal from which the author is requesting permission, or at the Copyright Clearance Center using the Purchase Permissions feature. In the request, whether done electronically or by hard copy, the author should include the complete citation of the original work; a description of the material to be reprinted, such as, portion of the text, table, figure, or other illustration including the page number(s) where it can be found; publication in which the material will be used; and how the original work would be adapted, if at all. For books, the publisher typically provides a permission form for the author to use for requesting permissions to reprint.

Authors will likely incur a fee, which may be significant, when requesting copyright permission. When seeking permission to reprint materials they have written, however, the fee may be waived. Another possibility is that permission to reprint may not be granted.

EXHIBIT 4.7

Sample Letter Requesting Permission to Reproduce Copyrighted Materials

Permissions Department
Publisher
Mailing or Email Address

Dear Permissions Department:

I am requesting permission to include Figure 4–12 Components of a Typical Graph in a manuscript I am writing for submission to *The Nurse Practitioner* or a similar scholarly journal. The figure was in: Lang, T. A. (2010). *How to write, publish, & present in the health sciences: A guide for clinicians and laboratory researchers*. Philadelphia: American College of Physicians, p. 90.

Thank you for your consideration of this request.

Sincerely,

[author's name, credentials
email and complete mailing address,
fax number and other contact information]

EXHIBIT 4.8

Sample Form for Requesting Permission to Reproduce Copyrighted Materials

Springer Publishing Company
11 W. 42nd Street, 15th floor
New York, NY 10036
Tel: 212.431.4370
Fax: 212.941.7842
www.springerpub.com

REQUEST FOR PERMISSION TO REPRINT
Date: _____
To: _____
From: _____
(Name)
Address: _____
City: _____State: _____ Zip: _____

I am requesting nonexclusive world rights in all languages and in all editions and formats to reproduce the following material from your publication. Please note that I intend to use this material in an upper-level scholarly publication for use in an academic market.

Full Title:
_____
Author: _____
Date of publication/copyright year: _____
Page numbers:_____

(Please give the precise details of the material desired, specifying page numbers, paragraphs, approximate number of words, and other identifying information.)

This material is to appear in the following volume:
Full Title:
_____
Author:_____Approx. no. of pages:_____Print run:_____
Publisher: _____
Date of Publication: _____
Form of Publication: _____
(book, journal, etc.)

The undersigned agrees as follows:
Full credit will be given the approving publisher where the reprinted material is used in Springer's publication, on every copy manufactured, in the form specified.

_____
(Signed)   (Date)

Continued

Exhibit 4.8   *Continued*

APPROVAL OF REQUEST
The foregoing application is hereby approved provided the following form
of credit and copyright notice is used:
Reprinted from [title of book] by [author] by permission of
_____

Date of approval: _____
Approved by: _____

Photographs

Patients, nurses, and other people shown in photographs need to provide written
permission for reproduction of the photograph in the manuscript. In the letter
asking their permission, the author should include the title of the manuscript,
possible journal in which it might be published, and when the photograph was
taken. The subject in the photograph must sign a release form that the author in
turns submits with the manuscript.

PLAGIARISM

When the literature review is completed and authors begin writing the paper,
they must be cautious to give proper credit to their sources. The exact words of
another should be placed in quotation marks. Paraphrasing refers to summarizing content, rearranging the order of words, or changing some words from source
material (APA, 2009). Many writers, especially students, believe that plagiarism
refers only to failure to indicate and cite properly a verbatim quotation. However,
any time authors present the ideas of another as their own, without giving proper
credit to their source, plagiarism has occurred. When parts of text are taken from
a publication, even if the number of words is small, that text should be credited to
the original author (Manogue, Rohlin, Baum, & Winning, 2009).
    Plagiarism can be considered a crime of theft of intellectual property. It is not
a victimless crime; plagiarism can harm the author of the original source material, the scientific community, and the plagiarizer.
    Authors can avoid plagiarism through adequate and appropriate documenta-
tion, but at times, this is not easy to do. All authors absorb and use the ideas of others, and a writer may forget the original source of an idea or even that there was an
original source. However, unless authors specifically acknowledge the sources of
ideas, they claim credit for them (AMA, 2007). Strategies to help avoid plagiarism
are careful note taking, record keeping, and documentation of data and sources
(AMA, 2007, p. 158). Authors should not cut and paste from an original source, a
Web site, or an electronic document. Over the months or longer of preparing the
paper, it may be difficult to remember that the text was from a source material and

not one's own ideas. Authors should not rely on only a few sources for an article because this tends to lead to duplication of words (Cronin, 2007).

Can an author plagiarize unintentionally? In some cases it is unclear whether the author lacked knowledge about proper documentation of sources or whether intentional plagiarism occurred, especially with students. Skillful paraphrasing without plagiarizing requires the writer to understand and synthesize the ideas and information from the original sources. Reading the materials and thinking about them before writing, and taking notes help authors to develop their own ideas about a topic. Exhibit 4.9 includes ways of preventing plagiarism when writing for publication.

EXHIBIT 4.9

Strategies for Preventing Plagiarism When Writing for Publication

1. Keep complete bibliographic citations of all works used in preparing the manuscript. If you make a photocopy of an article or portion of a book chapter, or download material from the Internet, attach a copy of the bibliographic information to it.
2. Read original source material thoroughly before starting to write. Express your understanding of the original authors' ideas, synthesizing thoughts and insights gained through reflection on the material. Avoid merely substituting similar terms and rearranging parts of sentences.
3. Use quotation marks when citing more than six words of original material. Note the page number of the original source in which you found the material. In deciding whether to quote or paraphrase material, consider the uniqueness and power of the original author's wording and your ability to express the same ideas in different ways.
4. Always give credit to the original sources of ideas, even when you paraphrase them.
5. Understand the difference between common knowledge and original material that must be cited. In general, information that appears in more than five sources can be considered common knowledge, but if all five sources cite the same original source, you should find, read, and appropriately cite that source as well.
6. Obtain written permission from the copyright holder for reproducing all copyrighted material, including tables, figures, diagrams, and other illustrations, and extensive verbatim quotations of text. Submit permissions with the manuscript.
7. If you are using even short verbatim quotations from your own previously published material, cite the original source. Seek permission from the copyright holder to re-use lengthier portions of your own previously

Continued

Exhibit 4.9   *Continued*

published material. If you want to publish ideas similar to those in previously published works in another form, consult the editor of the original publication.

Adapted from: Clark, A. J. (1993). Responsible dissemination of scholarly work. *Journal of Neuroscience Nursing, 25,* 113–117; Vogelsang, J. (1997). Plagiarism—An act of stealing. *Journal of PeriAnesthesia Nursing, 12,* 422–425; Cronin, S. N. (2007). The problem of plagiarism. *Dimensions of Critical Care Nursing, 26,* 244–245. doi: 10.1097/01.DCC.0000297407.98348.a6

Copying of one's own previously published material without proper citation of the source is also an example of plagiarism. Remember that once a publisher holds a copyright for published material, that material cannot be reused without permission. Even short verbatim quotes from an author's previously published content should be referenced back to the original source, and the author should seek permission from the copyright holder to reproduce lengthier portions.

SUMMARY

A literature review is a critique and summary of current knowledge about a topic, for research and for use in clinical practice, teaching, administration, and other areas of nursing. Literature reviews are conducted when writing a paper for a course, a thesis, a dissertation, grants, projects in which the nurse may be involved, and manuscripts.

There are three main purposes of reviewing the literature. The first purpose is to describe what is known already about a topic. The literature review provides the background needed for developing a research study, answering questions about clinical practice, developing new projects and initiatives, and making other decisions. It reveals existing knowledge about a topic and related areas. The second purpose is to identify gaps in knowledge and where questions still remain. The third purpose is to determine how the proposed study, project, innovation, or paper will contribute new knowledge to nursing.

The author first identifies the topic of the paper and then searches the literature. There are varied bibliographic databases for conducting literature searches in nursing. The two databases that are most useful for nurse authors are MEDLINE and CINAHL.

Each article in a bibliographic database is indexed similarly. It has a single record with specific information about that article. The record has fields that include information such as the author's name, title of the article, journal in which published, publication date and information, and terms or phrases that describe the content of the article. MeSH is used for MEDLINE indexing and other databases produced by the NLM. CINAHL has its own controlled vocabulary thesaurus based on MeSH but with additional terms for nursing and allied health literature.

After choosing the topic and narrowing it down, the next step is to select the most appropriate database for the search. The author does a preliminary search to evaluate the effectiveness of the search terms. Searches can be modified by choosing other terms to search; by manipulating the fields such as limiting publication dates; and by using the Boolean connectors *and, or,* and *not.* These connectors indicate how the search terms should be combined and used in relation to one another.

The literature should be reviewed starting with the most recent references and working backwards. Reviewing literature published in the last five years is usually sufficient for most papers. Reference lists of articles, chapters, and books also can be examined to identify citations that might have been missed.

The author should keep a record of (1) each database searched, (2) terms used for the search, (3) years searched, (4) limitations placed on the search, and (5) resulting citations. Considering the large number of references retrieved in a search, authors need efficient ways of managing these references and retrieving them for research, writing, and other projects, such as with reference management software.

Authors need to critically examine each publication before using it as a basis for their own research and writing, and for decisions about clinical practice. Not every document retrieved from a literature review may be used for preparing a manuscript. Some papers are not used because of poor quality; other times the content is not relevant to the purpose of the paper. When multiple studies exist in an area, authors should synthesize the literature, noting similarities and consistent findings across studies. The critical appraisal of research studies and synthesis of findings are essential for evidence-based practice.

In writing the literature review, authors should identify explicitly how their paper closes a gap in the literature and extends earlier work. They should emphasize how their research replicates an important study and contributes new knowledge to nursing.

When authors are reviewing the literature and deciding on text, tables, figures, and other illustrations to include in their papers, they need permission from the copyright holder, for example, the publisher of the journal or book, to adapt or reproduce the copyrighted material in their manuscript. This is true even for the author's own article, chapter, or book because the copyright was transferred to and is then held by the publisher. Patients, nurses, and other people shown in photographs need to provide written permission for reproduction of the photograph in the manuscript. A general principle is whenever identifying information about patients, other individuals, and institutions is provided in a manuscript, they should review the manuscript and give written consent.

Plagiarism is presenting the ideas of another as one's own, without giving proper credit to their source. Many writers, especially students, believe that plagiarism refers only to failure to indicate and cite properly a verbatim quotation, but plagiarism also can involve paraphrasing without citing the source of the ideas. Careful note taking and documenting sources, and using multiple sources of information are strategies to avoid plagiarism.

▓ REFERENCES

Allen, M., Jacobs, S., & Levy, J. (2006). Mapping the literature of nursing: 1996–2000. *Journal of the Medical Library Association, 94*(2), 206–220.

American Medical Association. (2007). *AMA manual of style: A guide for authors and editors* (10th ed.). New York: Oxford Press.

American Psychological Association (APA). (2009). *Publication manual of the American Psychological Association* (6th ed.). Washington DC: Author.

Brahmi, F. A., & Gall, C. (2006). EndNote and Reference Manager citation formats compared to "instructions to authors" in top medical journals. *Medical Reference Services Quarterly, 25*, 49–57.

Burns, N., & Grove, S.K. (2005). *The practice of nursing research: Conduct, critique, and utilization* (5th ed.). St. Louis: Elsevier.

Copyright Clearance Center. (2009).*Copyright.com. Business.* http://www.copyright.com/viewPage.do?pageCode=bu1-n

Cronin, S. N. (2007). The problem of plagiarism. *Dimensions of Critical Care Nursing, 26*, 244–245. doi: 10.1097/01.DCC.0000297407.98348.a6

Cronin, P., Ryan, F., & Coughlan, M. (2008). Undertaking a literature review: A step-by-step approach. *British Journal of Nursing, 17*(1), 38–43.

Elton B. Stephens Company (EBSCO). (2009a). *The CINAHL® Database.* Retrieved from http://www.ebscohost.com/thisTopic.php?marketID=1&topicID=53

EBSCO. (2009b). *CINAHL Databases.* Retrieved from http://www.ebscohost.com/cinahl/

Galvan, J. L. (2009). *Writing literature reviews* (4th ed.). Glendale, CA: Pyrczak Publishing.

Kessler, J., & Van Ullen, M. K. (2005). Citation generators: Generating bibliographies for the next generation. *Journal of Academic Librarianship, 31*, 310–316. doi:10.1016/j.acalib.2005.04.012

Larrabee, J. H., Sions, J., Fanning, M., Withrow, M., & Ferretti, A. (2007). Evaluation of a program to increase evidence-based practice change. *Journal of Nursing Administration, 37*, 302–310. doi: 10.1097/01.NNA.0000277715.41758.7b

Lawrence, J. C. (2007). Techniques for searching the CINAHL database using the EBSCO interface. *AORN, 85*, 779–791. doi: 10.1016/S0001-2092(07)60153-7

Manogue, M., Rohlin, M., Baum, B., & Winning, T. (2009). Editorial. *European Journal of Dental Education, 13*, 189. doi: 10.1111/j.1600-0579.2009.00602.x

National Center for Biotechnology Information. (2009). *PubMed Help.* Retrieved from http://www.ncbi.nlm.nih.gov/bookshelf/br.fcgi?book=helppubmed

National Library of Medicine. (2008a). *Fact Sheet MEDLINE®.* Retrieved from http://www.nlm.nih.gov/pubs/factsheets/medline.html

National Library of Medicine. (2008b). *Fact Sheet Medical Subject Headings (MeSH®).* Retrieved from http://www.nlm.nih.gov/pubs/factsheets/mesh.html

National Library of Medicine. (2009). *NLM Databases & Electronic Resources.* Retrieved from http://www.nlm.nih.gov/databases/

Oermann, M. H. (2007). Approaches to gathering evidence for educational practices in nursing. *Journal of Continuing Education in Nursing, 38*, 250–257.

Oermann, M. H., Cummings, S., & Wilmes, N. A. (2001). Accuracy of references in four pediatric nursing journals. *Journal of Pediatric Nursing, 16*, 263–268. doi: 10.1053/jpdn.2001.25537

Oermann, M. H., Mason, N., Wilmes, N. A. (2002). Accuracy of references in general readership nursing journals. *Nurse Educator, 27*, 260–264.

Oermann, M. H., Nordstrom, C., Ineson, V., & Wilmes, N. A. (2008). Web citations in the nursing literature: How accurate are they? *Journal of Professional Nursing, 24*, 347–351. doi: 10.1016/j.profnurs.2007.12.004

Oermann, M. H., & Ziolkowski, L. D. (2002). Accuracy of references in three critical care nursing journals. *Journal of PeriAnesthesia Nursing, 17*(2), 78–83.

Polit, D. F., & Beck, C. T. (2008). *Nursing research: Generating and assessing evidence for nursing practice.* Philadelphia: Lippincott Williams Wilkins.

Sandelowski, M. (1998). Writing a good read: Strategies for re-presenting qualitative data. *Research in Nursing & Health, 21*, 375–382.

Steele, S. S. (2008). Bibliographic citation management software as a tool for building knowledge. *Journal of Wound, Ostomy, and Continence Nursing, 35,* 463–466. doi: 10.1097/01. WON.0000335956.45311.69

Stevenson, D., & Bramson, J. (2009). Hospice care in the nursing home setting: A review of the literature. *Journal of Pain & Symptom Management, 38,* 440–451. doi: 10.1016/j. jpainsymman.2009.05.006

Taylor, M. K. (1998). The practical effects of errors in reference lists in nursing research journals. *Nursing Research, 47,* 300–303.

Thomson Reuters. (2009). *Science. EndNote.* Retrieved from http://thomsonreuters.com/products_services/science/science_products/a-z/endnote?parentKey=433713

Torraco, R. J. (2005). Writing integrative literature reviews: Guidelines and examples. *Human Resource Development Review, 4,* 356–367. doi: 10.1177/1534484305278283

Turner, A. M., Liddy, E. D., Bradley, J., & Wheatley, J. A. (2005). Modeling public health interventions for improved access to the gray literature. *Journal of the Medical Library Association, 93,* 487–494.

Vintzileos, A. M., & Ananth, C. V. (2009). How to write and publish an original research article. *American Journal of Obstetrics & Gynecology.* Advance online publication. http://dx.doi.org/10.1016/j.ajog.2009.06.038

WRITING RESEARCH, EVIDENCE-BASED PRACTICE, AND CLINICAL PRACTICE ARTICLES

5

WRITING RESEARCH ARTICLES

Research papers present the findings of quantitative and qualitative research based on original data. The chapter begins with a discussion of how to report research using the conventional format of an introduction and literature review; a methods section, including design and sample, measurements, and analytic strategy; a results section; and a discussion. This basic structure of research articles is known as IMRAD, i.e., **I**ntroduction, **M**ethods, **R**esults, and **D**iscussion. The chapter concludes by describing pitfalls to avoid when reporting research findings and revising academic papers as research manuscripts.

Research articles may be written for journals that publish mainly research articles, or they may be prepared for clinical journals that report research in that practice specialty. Many journals publish both research articles as well as other types. When developing research papers for clinical journals, the IMRAD format may not be explicit, but it serves as a framework for the author to use in deciding how to organize the content.

Chapter 5 does not explain the research process or different types of research that might be reported in the literature. Instead, it offers general principles for writing research papers. The author needs to adapt these principles for the type of journal to which the manuscript is submitted.

▦ RESEARCH DISSEMINATION

Research projects are not complete until the findings are communicated to others. All too often nurses conduct important research studies but fail to disseminate the results of their work. Some nurses are not prepared for their role as an author and are unsure how to proceed; others may believe that their work does not warrant publication. However, rigorous research is important to communicate to others, regardless of whether the findings were anticipated or not. Findings that do not support the hypothesis may be as important as ones that do, for other researchers and clinicians need this information as they plan studies and make decisions about clinical practice.

There are many reasons for disseminating the results of research in the literature. First, nursing research is of little value if the findings are not made available for use by clinicians and others who need the research results for their work. Nurses who conduct research are responsible for reporting the results in journals that are read by nurses who can use the information in their practice, teaching, management, and other roles. Research findings must be disseminated for them to have an effect on patient care and service delivery (National Institutes of Health [NIH], 2007).

Second, by publishing the findings of research, nurses advance the body of knowledge of nursing and contribute to the scientific basis of nursing practice. Research is essential for professional practice because it generates the knowledge that defines that practice.

Third, communicating the findings of research promotes the critique and replication of studies (American Medical Association [AMA], 2007). Researchers can build studies on one another, extending and refining what is known about the topic and enabling nurses to apply findings to other groups and settings. By reading research reports, nurses also ask new questions that lead to further studies.

Fourth, nurses also need research data to establish evidence for their decisions and interventions. Evidence-based practice involves the use of the best evidence available for making decisions about patient care (Tagney & Haines, 2009). This evidence includes clinically relevant research combined with individual clinical expertise. Summarizing research for evidence-based practice recommendations is described in chapter 6.

Fifth, disseminating the findings of research is essential for research utilization and evidence-based practice in nursing. Research utilization is the process by which knowledge from research is incorporated into clinical practice (Meijers et al., 2006). While there are varied research utilization and evidence-based practice models, they all involve the critique of research findings and subsequent use of those findings in practice. Improving the quality of care requires a commitment to provide nursing care that is based on sound research. Writing a manuscript on a review of research findings, such as a systematic review paper, and use of research for evidence-based practice are discussed in chapter 6.

Sixth, dissemination of findings from studies supported by federal funding is the law. As of March 9, 2009, researchers supported by the National Institutes of Health must submit an electronic copy of their final peer-reviewed manuscripts to the National Library of Medicine's PubMed Central, so that their work is available to the public within 12 months of publication, consistent with copyright law (U.S. Department of Health and Human Services, 2009). Compliance is a condition of the award of funding. Copyright law regarding scientific publications is discussed in chapter 15.

RESEARCH REPORTS

Writing about research is similar to making a reasoned argument—the author's goal is to demonstrate to readers that the study was important to do and follows logically from previous research, the methods were appropriate for examining the problem, the findings are valid, and the implications for practice are consistent with the data. The research report or paper summarizes the study and its purpose, methods, and findings. This report is the document that presents key aspects of the study for readers. Research reports vary in length ranging from manuscripts, which are about 15-20 pages, to master's theses and doctoral dissertations, which are significantly longer, ranging from approximately 50-200 pages depending on the study.

Writing Research Papers for Research Journals

The format for the research report follows the same format as the research process. It begins with an introduction and the purpose of the study, proceeds through a description of its methods and results, and concludes with a discussion of the findings. There are differences though in the extent of detail of the paper across journals. When writing a report for a research journal, the author explains each component of the research study with sufficient detail for others to understand the problem, methods, and findings, and to replicate it if desired.

For example, Crist and her colleagues (Crist et al., 2009) tested a conceptual model of proposed relationships among acculturation, familism, objective and subjective burden, and home care services among Mexican-American older persons. The article was organized using the traditional format of a research report: introduction, method, results, and discussion. In the introduction the researchers presented an extensive critique of related research on each of the concepts in the model; in the method section they described the study's design, sample, measures and analytic strategy; and in the results they presented the descriptive findings and model testing of study data, based on complex statistical analyses, followed by a discussion of the importance of the results of their study. The article described in detail each component of the research study and was organized in this same way.

Writing Research Papers for Specialty Journals

The author may decide to prepare the research report for a journal that publishes research in a clinical specialty, for nurse educators, or nurses practicing in specialty roles in management, law, or other fields. In research reports in specialty journals, the literature review may be less extensive than for a research journal, and there may be less discussion on the research methods themselves. Readers of specialty journals may not be interested in elaborate discussions of the statistical analyses used in the study nor have the background to understand this discussion. Instead their focus is on how the research findings should guide their practice and their work in other nursing roles. These manuscripts should emphasize the practical implications of the study. As discussed in earlier chapters, the author needs to gear the paper to the journal and audience.

Evangelista and colleagues (Evangelista, Dracup, Doering, Moser, & Kobashigawa, 2005) developed a research report for *Journal of Cardiovascular Nursing* on physical activity patterns in women after heart transplantation. In a brief introduction, the author reviewed the literature on functional ability and limitations after transplant surgery. The literature review discussed key research studies and descriptive articles about the persistent of activity limitations after the initial post-surgical period. In the next section of the manuscript,

Evangelista and colleagues described the benefits of regular physical activity for this patient group and the dearth of long-term follow-up studies beyond the recuperation period. The introduction concluded with a statement of the overall goal of the study: "to examine the prognostic value of different measures of daily activity and compare these with biobehavioral and clinical variables that may predict patient outcomes" (p. 335). The Methods section focused primarily on the procedures for measuring physical activity. The remaining section of the research report included the results of her study of 27 women who were 1-4 years post-transplant, the discussion, future considerations for research and clinical practice, and recommendations for long-term assessments of women having undergone transplantation. While the research format is apparent in the article, the emphasis is placed on understanding the nature of the patients' quality of life with respect to following exercise guidelines, and content is included to improve nurses' understanding of the important dimensions of post-transplant assessments.

For some research projects the author might write about the research itself for a research journal and the implications for practice for a specialty journal. A clinical specialty manuscript would build on the research report by describing how nurses can use the findings. Strategies for writing clinical practice articles are described in chapter 7.

Research projects that assess students or educational initiatives are subject to the same formatting guidelines as studies of patients, families, and communities. If the author is targeting an education journal that is research-oriented, then a full description of background literature, research methodology, and implications for future research should be provided in IMRAD format. If on the other hand, the target audience is primarily nurse educators who will be interested in the implications of the research findings for curriculum development, student support, or other applications, then the author should focus the manuscript on these elements.

Writing Randomized Controlled Trial Papers

Authors of randomized controlled trials (RCTs) are subject to stringent rules for publishing their study. The rules were designed for reports of simple two-group parallel-arm studies. The rationale for these rules is that RCTs, which represent the most rigorous testing of interventions prior to widespread implementation in human populations, must be described with complete transparency in order to avoid biased, unreliable, or irrelevant interpretation of the results.

To this end, an international body of scientists and editors developed the *Con*solidated *S*tandards *o*f *R*eporting *T*rials (CONSORT) statement (Moher, Schultz, & Altman, 2001). The CONSORT statement includes a checklist of elements to include in the title, abstract, introduction, methods, results, and discussions sections of the manuscript. For example, both the title and abstract should include "how participants were allocated to interventions (e.g., 'random allocation,' 'randomized,' or 'randomly assigned')" (p.659). Furthermore, the authors should include a flow diagram that presents how participants passed through the RCT in each of four stages: enrollment, intervention allocation, follow-up, and analysis. The template for the CONSORT flow diagram, shown in CHAPTER 12, Figure 12.2, allows readers to judge whether the analysis was performed based on intention-to-treat. The intent of the checklist and diagram is to improve reporting of RCTs in the scientific literature, but the checklist and diagram may be more broadly useful for authors of all intervention studies when choosing elements to present to readers.

Writing About Other Types of Research Projects

The research to be reported in the literature does not have to involve complex studies with large samples. There are many studies done by nurses on a smaller scale that are important for others to know about. These include studies of small patient groups or communities to which the nurse has ready access. The knowledge gained from research questions or program evaluations done by nurses of interventions and new initiatives for patient populations, for instance, may be important for advancing nursing practice and answering questions about one's own clinical practice. Reports of clinical studies conducted in one setting may guide replication research by nurses in another setting, which expands general understanding about care of patients across settings. Researchers can use findings from these smaller studies to design larger ones that develop general nursing knowledge.

A good example of a research report of a pilot study was written by Johnson and colleagues (Johnson et al., 2009). In this article Johnson tests the feasibility of using 'centering prayer' in an outpatient chemotherapy center to assess its impact on mood, spiritual wellbeing, and quality of life over a six-month period. Although only 10 patients were studied, the research builds on earlier projects described in the literature review and clearly extends this line of research.

There are other situations in which the author initiated a research study but because of problems in implementation was not able to carry it out as planned. In developing a manuscript about the study, the author might develop a manuscript on the difficulties encountered in conducting this type of study and possible solutions. For example, researchers (Steinhauser et al., 2006) studying palliative care published a manuscript that described problems they encountered in recruiting and retaining seriously ill and dying patients, with recommendations for overcoming specific obstacles. Articles that describe research methods are described in chapter 8.

ELEMENTS OF A RESEARCH REPORT

Title

Every research paper needs a title. The title should be carefully worded to capture the objective of the study. The intent of the title is to inform readers exactly what information will be presented in the paper (Penrose & Katz, 2004). Unfortunately, research shows that most titles succeed in informing readers whether the article refers to research or clinical practice but fail to make clear the quality of the evidence, e.g., were findings based on a clinical trial or consensus guidelines, or only on a single study, non-systematic review, or editorial, letter, or animal study (Demner-Fushman, Hauser & Thoma, 2005).

Titles should be specific (AMA, 2007), using key words that represent the content of the article. Titles are used for indexing and compiled in reference works; therefore, authors should select keywords for the title based on words that their target audience will find the most informative. Authors should avoid overly general titles that omit key elements of the population that was studied.

Titles should be "fully explanatory while standing alone" (American Psychological Association [APA], 2009, p.23). The title should be easily shortened for a running head. One title may be written, or it may be developed with a subtitle that provides supplementary information about the paper. Subtitles should not be used to provide additional information for overly general titles. For example:

> **Avoid:** Home Care Service Use: Impact of Caregiving Burden, Acculturation, and Familism among Mexican American Elders.

> **Better:** Caregiving Burden, Acculturation, Familism, and Mexican American Elders' Use of Home Care Services (Crist et al., 2009).

Subtitles should be reserved for supplementary information that helps the reader retrieve needed information. Subtitles may contain information about the study's methodology, e.g., "A systematic review" or "A pilot study." Subtitles should be avoided where key elements can be arranged simply and with style (APA, 2009).

Titles should be concise. APA (2009) recommends titles with no more than 12 words and avoiding unnecessary phrases such as "A Study of" and "An Investigation of." By reading the title, the information conveyed in the article should be apparent to any interested reader.

Abstract

Abstracts are as important as are titles in directing readers to articles they will find important. The abstract provides a summary of the research. It describes the study purpose and background, methods used for the research, key findings, and conclusions. "A well-prepared abstract can be the most important single paragraph in an article" (APA, 2009, p. 26). A densely constructed abstract rich in keywords can convince the interested reader to read the entire article.

Abstracts should be accurate, non-evaluative, coherent and readable, and concise (APA, 2009). The abstract should specify the purpose of the study and report the content of the article's text, without expanding upon it. Good abstracts use simple sentences and the active voice. Effective abstracts employ key words that interested readers would logically employ as search terms in online searches. Abstracts should feature the most important results and the key conclusions. Quantitative and qualitative results reported in the abstract should not differ from the numbers or concepts in the manuscript's tables and graphics. The abstract should also not repeat the title of the article, cite references, or use abbreviations (AMA, 2007).

In some journals structured abstracts are required. The journal's author guidelines will specify the information to the included in the abstract, including labels to be used for the headings. Structured abstracts may include one or more sentences under the following headings:

- Purpose: clinical importance and research question(s) or hypothesis
- Design: structure of study including year(s) and duration
- Setting: community or practice setting
- Subjects: selection criteria, number of subjects (by group, if appropriate), key socio-demographic data
- Intervention (if appropriate)
- Measures: independent and outcome variables
- Results: main outcomes, including effect sizes and confidence intervals and/or statistical significance
- Conclusions: discussion of the results "taking into account limitations, along with implications for clinical practice, and avoiding speculation and overgeneralization" (AMA, 2007, p. 22).

Abstracts of an original research report are typically between 150 (APA, 2009) and 300 words (AMA, 2007), although journals often specify the length and format for their abstracts. If the author guidelines do not specify a maximum length, the author should keep to a 250-word limit, as few journals would allow longer abstracts.

A second reason for limiting the length of the abstract has to do with the indexing of the article. If the abstract is too long, the complete abstract may not be included in some bibliographic databases. For example, in the MEDLINE database there is a 4,096-character limit; where abstracts exceed that limit, they are truncated (U.S. Department of Health and Human Services, 1995, p. 18). If the entire abstract is not included in a database, it will indicate that the abstract was truncated, but some important content might be omitted.

Examples of abstracts for research reports are displayed in Exhibit 5.1. The first two examples are structured abstracts; although the third example is unstructured, it provides the same information about the study as the other two. More discussion about writing titles and abstracts for other types of articles is provided later in the book.

EXHIBIT 5.1

Sample Abstracts

Structured Abstract: Quantitative Study

Effectiveness of an Aspiration Risk-reduction Protocol

Background: Aspiration of gastric contents is a serious problem in critically ill, mechanically ventilated patients receiving tube feedings.

Continued

Exhibit 5.1 *Continued*

Objectives: The purpose of this study was to evaluate the effectiveness of a three-pronged intervention to reduce aspiration risk in a group of critically ill, mechanically ventilated patients receiving tube feedings.

Methods: A two-group quasi-experimental design was used to compare outcomes of a usual care group (December 2002-September 2004) with those of an Aspiration Risk-Reduction Protocol (ARRP) group (January 2007-April 2008). The incidence of aspiration and pneumonia was compared between the usual care group (n = 329) and the ARRP group (n = 145). The ARRP had three components: maintaining head-of-bed elevation at 30° or higher, unless contraindicated; inserting feeding tubes into distal small bowel, when indicated; and using an algorithmic approach for high gastric residual volumes.

Results: Two of the three ARRP components were implemented successfully. Almost 90% of the ARRP group had mean head-of-bed elevations of 30° or higher as compared to 38% in the usual care group. Almost three fourths of the ARRP group had feeding tubes placed in the small bowel as compared with less than 50% in the usual care group. Only three patients met the criteria for the high gastric residual volume algorithm. Aspiration was much lower in the ARRP group than that in the usual care group (39% vs. 88%, respectively). Similarly, pneumonia was much lower in the ARRP group than that in the usual care group (19% vs. 48%, respectively).

Discussion: Findings from this study suggest that a combination of a head-of-bed position elevated to at least 30° and use of a small-bowel feeding site can reduce the incidence of aspiration and aspiration-related pneumonia dramatically in critically ill, tube-fed patients.[1]

Structured Abstract: Qualitative Study

Assessing Palliative Care Needs: Views of Patients, Informal Carers and Healthcare Professionals

Aim. This paper reports a study to assess the palliative care needs of the adult population served by a healthcare provider organization in Northern Ireland from the perspectives of patients, informal carers and healthcare providers.

Background. Assessing palliative care need is a key factor for health service planning. Traditionally, palliative care has been associated with end-of-life care and cancer. More recently, the concept has been extended to include care for both cancer and non-cancer populations. Various approaches have been advocated for assessing need, including the exploration of professional provider and user perspectives of need.

Method. Semi-structured qualitative interviews were undertaken with a purposive sample of patients and lay carers receiving palliative care services (*n* = 24). Focus groups were also conducted with multi-professional palliative care providers (*n* = 52 participants) and face to face interviews were undertaken with key managerial stakeholders in the area (*n* = 7). The focus groups and interviews concentrated on assessment of palliative care need. All the interviews were transcribed verbatim and analyzed using Burnard's framework.

Findings. Professional providers experienced difficulty in defining the term palliative care. Difficulties in communication and information exchange, and fragmented co-ordination between services were identified. The main areas of need identified by all participants were social and psychological support; financial concerns; and the need for choice and information. All participants considered that there was inequity between palliative care service provision for patients with cancer and non-cancer diseases.

Conclusion. All patients, regardless of diagnosis, should be able to access palliative care appropriate to their individual needs. For this to happen in practice, an integrated approach to palliative care is essential. The study methodology confirms the value of developing a comprehensive approach to assessing palliative care need.[2]

Unstructured Abstract: Quantitative Study

Caregiving Burden, Acculturation, Familism, and Mexican American Elders' Use of Home Care Services

Caregiving burden has been shown to predict use of home care services among Anglo-Americans. In a previous study, only one of two dimensions of caregiving burden predicted such use among Mexican American caregivers. Because acculturation and familism may affect burden, we conducted analyses to test three hypotheses: increased acculturation decreases familism; decreased familism increases burden; and increased burden increases use of home care services. Among 140 Mexican American family caregivers, acculturation was positively correlated with familism; familism was not significantly correlated with burden; objective burden was positively correlated with use of home care services, and objective and subjective burden significantly interacted in their effect on the use of home care services. Targeted interventions may be needed to increase use of home care services and preserve the well-being of Mexican American elders and caregivers.[3]

[1]From Metheny, N. A., Davis-Jackson, J., & Stewart, B. J. (2010). Effectiveness of an aspiration risk-reduction protocol. *Nursing Research, 59,* 18. doi: 10.1097/NNR.0b013e3181c3ba05. Reprinted by permission of Lippincott Williams & Wilkins, 2010.

[2]From McIlfatrick, S. (2007). Assessing palliative care needs: views of patients, informal carers and healthcare professionals. *Journal of Advanced Nursing, 57,* p. 77. doi: 10.1111/j.1365-2648.2006.04062.x. Reprinted by permission.

[3]From Crist, J. D., McEwen, M. M., Herrera, A. P., Kim, S-S., Pasvogel, A., & Hepworth, J. T. (2009). Caregiving burden, acculturation, familism, and Mexican American elders' use of home care services. *Research and Theory for Nursing Practice: An International Journal, 23,* p. 165. doi: 10.1891/1541-6577.23.3.165. Reprinted by permission of Springer Publishing Co., 2010.

IMRAD Formatted Reports

The conventional format for writing research papers is the IMRAD format: Introduction, Methods, Results and Discussion, or an adaptation of this depending on the journal and type of research (AMA, 2007; International Committee of Medical Journal Editors [ICMJE], 2008) (Exhibit 5.2). IMRAD provides a structure for organizing the paper and specifies in advance the headings for it.

EXHIBIT 5.2

IMRAD Format

Introduction
    Why was the study done?
 Methods
    What was done?
 Results **a**nd
    What did the researcher find?
 Discussion
    What does it mean?

Some authors choose to include a separate section in the paper for the literature review rather than incorporating it in the introduction, and additional subheadings might be included to highlight more specific components of the background literature, measurement scales, or discussion of hypotheses. Even when more specificity is added in the form of subheadings, the overall IMRAD format is helpful because it follows the process used for the research study and provides a clear structure for the manuscript. The IMRAD format also is useful in writing research reports for clinical journals even if the structure is not explicit in the paper.

The IMRAD format follows the research process and answers four important questions of interest to readers:

- Why was the study done?
- What was done?
- What did the researcher find?
- What does it mean?

Why was the study done? The first question to be answered in the manuscript is why the study was done. A manuscript written for a research or specialty journal should begin with an explanation of the nature and extent of the problem and its importance to nursing, leading to the questions that need answers or hypotheses to be tested. Presenting *why* the study was undertaken and its importance is an effective strategy for gaining reader interest in the topic and convincing them to read the article. Answering why the study was done provides the basis for the introduction, which includes information about the background research on the problem, its significance for human health, and the logical next steps of research reflected in the research questions or hypotheses.

What was done? Once the reader understands the problem, its importance, and the purpose of the study, the next question is what did the researcher do? How were the study questions answered or hypotheses tested? What procedures did the researcher use? This content reflects the methods section of the paper.

What did the researcher find? Once readers know the problem and how it was studied, the next question is what was learned? What were the findings of the study? In answering these questions, the author presents the data that were analyzed, observations, interview results, statistical findings, and so forth, in the results section of the paper. This part of the paper provides the evidence based on the stated methodological procedures that answer the research questions.

What does it mean? In this last section of the research paper, the discussion, the researcher briefly summarizes the answers to the research questions, compares the new findings to previous findings from other related studies, and specifies the limitations and strengths of the current study. Finally, the authors answer the important question for readers, "What do these findings mean for clinical practice, teaching, clinical management, or future research?"

Introduction

The first section of the manuscript is the introduction, which is the author's opportunity to explain the nature and background of the study, its purpose, and its importance. The goals of the introductory section are to explain to the reader the need for the study and why it was done. This section of the manuscript provides a framework for reading the related literature; determining how the study builds on previous research on the topic; and understanding how the study leads logically to the purposes, questions, and/or hypotheses to be addressed. Introducing the problem statement early in the manuscript also clarifies why certain concepts and theories were used to guide the research.

In the beginning sentences, readers should learn about the problem that prompted the study and why the research is important to the readers and their constituencies. The author should begin the introduction with a discussion of the magnitude of the specific problem, using published data on its nature and scope. Who suffers from the problem? How extensive is the problem? What barriers exist to solving the problem? When writing for a research journal, a good introduction clearly identifies research related to the health outcome and what is understood about its causes. When writing for a specialty journal, the author should be specific about how the study is linked to the nurse's own clinical, educational, or other specialty role practice. These strategies not only set the stage for the remainder of the manuscript but also capture the reader's interest. After reading the introduction, the audience should be convinced that there is a genuine need for specific information and that the remainder of the manuscript will address that need in a focused way that will help the reader.

When the research project was originally planned, the author reviewed the literature and identified gaps in the research. In the introduction the author should refer very briefly to these gaps in knowledge and how the current study addressed them. Exhibit 5.3 is an example of an effective introduction because it presents the problems with institutionalization for long term care early in the discussion and suggests gaps in the research about the rapidly growing Mexican American population that the study addressed. The first paragraph focuses on the epidemiologic data that frames the problem; the second paragraph focuses on key quality of life literature concerning care of frail elders and identifies the gap in this literature.

Some authors include too much discussion of the background of the study before they identify the specific problem under investigation. Instead, the statement of the problem should be clear to readers early in the introduction. In Exhibit 5.3, the authors provide a succinct introduction to the problem and gap by the end of the first two paragraphs. They then expand on the dimensions of the problem and what is already known about it in subsequent paragraphs of the literature review.

EXHIBIT 5.3

Sample Introduction

The "parent support ratio" (people aged 80 and over per 100 persons aged 50–64) is forecast to increase rapidly—from 11 in 1990 to 36 in 2050 (Covinsky et al., 2001). This fact, together with the high cost of institutionalization, has raised priority for home care and support for family caregivers in national policy. Minority groups, such as the rapidly growing Latino population, are another high priority in national policy. Latino elders (age 65 and older) comprise 12.5% of the general population but comprise only 5.5% to 6.2% of home care clients (Centers for Disease Control and Prevention [CDC], 2007; Madigan, 2007; Valle, Yamada, & Barrio, 2004). Latino elders' limited use of home care services is made more concerning considering that they are more functionally impaired at younger ages than other elders (Laditka, Laditka, & Drake, 2006). Thirty-six percent of Latino households provide care to an elder, compared to 21% of all other households in the United States (National Alliance for Caregiving, 2008). Latino elders, of whom Mexican American elders comprise the largest percentage, may therefore be in greatest need of home care services. Trends in underutilization of home care services by this population are symptomatic of a significant health care disparity.

Several reasons exist to consider home care services as an option in the care of elders (Covinsky et al., 2001). First, institutionalization is costly and home care can delay or forestall institutionalization. Second, elders who use home care services have better health outcomes such as prevention or delay of onset of acute illness, control of acute illness episodes, and management of chronic conditions (Anderson & Horvath, 2002; Madigan, Tullai-McGuinness, & Neff, 2002). Third, home care services provide needed assistance and education to distressed family caregivers and reduce caregiving burden (National Family Caregivers Association & Family Caregiving Alliance, 2006). Empirical studies with primarily Anglo American samples have shown that higher caregiving burden leads to more admissions to long-term care facilities (Bass & Noelker, 1987; Houde, 1998) or to greater use of home care services (Crist, Kim, Pasvogel, & Velázquez, 2009). The purpose of this study was to examine factors that predict use of home care services by Mexican American elders.

From Crist, J. D., McEwen, M. M., Herrera, A. P., Kim, S-S., Pasvogel, A., & Hepworth, J. T. (2009). Caregiving burden, acculturation, familism, and Mexican American elders' use of home care services. *Research and Theory for Nursing Practice: An International Journal, 23*(3), pp. 165-166. doi: 10.1891/1541-6577.23.3.165. Reprinted by permission of Springer Publishing Co., 2010.

Literature Review   The literature review describes what is already known about the topic and what needs to be studied, thereby justifying the current project. The literature review is critical to validate the need for the research. In the literature review the author synthesizes related research, summarizes major findings from the studies, indicates when they are consistent, and suggests reasons for conflicting results. Gaps in knowledge and limitations of prior studies are emphasized to provide support for the current study. Continuity between previous research and the current study should be made explicit (APA, 2009). The author also may address methodological issues in the research, particularly when the design of the current study sought to resolve these. How to review the literature and write the literature review was presented in chapter 4.

Typically, for research papers, only research studies are included in the literature review section. Exhibit 5.4 depicts a portion of a literature review that demonstrates how to organize studies for a research manuscript. Note that the studies are organized around topics rather than the findings of individual researchers. Descriptive articles, anecdotal reports, and other non-research papers may be used in the beginning of the manuscript to introduce the problem, but generally only research is incorporated in the literature review.

EXHIBIT 5.4

Sample Literature Review

Acculturation

Acculturation is a blending of behaviors and attitudes between a minority and majority culture (Cuéllar, Arnold, & Maldonado, 1995). Researchers have predicted that as North American society becomes more complex, shifts toward individualism would be seen (Triandis et al., 1988). These shifts may become apparent in changing traditional values such as familism.

Continued

Exhibit 5.4 *Continued*

Familism

Within the collectivist worldview, traditional cultural values important to Mexican American elders include *familism* (the obligation of relatives, particularly children, to provide material and emotional support to family members), *simpatia* (establishing warm interpersonal relationships), *respeto* (respect), and *personalismo* (pleasant social exchanges, cooperation, conformity, and reduction of conflict; Bassford, 1995). These values help group members to work together harmoniously toward common goals. Familistic values also include respecting the *dignidad* (dignity) of others (Marin & Marin, 1991), especially toward an elder family member who holds a position of prominence and authority....

Caregiving Burden

Caregiving burden has been conceptualized as family caregivers' perceptions of the degree of difficulty they experience due to elders' impairments (Poulshock & Deimling, 1984). Without skilled or supportive services, elder care at home places an enormous responsibility on caregivers. Elders' dependence and impairment may be overwhelming for caregivers. Burden can have negative physical and psychological outcomes for the family caregiver, such as cellular immune responses, weight change, problems with health and medical conditions, depression, negative affect (Gitlin et al., 2003; Nelson, Smith, Martinson, Kind, & Luepker, 2008), and stress in relationships with the elder or with other family members (Poulshock & Deimling, 1984)....

Use of Home Care Services

Home care services consist of skilled care that includes assessment, teaching, and procedures by licensed providers (e.g., registered nurses or physical therapists) for healing, secondary prevention, and rehabilitation for homebound clients. Use of home care services decreases elder functional impairment and use of other health care services, and reduces the indirect costs of caregiver illness, burden, depression, and mortality (Felix, Dockter, Sanderson, Holladay, & Stewart, 2006; Valadez, Lumadue, Gutierrez, & de Vries-Kell, 2005).

Note: Selected part of literature review.
From Crist, J. D., McEwen, M. M., Herrera, A.P., Kim, S-S., Pasvogel, A., & Hepworth, J. T. (2009). Caregiving burden, acculturation, familism, and Mexican American elders' use of home care services. *Research and Theory for Nursing Practice: An International Journal, 23*, pp. 167-169. doi: 10.1891/1541-6577.23.3.165. Reprinted by permission of Springer Publishing Co., 2010.

The intent of the literature review is to present the most relevant and recent studies that show why the current study is of critical importance to conduct. It is not an exhaustive review of the research, nor is the author attempting to give an historical perspective to the field of study. Avoid citing research that is tangential to the primary question of the study. At the same time, the review of the literature should not be so brief as to be intelligible only to specialists. The most recent and relevant published research should be featured, with exceptions for classic studies that defined the field. A literature review developed prior to the study should be updated with newer studies that may have emerged during the conduct of the study. Readers will gain a sense of the development of the research by reviewing the progression of studies.

The literature review may be incorporated into the introduction as suggested by the IMRAD format or presented as a separate section in the manuscript. This differs across nursing journals. The author should read selected articles from the target journal and follow guidelines for authors to gain a sense of how specific journals handle the literature review.

When writing research reports for clinical journals, the literature review is generally less extensive than for a research journal and is often incorporated into the introduction rather than presented as a separate section. Generally, readers of clinical journals are interested in whether the background literature and research methods are relevant for their patient populations. Some biomedical journals confine the entire introduction to 2-3 paragraphs (AMA, 2007).

Theoretical Framework The literature review may contain the discussion of the conceptual or theoretical framework that guided the study, or the framework may be included in a separate section. In the example in Exhibit 5.5, the conceptual framework is discussed within the literature review. Presenting the framework is one way of organizing the literature because the framework includes the variables and their relationships that are relevant to the research study.

Exhibit 5.5 provides two examples of theoretical frameworks incorporated into the introductions of research reports. The length and complexity of the description of the conceptual or theoretical framework vary across research reports. With some manuscripts, authors discuss the framework in detail particularly when the research tested a model. In other research reports, often those prepared for clinical journals, the discussion of the framework may be limited or not even included in the manuscript. These discussions may or may not include a visual depiction of the framework.

EXHIBIT 5.5

Sample Theoretical Frameworks

Example 1

Euro-American individualism has served as the basis of previous U.S. studies on caregiving burden (Bella, Madsen, Sullivan, Swidler, & Tipton, 1996; Phillips & Crist, 2008). We examined caregiving burden along the individualism–collectivism continuum (Triandis, 1995) in a Mexican American community, generally described as collectivistic (Marin & Marin, 1991). The

Continued

Exhibit 5.5 *Continued*

individualistic worldview exists when members of a culture primarily exhibit independence from groups or organizations (Hofstede, 1980), emphasizes personal freedom and expression in an individualistic context (Dutta-Bergman & Wells, 2002; Lam, Chen, & Schaubroeck, 2002), and is characterized as independent and self-reliant (Bordia & Blau, 2003; Triandis, 1994). In contrast, members in a collectivistic culture prefer tightly knit social networks, are largely influenced by group-defined norms and roles (McCarthy & Stadler, 2000; Sato, 2007), and subordinate personal goals for the benefit of the group to maintain interpersonal harmony (McEwen, Baird, Pasvogel, & Gallegos, 2007; Triandis, Bontempo, Villareal, Asai, & Lucca, 1988).[1]

Individualism or collectivism may coexist in individuals in varying degrees in given cultures (Walumbwa, Lawler, & Avolio, 2007). Common societal influences tend to strengthen either individualism or collectivism in any particular culture. Acculturation, which can vary substantially within Mexican American communities, can move individuals along this continuum from collectivism toward individualism, and, we hypothesize, can alter perceptions of caregiving burden.

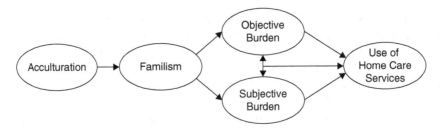

Figure 1. Conceptual Framework: Example 1[1]

Example 2

The concept of QOL grew out of the World Health Organization's definition of health as "a state of complete physical, mental, and social well-being and not merely the absence of disease or infirmity" (World Health Organization, 1947, p. 29). Lawton proposed that QOL subsumed "all legitimate personal and social goals...including every aspect of behavior, environment, and experience" (Lawton, 1983, p. 349). His approach highlighted two themes relevant to the presence or absence of APOE ε4: environmental fit and personal agency. How persons function in their environments may well be influenced by APOE ε4, given its association with cognitive impairment. Exposed individuals may have more difficulty managing a wide range of complex activities, environmental demands, and interpersonal relationships, compared to those who are not exposed. If that is indeed the case, its relevance for long-term care planning becomes critical. In light of Lawton's emphasis on environmental fit and personal goals, we were guided in this study by his quadripartite QOL model of the good life (Lawton, 1983, p. 355).

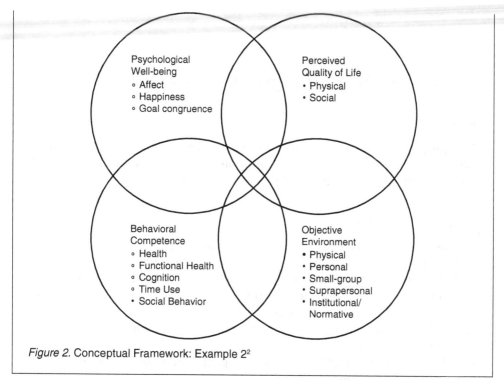

Figure 2. Conceptual Framework: Example 2[2]

[1]From Crist, J. D., McEwen, M. M., Herrera, A. P., Kim, S-S., Pasvogel, A., & Hepworth, J. T. (2009). Caregiving burden, acculturation, familism, and Mexican American elders' use of home care services. *Research and Theory for Nursing Practice: An International Journal, 23*, pp. 166-167, 170. doi: 10.1891/1541-6577.23.3.165. Reprinted by permission of Springer Publishing Co., 2010.
[2]From Hays, J. C., Burchett, B. M., Fillenbaum, G. G., & Blazer, D. G. (2004). Is the APOE e4 allele a risk to person-environment fit? *Journal of Applied Gerontology, 23*, pp. 248-250. Reprinted by permission.

In the first example in Exhibit 5.5, the authors base their research hypotheses on the premise that previous studies have assumed individualism over collectivism as the dominant value system in family decision-making. Their section on the conceptual framework that guides their study discusses the background literature on each element and their interrelationships. Whether to discuss the framework, and in how much depth, depends on the journal, goal of the paper, and objective of the research study.

Purpose The last part of the introduction includes the statement of the approach that the current study will take to address the problem as described in the preceding paragraphs. This should be the closing paragraph of the introduction (APA, 2009). The author may include a statement of the: (1) purposes of the study, (2) questions the research was designed to answer, and/or (3) hypotheses that were tested. An example of each of these is shown in Exhibit 5.6. A clear statement of the purpose of the research is essential to provide a rationale for the method chosen for the study and serves to link the background concepts with the specific procedures and variables discussed in the next section of the manuscript.

EXHIBIT 5.6

Sample Purpose, Research Questions, and Hypotheses

Purpose

The purpose of this study was to evaluate the effectiveness of a three-pronged intervention to reduce aspiration risk in a group of critically ill, mechanically ventilated patients receiving tube feedings.[1]

Research Questions

1. Does increased acculturation decrease familism?
2. Does decreased familism increase caregiving burden?
3. What is the relationship between objective and subjective burden?
4. Is objective burden significantly related to the use of home care services if subjective burden is controlled for?
5. Is subjective burden significantly related to the use of home care services if objective burden is controlled for?
6. What are the interactive effects of objective and subjective burden on use of home care services?[2]

Hypotheses

In a biracial sample of community-dwelling elders living in the Piedmont region of North Carolina, we hypothesized that, compared to sample members without an ε4 allele, sample members with an ε4 allele would:

- not differ with respect to elements of their objective environment at baseline;
- report fewer contacts with non–coresident family and friends and less frequent assistance given to others;
- report more negative perceptions of their physical and social environment; and
- report more social and residential discontinuity in the past and during 10 years of follow-up.[3]

[1]From Metheny, N. A., Davis-Jackson, J., & Stewart, B. J. (2010). Effectiveness of an aspiration risk-reduction protocol. *Nursing Research, 59*, 18. doi: 10.1097/NNR.0b013e3181c3ba05.
[2]From Crist, J. D., McEwen, M. M., Herrera, A. P., Kim, S-S., Pasvogel, A., & Hepworth, J. T. (2009). Caregiving burden, acculturation, familism, and Mexican American elders' use of home care services. *Research and Theory for Nursing Practice: An International Journal, 23*, p. 170. doi: 10.1891/1541-6577.23.3.165.
[3]From Hays, J. C., Burchett, B. M., Fillenbaum, G. G., & Blazer, D. G. (2004). Is the APOE e4 allele a risk to person-environment fit? *Journal of Applied Gerontology, 23*, p. 251. doi: 10.1177/0733464804267565.

While the study's original (*a priori*) questions or hypotheses must be included in the introduction, subsidiary research questions may be presented in the results section of the manuscript. For instance, in a study comparing exercise interventions for older persons, the researcher might find evidence of gender differences in use of the interventions. These effects might be tested subsequently as interaction effects and reported in the Results section as exploratory findings, but the effect would not be listed as a primary research question in the introduction. The main research questions should be presented in the introduction, keeping the report focused on the effectiveness of those treatments. Exploratory findings should be noted in the discussion section as being important lines of future research.

The introduction should not contain a statement about the research design unless the study was explicitly designed to refine a methodological limitation of previous studies. For example, if the current study is the first prospective cohort study, following up on several published case control studies, this should be highlighted as a purpose of the study in the introduction.

Methods

The next section of the manuscript is methods. How did the researcher carry out the study? What was done? In the methods section information about the study design, subjects, measures, procedures, and data analysis is presented in this order. Often, each subsection is labeled accordingly, making it easy for the reader to follow the methodology of the research.

The methods section needs to be detailed to demonstrate the appropriateness of the procedures to the purpose of the study and the validity and reliability of the methods for a quantitative study (APA, 2009). Enough detail should be provided such that researchers can replicate the study if desired and so that clinicians can evaluate the relevance of the findings for their patient population.

This section is written in the past tense since the study has been completed. Often the material from a research grant, thesis, or dissertation may be used in the manuscript if changed to the past tense, updated (where procedures changed from the original proposal), and shortened to comply with the page limits of the journal. Material written for research proposals and academic assignments may include a rationale for each concept that will be measured. In a scientific manuscript, this rationale is not necessary to include unless the study addressed methodological issues or tested new methods for examining the problem.

If the research is an extension of an earlier study, the author can refer the reader to a previously published article for more detailed information about the methodology. For example:

"The sample consisted of participants in the Established Population for Epidemiologic Studies of the Elderly at Duke University (Duke EPESE: Cornoni-Huntley et al., 1990)" (Hays, Burchett, Fillenbaum, & Blazer, 2004, p. 251).

Design The first subsection is the study design. The design should follow logically from the background literature on the problem and be consistent with the purposes, questions, and/or hypotheses presented in the introduction. For designs that are well known, such as descriptive and experimental, no further information is needed other than indicating the design used for the research. Dates and period of study should be included, in addition to notation of approval by committee or board overseeing protection of human subjects (AMA, 2007). Sample statements of the design are found in Exhibit 5.7.

EXHIBIT 5.7

Sample Design Statements

Quantitative Study

The Duke (North Carolina) EPESE is a 10-year prospective cohort study with a baseline interview (P1) conducted in 1986 and 1987 and three additional in-person contacts with sample members in 1989 and 1990 (P2), 1992 and 1993 (P3), and 1996 and 1997 (P4). Telephone follow-ups were conducted in 1987 and 1988, 1988 and 1989, 1990 and 1991, and 1991 and 1992. The design of the current study was a retrospective-prospective cohort study. All Duke EPESE sample members who participated in the third inperson interview (6 years after baseline) and gave personal consent to draw a blood sample were assessed for APOE genotype. Approximately 4 years later, cheek swabs were sought from survivors who had been unwilling to undergo the blood draw.... Data collection and analysis procedures were approved by the Institutional Review Board of the Duke University Medical Center.[1]

Intervention Study

A two-group quasi-experimental design was used to compare outcomes of a usual care group with those of an Aspiration Risk-Reduction Protocol (ARRP) group. Both groups included critically ill, mechanically ventilated tube-fed patients cared for in the same intensive care units (ICUs). The primary outcomes of interest were the frequency of aspiration and the incidence of pneumonia. A secondary outcome was the use of hospital resources (length of hospitalization, length of intensive care stay, and number of days of mechanical ventilation). The study was approved by the appropriate institutional review boards.[2]

Qualitative Study

The study had a mixed method approach, incorporating quantitative analysis of demographic data and qualitative exploration of perception of need (see Figure 1). This paper reports the qualitative aspects of two phases of this work. The first phase, focusing on the professional perspective, incorporated professional providers of care and key managerial stakeholders in the area. The second phase focused on informal carers' and patients' perspectives.... Approval for the project was gained from the Office for Research Ethics Committees Northern Ireland.[3]

Note. Selected portions of published manuscripts.
[1]From Hays, J. C., Burchett, B. M., Fillenbaum, G. G., & Blazer, D. G. (2004). Is the APOE e4 allele a risk to person-environment fit? *Journal of Applied Gerontology, 23,* pp. 251-252. doi: 10.1177/0733464804267565
[2]From Metheny, N. A., Davis-Jackson, J., & Stewart, B. J. (2010). Effectiveness of an aspiration risk-reduction protocol. *Nursing Research, 59,* 19. doi: 10.1097/NNR.0b013e3181c3ba05.
[3]From McIlfatrick, S. (2007). Assessing palliative care needs: views of patients, informal carers and healthcare professionals. *Journal of Advanced Nursing, 57,* pp. 79-81. doi: 10.1111/j.1365-2648.2006.04062.x

For intervention studies, it should be clear to the reader how the study groups were determined and how the interventions differed across the groups. An example of this is seen in Exhibit 5.7.

For qualitative manuscripts, the method of the study, such as grounded theory, phenomenology, ethnography, and historical research, would be described. Exhibit 5.7 includes an example from an article on a qualitative study.

Subjects or Sample The next subsection deals with the subjects who were studied. The description of the participants in the research is important for making comparison across groups, generalizing the findings, and replicating the study (APA, 2009). Results can only be interpreted accurately when there is sufficient information provided about who was studied and their characteristics.

In writing the description of the subjects, the author can refer to the following list for information that may be included in this section, depending on the type of study:

- Source of subjects
- Number of subjects recruited, number who participated, and number in each study group if relevant
- How subjects were recruited
- Criteria for including and excluding participants
- How subjects were assigned within the study
- Randomization method if random assignment used
- Basis for decisions about sample size
- Procedures when subjects withdrew from study and actions taken, including how many and why
- Payments or other incentives provided to subjects.

In Exhibit 5.8 the sample is described in the beginning of the methods section to give the reader an understanding of patients who participated in the research. Demographic information about the subjects such as age, gender, racial and ethnic background, and educational level, among others, is usually reported in the beginning of the results section of the manuscript, particularly when these are variables in the study.

However, Crist et al. (2009) elected to include information on the subjects in the Methods section in order to focus the Results section on the findings about the main concepts of their theoretical framework.

EXHIBIT 5.8

Sample Methods

METHOD

Design

The data used in this study were taken from a larger cross-sectional study (Crist et al., 2009). Surveys in English or Spanish were completed by care-givers who were recruited at community settings such as health fairs and neighborhood associations. The University of Arizona Human Subjects Committee approved the study (2004).

Sample

Inclusion criteria were: female, 21 years of age or older, primary caregivers of elders 55 years of age or older, of Mexican descent, able to read or speak Spanish or English, and living with the elder or within a 30-minute drive of the elder's home. The average age of the 140 Mexican American caregiv-ers was 49.75 years (SD = 13.84); according to the U.S. Census categories, all were of Latino ethnicity (100%; n = 140); most were of the Hispanic White race (90%, n = 126), elders' daughters (60%; n = 84), married (59%; n = 83), Catholic (76%; n = 107); and had more than a high school education (42%; n = 59). Sixteen percent (n = 22) of the caregivers indicated their elders had used home care.

Measures

Well-known and widely tested instruments used in this study have been tested over time in both Spanish and English in the Mexican American cul-ture. (See, for example, Crist et al., 2009; Crist et al., 2007; Lim et al., 1996). Bicultural–bilingual research assistants assisted participants in completing self-administered questionnaires.

Acculturation was measured with the Acculturation Rating Scale for Mexican Americans (ARSMA II; Cuéllar et al., 1995). The scale had two dimensions to be measured (Mexican American and Anglo American), which could be combined for a total acculturation score by subtraction. We used the total acculturation measure. Cuéllar and colleagues reported

Cronbach's alphas of .81 and .88 and test–retest reliabilities of .72 and .80 for the Mexican American and Anglo American dimensions respectively. In the current study, alpha for the Mexican American dimension was .84 and for the Anglo American dimension was .92. There were 30 items; the range on the Likert-type scale was 0–5. Higher scores indicated the respondent was more acculturated toward the Anglo American culture.

Familism was measured with the Familism Scale, with Sábogal et al. (1987) reporting alphas that ranged from .64 to .72. There were 14 items; the range on the Likert-type scale was 0–56. Higher scores indicated more influence by the familistic norm. Alpha in the current study was .80.

To measure *caregiving burden*, we used the Activities of Daily Living (ADL) scale (Fillenbaum, 1988) for objective burden and the Caregiving Burden Scale (Poulshock & Deimling, 1984) for subjective burden....

Specifically, objective caregiving burden was measured by the ADL scale, (Fillenbaum, 1988), with Fillenbaum reporting test–retest reliability as .88–1.0. There were 15 items; the range on the 0–4 Likert-type scale was 0–60. Higher scores indicated greater functional ability, or lower objective burden. Alpha in the current study was .90.

Subjective burden was measured by Poulshock and Deimling's (1984) Perceived Burden subscale of the Caregiving Burden Scale, adapted by Crist et al. (2009) and Lim et al. (1996), with Poulshock and Deimling reporting alphas ranging from .67 to .70. To complete the questionnaire, each item on the ADL scale (Fillenbaum, 1988) was scored according to how "tiring, difficult, or upsetting" each item was, with a range of 0–3; the range on the Likert-type scale was 0–45. Alpha in the current study was .95....

Use of home care services was measured using the Utilization of Services Scale (Fillenbaum, 1988). Nine items were tabulated; sums were scored dichotomously for analysis as no use (0 or 1 visit) and use (2 or more visits)....

Data Analysis

Correlations were used to test the relationships between acculturation and familism and between familism and objective burden. ANOVAs were used to assess differences in familism and objective burden at three levels of subjective burden. Logistic regression was used to assess the relationships between use of home care services and objective and subjective burden, and the interaction of objective and subjective burden. A logistic regression model predicting the dichotomous use of home care services variable from the continuous objective burden and the categorical subjective burden variables was run.

Note: Selected part of methods.
From Crist, J. D., McEwen, M. M., Herrera, A.P., Kim, S-S., Pasvogel, A., & Hepworth, J. T. (2009). Caregiving burden, acculturation, familism, and Mexican American elders' use of home care services. *Research and Theory for Nursing Practice: An International Journal, 23*, pp. 170–172. doi: 10.1891/1541-6577.23.3.165. Reprinted by permission of Springer Publishing Co., 2010.

An explanation should be included about human subjects requirements met for the research. This includes a statement about informed consent, review and approval of the research proposal by the institutional review board, and its review and approval by the institutions where the subjects were recruited. Frequently, one statement will suffice, such as, "The study was approved by the institutional review boards of the university and participating hospitals prior to subject selection. Each subject signed an informed consent." For other studies, though, more information may need to be provided. This statement may be included in the description of the design, the subjects, or under a separate sub-heading, depending on the journal's guidelines for authors.

Interventions For intervention studies, the groups and treatments can be briefly described as part of the design or, if more explanation is needed, under a separate subheading (Exhibit 5.9).

EXHIBIT 5.9

Sample Description of an Intervention

The independent variable consisted of the two treatment conditions (usual care and the Aspiration Risk-Reduction Protocol [ARRP]. Usual care was defined as the absence of a systematic approach to minimize risk for aspiration. In 2002-2004, standing medical orders on the ICUs did not routinely include information about head-of-bed elevation, and nurses did not chart head-of-bed angles on the patients' flow sheets. Further, no formal program was in place to teach ICU nurses how to place small-bowel feeding tubes. Finally, there was no standardized approach for dealing with high gastric residual volumes (GRVs).

The ARRP had three components: (a) maintain head-of-bed elevation at 30° or higher, unless medically contraindicated; (b) insert feeding tube into distal small bowel, when requested by the attending physician; and (c) initiate an algorithmic approach for high GRVs.

Maintain Head-of-Bed Elevation at 30° or Higher, Unless Medically Contraindicated

Attending physicians were encouraged to write orders for the desired head-of-bed elevation, and this action promoted appropriate patient positioning. Also, bedside nurses were encouraged to record head-of-bed angles at hourly intervals on the patients' ICU flow sheets; this action reminded the nurses to check the bed position frequently and make corrections as necessary.

Insert Feeding Tube Into Distal Small Bowel, When Requested by Attending Physician

Physicians were informed that the advanced practice nurse would assist ICU nurses with small-bowel tube insertions at the bedside. Thus, physicians were able to write orders more freely for bedside small-bowel tube insertions when they were deemed important for high-risk patients. The advanced practice nurse demonstrated small-bowel tube insertion to bedside nurses who were unskilled in this procedure and coached these nurses during small-bowel tube insertions until they gained proficiency in the procedure. A videotape of a successful tube insertion was made available in all of the ICUs for nurses to view at their discretion to facilitate learning further.

Detect and Manage High GRVs

The algorithmic approach used to manage high GRVs during gastric feedings is depicted in Figure 1.

From Metheny, N. A., Davis-Jackson, J., & Stewart, B. J. (2010). Effectiveness of an aspiration risk-reduction protocol. *Nursing Research, 59*, 19-20 doi: 10.1097/NNR.0b013e3181c3ba05. Reprinted by permission of Lippincott Williams & Wilkins, 2010.

Interventions may also be highlighted in a figure and summarized in the body of the methods section. A visual aid with supplemental description may be particularly helpful when reporting research for clinical journals because readers may be particularly interested in the detailed descriptions of promising interventions designed to enhance patient care. An example of a visual aid for intervention studies is present in Exhibit 12.2.

APA (2009) offered these suggestions when writing a complete description of an intervention study. Authors should explain:

- All groups, including the screening criteria for each;
- Content of interventions, including a summary of instructions to participants or, if unusual or represent a manipulation, verbatim in an appendix or a supplemental online section;
- Procedures of manipulation or data acquisition, including equipment model, manufacturer, and settings, if any;
- Persons who delivered the intervention, including their numbers, ratio to participants, professional training, and training in the intervention;
- Setting, including quantity and duration of exposure, time frame of each intervention and between first and last intervention;
- Incentives for participation.

Procedures For non-intervention studies, if the procedures used in carrying out the research were complex, a separate subsection on procedures may be included in addition to sub-sections on design and subjects. Therein, the author presents each step in detail. This section might include how surveys were distributed to subjects and returned to the investigator; how instruments and other measures were administered to subjects; the explanations given to participants; the qualifications of those who administered instruments or interventions; how groups were formed and interventions implemented; the setting, duration, and repetition of elements of the study; and other steps in collecting the data and carrying out the research. The principle for writing the procedures section is to describe what was done in enough detail for others to replicate it. For example, the complex procedures used to measure physical activity among heart transplant patients were explained in a separate section of a manuscript by Evangelista and colleagues:

> Physical activity of participants was measured using an accelerometer (Actiwatch 2, Mini Mitter Company, Bend, Ore[sic]) for one continuous week. The Actiwatch 2...is worn on the nondominant hand and programmed to quantify physical activity at 15-minute intervals.... Participants were instructed to wear the Actiwatch 2 at all times of the day and night from the time it was placed on their wrists until the researcher removed it a week later. We used a sampling period of seven days to minimize variability (Evangelista, Dracup, Doering, Moser, & Kobashigawa, 2005, p. 335).

Measures In the next subsection the author describes the measures used for the study. This includes a discussion of the instruments, observations, and other measures for collecting the data. Widely used measures should be accompanied by a citation where the reader can find a description of the scale's content, validity and reliability. For previously unpublished measures, full information about their validity and reliability should be provided. If the research involved the use of equipment, this should be indicated, including its manufacturer.

Exhibit 5.8 presents an abbreviated portion of the methods section from the study by Crist and colleagues (2009) on caregiving burden, acculturation, familism, and use of home care services among Mexican American elders. It is easy to see how the researchers collected data for this study and how the instruments relate to the purposes of the research. Note the consistency between organization of the literature and the order used to present the instruments. This type of organization is essential in a research report so readers can see the relationships among the components of the study.

Qualitative manuscripts would emphasize methods and sources of data collection, such as interviews and field notes, and how these data were recorded, transcribed and then analyzed.

Data analysis The final subsection in methods deals with the procedures used for data analysis. In this section the author describing a quantitative study lists the statistical methods, the alpha level considered acceptable, how variables were modeled and analyzed, and computer programs used for the analysis. The goal of this section is to explain to readers how the data were analyzed. In qualitative reports the author provides a detailed explanation of how the data were analyzed, what software program was used if any for organizing the analysis, coding strategies, how saturation was determined, and how the validity and reliability of the data were addressed.

Exhibit 5.10 provides examples of data analysis sections. In the first example, from a quantitative study, the statistical methods are listed for the reader; since these are common procedures, no further discussion is indicated. The second example is from a qualitative study.

EXHIBIT 5.10

Sample Statements of Data Analysis

Quantitative Study

Simple descriptive statistics were used to describe the sample. To determine the effect of the ARRP on frequency of aspiration, we used a t test for independent groups to compare patients in the usual care and ARRP groups on the mean percentage of pepsin-positive tracheal secretions. To determine the effect of the ARRP on the incidence of pneumonia, we used a z test for comparing proportions in independent groups to compare the proportion of usual care patients with the proportion of ARRP patients with a positive CPIS for pneumonia on Day 4. Significant baseline differences between the two groups were controlled for in the analyses. To evaluate the effect of the ARRP on hospital resources, we compared usual care and ARRP groups using a z test from the Mann-Whitney U test because the secondary outcomes of hospital length of stay, ICU length of stay, and days of ventilator use had skewed distributions.[1]

Qualitative Study

All interviews and focus groups were tape recorded and transcribed verbatim. Using the guidelines for data analysis described by Burnard (1991, 1996), the following stages were undertaken:

- Each transcript was read a number of times.
- Transcripts were then organized into general themes, based on the aims of the study and the interview topics.
- Categories of data were allocated to each theme: meaning units were then identified for each category.[2]

[1]From Metheny, N. A., Davis-Jackson, J., & Stewart, B. J. (2010). Effectiveness of an aspiration risk-reduction protocol. *Nursing Research, 59*, 22 doi: 10.1097/NNR. 0b013e3181c3ba05. Reprinted by permission of Lippincott Williams & Wilkins, 2010.
[2]From McIlfatrick, S. (2007). Assessing palliative care needs: views of patients, informal carers and healthcare professionals. *Journal of Advanced Nursing, 57*, p. 81. doi: 10.1111/j.1365-2648.2006.04062.x. Reprinted by permission.

Results

In the results section the author presents the findings of the study. What was learned directly from the procedures just described? What new evidence was gathered? The findings should address the original purposes of the study and should answer each of the research questions or shows results of hypothesis-testing. This is the section in which the author presents the data and its analysis but without discussion of the findings. Authorial comments about their meaning, importance, implications, strengths, and weaknesses are held for the subsequent section. The reader needs an understanding of the results before considering their relationship to previous research and their implications. An example of how to present the results can be found in Exhibit 5.11.

The author is obligated to present all of the findings even (and especially!) when they run counter to what was anticipated or do not support the hypotheses. In those cases the author examines, in the discussion section, possible reasons for the findings.

EXHIBIT 5.11

Sample Results

Results

Acculturation and Familism

There was a positive correlation between acculturation and familism ($r = .275$, $p = .001$). Individuals with higher scores on acculturation tended to have higher scores on familism.

Familism and Caregiving Burden

There was no difference in familism at three levels of subjective caregiving burden. ($F(2,137) = .300$, $p = .742$). Objective caregiving burden was not related to familism ($r = .012$, $p = .891$).

Objective and Subjective Caregiving Burden

Objective burden was significantly different, $F(2,137) = 3.86$, $p = .023$, at each level of subjective burden, with means in the expected direction. With no subjective caregiving burden there was the highest level of functional ability (or lowest level of objective burden, $M = 23.04$); with moderate subjective caregiving burden there was a moderate level of functional ability ($M = 22.26$); and with high levels of subjective caregiving burden there was the lowest level of functional ability (or the highest level of objective burden, $M = 19.93$).

Caregiving Burden and Use of Home Care Services

The logistic regression for the overall model was significant, $\chi2$ (3, $N = 140$) $= 26.55$, $p < .001$, Cox & Snell $R2 = .173$, Nagelkerke $R2 = .297$. Subjective burden was not a significant predictor, Wald $= 3.49$, $df = 2$, $p = .175$. Objective burden was significant, Wald $= 16.45$, $df = 1$, $p < .001$. Exp(B) for objective burden (functional ability) was .819 with a 95% CI of .739–.900, indicating that a one point decrease in functional ability resulted in individuals being

22% more likely to use home care services. Thus, objective burden was significantly related to the use of home care services when controlling for subjective burden; but subjective burden was not significantly related to the use of home care services when controlling for objective burden.

A logistic regression was also conducted to evaluate a model predicting use of home care services from objective burden, subjective burden, and their interaction. The overall model was significant ($\chi2(5$, $N = 140) = 33.84$, $p < .001$, Cox & Snell $R2 = .215$, Nagelkerke $R2 = .370$). A significant interaction was found, ($\chi2(2, N = 140) = 7.29, p = .026$). The relationship between use of home care services and objective caregiving burden differed depending upon the level of subjective caregiving burden.

Note: Selected part of results.
From Crist, J. D., McEwen, M. M., Herrera, A. P., Kim, S-S., Pasvogel, A., & Hepworth, J. T. (2009). Caregiving burden, acculturation, familism, and Mexican American elders' use of home care services. *Research and Theory for Nursing Practice: An International Journal, 23*, pp. 172-173. doi: 10.1891/1541-6577.23.3.165. Reprinted by permission of Springer Publishing Co., 2010.

Describe Subjects With some manuscripts, the participants in the study may be described adequately in the method, allowing the author to begin the results with the findings related to the research questions. For most research papers, though, the results section begins with a description of the study population, its demographic characteristics, the number of subjects who began the study, and the number who were excluded or were not included in the research because they withdrew, were lost in the follow-up, or for other reasons. If there were subgroups, the demographics characteristics of each group should be presented in the beginning of the results. With extensive demographic data, a table is helpful to summarize this information. When the results section begins with the report of the demographic data, the author should be careful not to replicate the information provided earlier in the methods section.

Present Main Findings First After describing the subjects, the author presents the main findings, followed by other findings based on exploratory follow-up analysis. The order used to present this information should be consistent with the organization of the introduction and the way the purposes, questions, and/ or hypotheses were listed earlier in the paper. This makes it easy for readers to relate the findings to the original questions for the study.

If there were subgroups in the study, the main findings should be reported first, then the data and related analyses for the subgroups. Along the same line, if varied outcomes measures were used, the most important outcomes should be addressed first.

Use Subheadings Subheadings in the results section clarify the relationship of the findings to each research question or hypothesis. This is particularly important when the results are complex and extensive. If the section is short, though, subheadings are not necessary.

Be Accurate and Precise While all researchers acknowledge the need for accuracy in conducting the research and reporting the findings, the author must be careful that the writing conveys the true results. Analysis results from every variable described in the measures subsection and every model or other analysis described in the analysis section should be described in the results section. Missing information confuses the readers and may suggest the unreliability of the overall report. While some evidence may support the hypotheses, other data may not. The author is responsible for presenting all of the data and discussing any conflicting evidence in the discussion section of the manuscript. Data presented in the text should be consistent with the tables and figures.

Scholarly writing requires accuracy, lack of bias, and completeness (APA, 2009). Accuracy is essential in carrying out the research and in presenting the results. Missing information about subsets of the subjects and strategies used to minimize its impact should be clearly shown, such that readers can evaluate the potential effects.

The author should also be precise in reporting the data. Rather than indicating that the data showed "promising trends in the directions hypothesized" or the findings "tended to support the model," the author should state exactly what were the findings of the study.

Report Data With Related Analyses The data and the related statistical analyses are reported together. For means and other descriptive statistics, the author includes the standard deviations; for inferential statistics, the use of confidence intervals is strongly recommended and often required by journal editors (APA, 2009). The author should always check a manual of style if unsure what information to include when reporting statistics in the paper. Two helpful style manuals are: *Publication Manual of the American Psychological Association* (APA, 2009) and *American Medical Association Manual of Style* (AMA, 2007). Both of these references provide numerous examples of how to report statistics in a manuscript.

Most manuscripts are prepared using word processing software. Statistical symbols are prepared with standard type, **boldface**, and *italics* (APA, 2009, p. 118) . For example, Greek letters, such as α (alpha) and β (beta), subscripts, and superscripts use standard type. Symbols for vectors and matrices are bold, and the symbols N, M, and p are in italic type. Appendix 1 lists common statistical abbreviations and symbols.

There are a few other points that should be noted when reporting statistics in the results of research papers. When citing a statistic in the narrative, the statistical term is used, not the symbol. For example, "The M score was 25" should be written as "The mean score was 25." Remember also in preparing the manuscript that an upper case N refers to the total sample, whereas a lower case n refers to a part of the sample. The actual p value should be reported (e.g., $p = .04$) rather than $p < .05$ or $< .01$, unless $p < .001$. In that case it should be reported as $p < .001$ (AMA, 2007). P-values should not be listed as non-significant (NS) since the actual value is needed for eventual meta-analyses (AMA, 2007).

Develop Tables for Numerical Data Tables are an effective means of presenting detailed and complex information succinctly and clearly. In the text the author can describe the main findings and then use a table to display specific quantitative or qualitative data that supplements the statements in the text. Tables *support* the text and therefore should not duplicate that information. For intervention studies, tables are particularly valuable in comparing groups and how differences across groups were analyzed.

As an example of how tables are useful in presenting the results, consider the need to report demographic data. Including this information in the text would require a large amount of space, would be cumbersome to report, and more than likely would not maintain reader interest. The author should provide numerical data with as much nuance as is available. For example, if data are available on exactly how many years of school the subjects, the author should show the mean, median, and range and then may want to report the number and percent of subjects who completed education at intuitively logical levels:

1. Less than 12th grade
2. High school graduate
3. Trade school (2 years or less after high school)/some college
4. College graduate (bachelor's or other 4-year degree)
5. Post-graduate or professional program (e.g., master's degree, law degree).

Data such as these can be reported more efficiently in the form of a table.

Tables and figures, which include graphs, charts, diagrams, and other illustrations, have the advantage of allowing readers to visualize trends and patterns in the data more easily than when written in the narrative. Figures are particularly useful to show trends, make general comparisons, and help readers understand complex data.

Tables and figures are expensive to produce in a publication and should be used wisely by authors. Many journals limit the number of tables and figures submitted with a manuscript. While tables are valuable for presenting the findings of a study, they should not be used when the data may be presented more easily in the text. Chapter 12 explains how to develop tables, figures, and other illustrations. In that chapter examples are provided of how best to design a table and figure and use them in a manuscript. The AMA (2007) and APA (2009) style manuals are also excellent references for development of tables and figures.

Do Not Report Individual Scores. In most research reports, the author should not include the scores of individual participants or the raw data. Instead, summary statistics such as the mean and standard deviation are reported. For example, researchers presented results from a palliative care study of eight patients-caregivers and eight clinician focus groups in two tables. In one table, data for patients, caregivers, and caregivers' previous experience of death was tabulated in three columns, e.g., 88-year-old female with colon cancer, 55-year-old daughter, and daughter's husband who died of melanoma when she was 41 years old. In a second table, focus group data were presented in five columns: group number (e.g., 1-8), description (e.g., primary care providers), age range (e.g., 29-46), length of time qualified (e.g., 6-22 years), and number of participants (e.g., 8). Although the study was small and the geographical area identifiable, participants in the study would not be identifiable using the summary data reported.

An exception to this rule is the case report, which is discussed in chapter 8. Principles of confidentiality and autonomy govern what data on individual participants may be published. The rights of research subjects to privacy are further discussed below.

Discussion

The discussion section provides an opportunity to interpret the results and explain what the findings mean in relation to the purpose of the study (Exhibit 5.12). In the discussion the author begins by making a clear statement of the answer to the research question or support or lack thereof for the research (APA, 2009). The author should not repeat what was already described in the results section.

In this section, the author discusses whether it is consistent or not with prior research. While it may be tempting to cite only studies that support the findings of the current research, it is equally important to report studies with different conclusions. In those cases the discussion includes potential reasons for differences in findings. Perhaps there were varied subjects or settings, the instruments and measures may have differed, or the data may have been analyzed using different statistical methods. The responsibility of the author is to evaluate possible reasons for these conflicting findings in order to refine what is known about the problem. The author should not repeat what was stated in the introduction but rather reflect on previous work in light of the new findings of the current study and how understanding of the problem is refined with new information.

The discussion also allows the researcher to present implications of the study for clinical practice, teaching, administration, and others. What do these findings mean in terms of nursing practice? How can readers use this information in

EXHIBIT 5.12

Sample Discussion

Discussion

In the following sections we discuss our findings vis-à-vis what has been reported in the literature. Specifically, we suggest possible explanations of how acculturation, familism, caregiving burden, and use of home care services were related, discuss practice and research implications, and identify study limitations.

Acculturation and Familism

We found that acculturation and familism were associated but not in the predicted direction. That is, acculturation was higher, rather than lower, for the caregivers who scored more highly on familism. The proposed theory was that as caregivers became more acculturated, their familism would decrease. One possible explanation might be that Mexican American care-givers do not lose their sense of dedication to the family (familism) as they become more acculturated. Perhaps even as they become more acculturated, but also find themselves still in the role of caregiver, they are more cogni-zant of, and thus report higher, familism. Also, as individuals become more skilled at navigating the individualistically dominant culture (i.e., become more acculturated), they may also value the family even more strongly to maintain a sense of continuity with their original culture, familiar com-fort, and safety. This relationship should be examined with other Mexican American caregivers and noncaregiving individuals.

Familism and Caregiving Burden

Familism was not significantly associated with higher burden, as had been anticipated. Lack of associations between familism and caregiving burden may indicate ineffective measures of familism or burden. Steidel and Contreras (2003) have developed a new familism scale for Latino popula-tions, for use especially with less acculturated Latino individuals. Escandón is testing the Intergenerational Caregiver Familism Scale, designed with and for Mexican American caregivers (S. Escandón, personal communica-tion, December 5, 2008). This may be a better instrument to use because it will measure the structure, attitudes, and behavior of Latino family care-givers in a possibly shifting collectivist orientation....

Caregiving Burden and Use of Home Care Services

Results of the ANOVA showed that level of subjective burden accounted for only about 5% of the variance of objective burden. Substantial unac-counted for variance suggests that, as measured in this study, two distinct constructs were assessed in this sample. This interpretation is consistent with the discussion of caregiving burden presented above.

In a previous study only objective burden was associated with use of home care services (Crist et al. 2009). However, in this study, when we categorized subjective burden, we found that objective and subjective burden interacted in their effect on the use of home care services. Bass and Noelker's (1987) work with Black and Anglo American participants tested and found asso-ciations between subjective burden and use of home care services. Houde's (1998) work with Anglo American participants tested and found associations between objective burden and use of home care services. Our study allowed for not only an assessment of the main effect of subjective and objective burden on use of home care services but also their interaction....

Implications and Future Research

The relationship between objective caregiving burden and use of home care services when subjective caregiving burden is low should be tested

Continued

Exhibit 5.12 *Continued*

further. The small percentage (15%) that reported use of home care services warrants using caution when drawing conclusions from these results. If the relationship continues to be supported, important practical implications for this subgroup could be projected. For example, interventions for individuals with low subjective burden could be designed to prevent them from setting themselves up to attempt to deal with more objective burden than they are able, inadvertently resulting in unhealthy consequences. We may design interventions for subgroups, such as caregivers reporting low burden, who may need but not recognize the need for home care services....

Limitations

As stated previously, the small percentage (15%) mentioned above who reported use of home care services warrants using caution when drawing conclusions from these results. An additional consideration is trying to measure caregiving burden with Mexican American caregivers. As discussed previously, these caregivers may refuse to report burden or they may not even recognize or acknowledge it as an experience. However, the overall moderate association of subjective burden with use of home care services reported in the current study could be related to a relatively ineffective measure of burden. As discussed previously, we used the Poulshock and Deimling (1984) scale. We may need to explore ways to improve the use of the current burden instrument. Further exploration would include examining how each subcategory (i.e., how tiring, difficult, upsetting) behaves in relation to variables such as use of home care services, acculturation, and familism, as well as contextual realities such as fluctuating caregiver health. To explore and compare the use of other existing burden instruments in collectivistic cultures might also be fruitful. New instruments should be tested.

Summary

Families' decisions to access home care services are often driven by underlying cultural and social norms that can be manifested by acculturation, familism, and caregiving burden (subjective and objective). These phenomena can alert clinicians to family caregivers who may be approaching their personal threshold and flag them for appropriate intervention, including exploring the use of home care services. Home care services can delay costly institutionalization, provide respite to stressed caregivers, and is congruent with Mexican American elders' cultural preferences to be cared for at home. Moreover, the effective use of home care services can offset posthospital care costs in the billions of federal dollars each year (Murtaugh, McCall, Moore, & Meadow, 2003).

As the current study demonstrated, relationships among the phenomena studied continue to show inconsistency in their predictive behavior. For instance, acculturation was positively correlated with familism; familism was not significantly correlated with burden; objective burden was positively correlated with use of home care services; and objective and subjective burden significantly interacted in their effect on use of home care services. These phenomena and their relationships and measures require further exploration. Targeted interventions may be needed, depending upon caregivers' level of burden, to increase use of home care services and preserve the well-being of Mexican American elders and caregivers.

Note: Selected part of discussion.
From Crist, J. D., McEwen, M. M., Herrera, A. P., Kim, S-S., Pasvogel, A., & Hepworth, J. T. (2009). Caregiving burden, acculturation, familism, and Mexican American elders' use of home care services. *Research and Theory for Nursing Practice: An International Journal, 23,* pp. 173-177. doi: 10.1891/1541-6577.23.3.165. Reprinted by permission of Springer Publishing Co., 2010.

their work in nursing? Some journals have a separate section that discusses the implications of the research for practice.

It may be tempting for novice authors to overstate the implications of the study. The author should avoid unqualified statements and conclusions that are not completely supported by the data analysis, such as making comments about social, economic, health, or cost benefits, unless these outcomes were measured as part of the research (ICMJE, 2008).

The author should clarify for readers if the findings can be generalized to specific populations and settings. The findings are likely to be applicable only to patients or populations similar to the subjects in the research. If a study was conducted with acutely ill adults in a hospital setting, the findings may have limited or no implications for healthy adults; research on teaching methods for use with basic students may not be applicable to teaching graduate students or staff nurses. Many other examples could be cited. While the implications are an important part of the discussion, they need to be based on the results of the study considering its methods and limitations.

Limitations of the research should be addressed along with needs for further study. It is useful to suggest how the research should be extended.

Many research papers end with the discussion section, but the author may choose to include a short summary paragraph at the end highlighting major findings and what they mean for readers. This can be labeled "conclusions."

Other Parts of a Research Paper

For some research papers the author includes an acknowledgment section to recognize the support of others in the research and preparing the manuscript. Every research paper, and nearly every other manuscript written, has a reference list. This is an important section in a research paper because it represents the literature used to establish why the study was conducted and its importance; a good reference list provides the critical work done previously on the topic.

Acknowledgments

For funded research, the acknowledgment specifies the financial and material support provided for the project, as discussed in chapter 3. The Acknowledgements section also expresses appreciation for individuals who assisted with preparation of or feedback to the manuscript but who did not meet the criteria for authorship, also described in chapter 3. When an acknowledgment is included in print copy, it is placed between the text and references. For online submissions, directions will often specify a data-entry field where the acknowledgements should be cut and pasted.

References

As discussed in the prior chapter on reviewing and reporting the literature, the references should be current, except for classic works that may be cited in the paper, and should be primary rather than secondary sources. The reference list is not exhaustive but instead represents the most recent and relevant work on the topic.

The format for reference lists varies with the journal. The journal's information for authors indicates the format to use for the journal and usually contains examples of preparing different types of references. When unsure, the author should refer to the manual of style used for that journal. Varied reference formats are discussed in chapter 11, with examples of common ones the author might use when writing for nursing and healthcare journals.

The reference list should be consistent with the references cited in the paper. All citations in the text should be on the reference list, and every reference on this list should be cited in the paper. With APA format, the author should check that the names and years of publication cited in the manuscript are the same as on the reference list. With numbered references, the author should check that the number cited in paper correctly matches the corresponding publication on the reference list.

Exhibit 5.13 provides a summary of the parts of the research manuscript discussed in this chapter and their order. Not every manuscript, however, will have each of these sections, but the order is consistent across journals. Use Exhibit 5.13 as a checklist when submitting a research paper.

▥ QUALITATIVE RESEARCH REPORTS

The IMRAD format may be used as a structure for organizing qualitative research papers similar to quantitative studies. With this format the author begins with an introduction to the study, establishing its need and importance. As with quantitative studies, the choice of a qualitative design should be a logical extension of the state of the science on the topic, as presented in the review of background literature. The literature review might establish an unmet need to generate, modify or extend a theory; describe, interpret, or understand some phenomenon; or describe a group, culture or community (Ryan, Coughlan, & Cronin, 2007). Other sections of the manuscript are methods, which include the setting, participants, procedures, and how data were collected and analyzed; results; and discussion.

EXHIBIT 5.13

Order of Sections of Research Manuscript

Cover letter
Copyright transfer page (if submitted with manuscript)
Title page (numbered as page 1)
Abstract (and key words if requested by journal)
Text
   Introduction
   Methods
   Results
   Discussion
Acknowledgment
References
Tables (with titles and footnotes)
Figures (with captions)

Hamilton and colleagues (2009) conducted a grounded theory study of the adaptation of non-symptomatic individuals to knowledge of the results of genetic tests for hereditary breast and ovarian cancer. They used an IMRAD format to organize the research report. In the introduction they described the epidemiology, screening, and follow-up protocols for breast cancer mutations, a proposed model to explain their expression in family systems, and the gaps in observational research on life after genetic testing. The second section of the paper presented their methods. Here the authors described the sample, procedures for their recruitment and data collection, wording of the probes, and how the qualitative data were analyzed. Under data collection they presented how and when interviews were conducted and data analysis consistent with grounded theory methods. In the next section they presented the findings followed by discussion. The discussion section included implications for research and clinical practice. This example illustrates how the conventional format for reporting research may be used with qualitative papers although differences will be apparent in the methods and how the findings are presented.

Presenting Findings of Qualitative Studies

The format of a qualitative research article necessarily depends on the purpose of the research, methods, and data. This is an important difference between writing quantitative and qualitative research manuscripts. When presenting the results of quantitative studies, the findings and related discussion are organized according to the purposes, questions, and/or hypotheses. In a qualitative research report, however, the purpose of the study, qualitative method used for it, and the data determine how the findings are presented.

In a qualitative research study, McIlfatrick (2006) assessed palliative care needs of patients, informal caregivers, and healthcare professionals. Four care themes were identified in the qualitative analysis of data: psychological needs, financial needs, practical home care needs, and need for information and choice. In the article, the researchers provide examples of narratives that support each theme. The theme of practical home care needs reflected stories from informal caregivers in the home. One narrative that supported this theme was:

> The [formal caregivers] really are the, the connecting thing. They're the one ... they're the people that makes me feel more at ease, 'cause I know that they're coming in and they know what they're doing, ... They're the central people, to me anyway (p. 84).

In this paper, the objective of the authors was to describe the views of patients, informal caregivers, and healthcare professionals in their own voices. However, with a grounded theory method, in which the goal is to discover theoretical explanations about particular phenomena (Ryan et al., 2007), the data would be used in the paper to demonstrate how a theory of palliative care needs was developed from the interviews.

In presenting the findings of qualitative studies, the first step is to determine the approach to be taken with the wealth of data collected (Ryan et al., 2007). Qualitative researchers might use grounded theory, phenomenology, or ethnography as a useful approach in their study. Regardless of their overall purpose, authors still need to demonstrate that what they did was a valid way of studying the problem and interpreting the data (Porter, 2007).

Organizing Qualitative Research

Data from qualitative research may be organized in the paper according to several formats: (1) by time whereby the findings are organized as a narrative story of an experience; (2) by the frequency of occurring themes; and (3) as a description and interpretation of a phenomenon (Ryan et al., 2007). With any of these strategies, the data are framed in advance by evidence of a problem or gap in understanding that sets up the importance of the study and in conclusion by discussion of the findings as extensions of the available knowledge base. Ryan and colleagues underscore the need to avoid exaggerating the implications of qualitative findings for research and practice.

In reporting the data, the perspectives of the participants, as distinct from the researcher's point of view, should be apparent to readers. Bradbury-Jones warns against slipping into the role of a crusader for a particular perspective or cause, favoring novel or unorthodox conclusions, or rushing to judgment; rather, a pragmatic, sensible, and logical approach to presenting the data is optimal (Bradbury-Jones, 2007). One way of accomplishing this is to use the conventional form of research reports in which the participants' views, i.e., the data, are presented in the results, and the researcher's analysis and discussion of them are presented in the discussion section.

Qualitative research generates a lot of data that must be synthesized for readers. There are some studies in which multiple manuscripts might be written, and this decision should be made before the first manuscript is prepared. The author may have conducted a study on what it is like to care for a child with a chronic illness and the effect on the family. One manuscript might present the experiences from the parents' point of view and a second on how children cope with a chronic illness.

Data analysis is often poorly presented in qualitative research manuscripts (Ryan et al., 2007). Authors must provide enough details to convince readers that the findings should be accepted. Details to be provided to readers include the rigor of documentation, all procedures, and protection of the rights of human subjects. The manuscript should make plain that the experience of the informants was faithfully interpreted by the authors (credibility), what decisions the authors made in each stage of the research (dependability), the fittingness of the findings for other contexts (transferability), and the degree to which conclusions in the manuscript are directly traceable to the data (confirmability) (Ryan et al.).

The decision on the journal for submission of the manuscript also influences its preparation. When writing the research paper for a clinical journal, the findings of the study and their implications for practice would be emphasized. Less attention would be given to the qualitative method and analysis of the data.

HOW MANY MANUSCRIPTS ARE TOO MANY?

The author needs to avoid writing several manuscripts when one would be sufficient. Each paper should make its own contribution to the literature and should not overlap with one already published. Editors deserve to publish original papers, and readers assume what they are reading in their journals are original ideas.

While some projects lend themselves to writing more than one paper, others do not. An example of dividing a research study into separate manuscripts when one would suffice is with a study on the effectiveness of pressure ulcer treatments. In the study the researcher collected data on clinical outcomes, such as the location, stage, and size of the ulcer; hours of nursing care each patient received and level of education of nursing staff; and treatment costs. Separate manuscripts would not be appropriate in presenting the findings of this research because the author measured the effectiveness of the treatments based on clinical outcomes, staff variables, and cost. These measures are closely related and as a whole describe the treatments' effectiveness.

Some research studies and other projects, though, may be divided legitimately into more than one manuscript. The author may report the findings of research in one journal and a critical analysis of the literature in another. The implications of the findings for nursing practice may even be reported in yet a third article as long as each of the manuscripts has a clear message and presents new information not in the other articles.

When writing about a clinical project or an innovation in practice, a professional issue, and other non-research topics, the same question should be asked: Is it legitimate to divide the topic into separate manuscripts, or would one suffice? The author may be planning on writing a manuscript about nursing care for patients following a new surgical procedure recently initiated in the clinical setting. Separate manuscripts about care of these patients in the immediate postoperative period and home care would be inappropriate. The care of these patients would be better presented across the continuum, and neither manuscript would be too long to warrant separate papers.

Duplicate or Redundant Publication

The publication of essentially the same material in two or more publications is termed duplicate or redundant publication. Duplicate publication can range from disseminating the same content to different audiences in different forms to submitting duplicate manuscripts with identical content to different publishers (AMA, 2007).

The ethical issues associated with duplicate publication include the wasteful use of resources and the originality of scientific work. When an author submits the same material to two or more journals simultaneously, or attempts to divide one work into several publications, the resources of scientific publication are used inappropriately. The time and energy of peer reviewers and editors and the financial resources of publishers are invested in reviewing and preparing manuscripts for publication. A manuscript cannot be published in more than one journal due to copyright considerations; when the manuscript is accepted for publication in one journal and the author must withdraw it from consideration by others, the resources of the other journals are wasted, contributing to the ever-increasing costs of scientific publication (AMA, 2007). Duplicate publication can also result in double-counting or wrongly weighting data in meta-analyses and suggesting more evidence of replication than is actual, which distorts the scientific evidence (APA, 2009; Saver, 2006).

Publishers, editors, and readers of scientific papers assume that published material is original. Editors were more concerned about redundant publications than any other breach of authorial ethics (Wager, 2009). Therefore, editors typically require authors of manuscripts to certify that their submitted manuscripts are not under consideration for publication elsewhere and that, if accepted for publication, the materials would not be published elsewhere in the same form without the consent of the editors (ICEMJ, 2008).

Authors should guard against two specific forms of redundant and duplicate publication: shotgunning and salami slicing. Each practice has associated ethical issues.

Shotgunning

Shotgunning is submitting the same manuscript for review by two or more journals. An author who engages in shotgunning typically intends to wait until the manuscript is accepted for publication by one journal, and then withdraw it from consideration by others. However, the author has no control over the timing of review procedures and, at worst, this practice could lead to publication of the same material in more than one journal, violating the standard of originality of scientific publication. At a minimum, the author has inconvenienced the editor and reviewers of the journal from which the manuscript was withdrawn.

Shotgunning may be sanctioned as an inappropriate act according to the Uniform Requirements or specific journal policy. The Uniform Requirements suggest that, if duplicate publication occurs, a notice of redundant publication be published by the journal editor with or without the author's explanation or approval (ICMJE, 2008). Additional sanctions also may apply, such as notification of the author's dean, director, or supervisor (AMA, 2007). Notice of confirmed duplicated publications is placed on a numbered journal page and in the table of contents to facilitate linkage to the original articles in online searches.

Salami Slicing

Salami slicing (divided or fragmented publication) is the practice of breaking down findings from a single research study or project into a series of papers (known as "least publishable units") submitted to different journals or to the same journal at different times (Baggs, 2008). The intent of salami slicing usually is to increase the number of publications attributable to an author. Most editors consider it to be unacceptable, citing it as an example of wasteful publication and an abuse of scientific publication (Hoit, 2007).

Divided publication can obscure the true value of the findings of a research study, making them appear more important than they really are; may confound meta-analyses of research findings; and may misrepresent the true incidence of reported phenomena (Hoit, 2007; Saver, 2006). Divided publications may also blur the distinction between original research and secondary analysis and may lead to overgeneralization of implications for interventions that may adversely affect health outcomes of at-risk populations.

Acceptable Duplicate Publication

Duplicate publication does not include sending a manuscript rejected by one journal to another. When an author receives a notice that the manuscript was rejected, it may then be submitted to another journal for review. Other forms of publication not considered redundant include when a full manuscript follows (1) an abstract published as part of conference proceedings, (2) news media reports of study findings, or (3) detailed reports distributed to narrowly defined audiences (AMA, 2007; ICMJE, 2008).

The key to whether duplicate publication is acceptable or not is disclosure (AMA, 2007). It is unethical when authors do not notify editors about duplicate publications and do not include references to them. Authors should inform editors about duplicate publications, and copies of these articles should be sent with the submission. If there is any question about whether a manuscript reflects duplicate publication, the author should include a statement to the editor describing similar work. If the manuscript is based on the same subjects as one or more earlier publications, the author should cite the publications that inform the reader most completely about the data or report findings of relevance to the current manuscript. Earlier articles should always be referenced in a subsequent manuscript in both the text and reference list. Some journals such as *Applied Nursing Research* ask the author to specify any publication in which the same content or data set has been used and how the submitted manuscript differs.

Secondary Publication

Secondary publication is the republication or parallel publication of an article in more than one journal with consent of the involved editors (AMA, 2007, p.149). An example of a secondary publication is when an article is translated for publication in a journal of a different language than the original. Typically, secondary publications are released at least one week after the primary publication, are intended for a different audience than the original paper, do not modify the data nor conclusions of the original paper, and include a footnote on the title page that informs readers that the paper was previously published (ICMJE, 2008). The footnote should contain the full reference to the primary paper.

■ PROTECTING THE RIGHTS OF INDIVIDUALS IN PUBLICATIONS

In preparing a manuscript, the author needs to protect the rights of individuals to privacy and to avoid harming the reputations of others by defamation.

Privacy Rights

Publications in nursing, medicine, and other healthcare disciplines must protect the rights of certain individuals to privacy. Historically, this effort included omitting patient names, initials, and case numbers from published case reports; removing identifying information from x-ray films, digital images, and laboratory slides; deleting certain identifying details from descriptions of patients or participants in research studies; and concealing certain facial features of patients in published photographs (e.g., placing black bars over the eyes). However, masking facial features does not always disguise identities sufficiently, and since the late 1980s, its use has not been recommended. If a patient's or legally authorized representative's written informed consent to publish a photographic likeness has not been obtained, the photograph should not be published (AMA, 2007). Authors who have obtained such written consents should, of course, include them with other permissions when the manuscript is submitted.

To prevent patients and participants in research studies from recognizing descriptions of themselves in published reports, some authors omit certain descriptive data from the manuscript, including age, sex, and occupation. However, omitting such details may hinder future investigations and meta-analyses. For example, occupational information might be useful to a researcher who is conducting a study of occupational injuries. Altering some demographic details about patients or research participants may appear to be a harmless way to protect the identities of these individuals, but doing so allows falsified data to be published, a serious breach of scientific integrity (ICMJE, 2008). Altered or falsified data also can affect a subsequent investigation or meta-analysis, for example, changing the name of a city can contribute error to an epidemiological analysis of disease outbreak locations (AMA, 2007). The Uniform Requirements suggest that identifying information about patients should not be published unless it is essential for scientific purposes, and that the patient or legally authorized representative should be allowed to review the manuscript before giving informed consent for the information to be published (ICMJE, 2008).

Defamation

Although every citizen is guaranteed freedom of expression by the First Amendment to the Constitution of the United States, this right is balanced against the right to protect one's personal reputation. Therefore, authors, editors, and publishers must take care not to harm the reputations of others by defamation, thereby exposing them to public ridicule, contempt, hatred, or financial loss. Defamation can take the form of libel or slander, but it always includes a false public statement concerning another (AMA, 2007).

Libel is a false, negligent, or malicious statement about another person or existing entity, made in print, images, or signs; slander is defamation by oral expression or gestures. With the increasing use of digital publication that includes mixtures of print, audio, and video content, the distinction between libel and slander has become increasingly blurred (AMA, 2007).

The laws concerning defamation are complex, and it is beyond the scope of this book to offer specific advice about how to avoid defamation in the process of writing for publication. Authors are advised to consult the editors of the publications to which they submit manuscripts for specific guidance.

MOVING FROM THESIS AND DISSERTATION TO MANUSCRIPT

Generally sections of previously written grants, theses, and dissertations need to be rewritten to comply with expected manuscript formats, with references carefully selected. Rarely can these other written forms be used "as is" for manuscripts.

A thesis and dissertation cannot be "cut and pasted" as a manuscript; they need to rewritten as such. A common reason for manuscript rejection is it "reads like a thesis," often containing inappropriately long and extensive literature reviews. Even experienced researchers may find it difficult to revise a research grant into a manuscript.

Problematic manuscripts developed from theses and dissertations usually contain exhaustive literature reviews, extensive reference lists, and such a broad focus on the topic as to be inappropriate to the information needs of the audience of the journal to which submitted. They also may extend well beyond the page limits and may contain too many tables and figures. Dissertations and theses may also omit any implications for clinical practice.

What can be done to prepare a manuscript from a student research project that has a good chance of acceptance rather than a good chance of rejection? First, the author must decide what is the focus of the one or more manuscripts appropriate to the thesis or dissertation. Is the goal to present the findings of the study to advance research on the topic, to describe the clinical implications of the research for practitioners, or both? If the author can write more than one paper, how many and what types of manuscripts are planned? Second, the author needs to choose a journal that would provide an avenue for publishing the first intended manuscript. Clinical journals want manuscripts with practice implications. Research journals want manuscripts that describe the study methods and findings even if implications also are discussed. Third, think about the target audience so the manuscript is geared to the readers of the journal.

Once these preliminary decisions are made, the next steps involve adapting the research project to a manuscript format. Some techniques follow:

- Shorten the title if needed
- Develop a new outline that reflects the required format of the journal
- Write new subheadings to reflect the goals of the manuscript rather than using the subheadings required for the thesis or dissertation
- Shorten the background of the study and introduce the purpose of manuscript early in the introduction
- Synthesize the literature review, present the most important and relevant studies, and consider integrating the literature within the introduction (depending on the journal's format)
- Review sample research articles in the journal to determine if they include a separate section on the theoretical framework. If not, integrate a brief statement of the framework in the literature review. If articles include a section for the theoretical framework, shorten the one from the thesis and describe it briefly in the manuscript
- Shorten the methods section, omit the rationale for the methods, and shorten the discussion of psychometric properties of the measures unless submitting the manuscript to a research journal
- Revise the description of the sample and presentation of the demographic data to fit the journal being considered for submission
- Consider the extent of statistical analysis described in the manuscript and write for the audience
- If submitting to a clinical journal, emphasize practice implications
- Shorten the reference list to the most recent and relevant references
- Include only essential tables and figures up to a maximum of four
- Rewrite the manuscript consistent with the writing style of the journal and for its readers who need the information
- Shorten the manuscript to comply with the page limits specified by the journal.

■ SUMMARY

Nursing research is of little value if the findings are not made available for use by clinicians and others who need the research results for their work. Nurses who conduct research are responsible for reporting the results in journals that are read by nurses who can use the information in their practice, teaching, management, and other roles. By publishing the findings of research, nurses advance the body of knowledge of nursing and contribute to the scientific basis of nursing practice. Communicating the findings of research promotes the critique and replication of studies and is essential for evidence-based practice in nursing. Nurses also need research data to establish evidence for their decisions and interventions.

The conventional format for writing research papers is the IMRAD format: **I**ntroduction, **M**ethods, **R**esults **a**nd **D**iscussion, or an adaptation of this depending on the journal and type of research. IMRAD provides a way of organizing the paper and specifies in advance the headings for it.

The first section of the manuscript is the introduction, which is the author's opportunity to explain the nature and background of the study, its purpose, and its importance. The author begins the introduction with a discussion of the specific problem the research addressed and its significance. This discussion provides a framework for reading the related literature; determining how the study builds on previous research on the topic; and understanding the relationship of the purposes, questions, and/or hypotheses to the problem.

The literature review describes what is already known about the topic and what needs to be studied, thereby justifying the current project. Gaps in knowledge and limitations of prior studies are emphasized to provide support for the study. The literature review may be incorporated into the introduction or presented as a separate section in the manuscript. The literature review may contain the discussion of the conceptual or theoretical framework that guided the study, or the framework may be included in a separate section.

The last part of the introduction includes the purposes of the study, questions the research was designed to answer, and/or hypotheses that were tested. The author should review sample articles in the target journal before beginning the manuscript.

The next section of the manuscript is methods. In this section information is presented about the study design, subjects, measures, intervention or procedures, and data analysis in that order.

In the results section the author presents the findings of the study. The findings should answer each of the research questions and address the original purposes of the study. This is the section in which the author presents the data and its analysis but without discussion of the findings.

The discussion section provides an opportunity to interpret the results and explain what the findings mean. In the discussion the author begins by stating the main conclusion that can be drawn from the results. The discussion allows the researcher to present implications of the study for clinical practice, teaching, administration, and other areas. Limitations of the research should be addressed along with needs for further study.

The IMRAD format also may be used as a broad structure for organizing qualitative research papers. With this format the author begins with an introduction to the study, establishing its need and importance. Other sections of the manuscript are methods, which include the setting, participants, procedures, and how data were collected and analyzed; results; and discussion. The content in each section, however, reflects the purpose of the study, qualitative method, and data.

Ethical considerations when writing research papers include deciding the appropriate number of articles to write from a single study and avoidance of redundant or duplicate publications, except as approved by journal editors. Authors should take care to protect the privacy rights of their subjects and to avoid defamation of other members of the research community.

A thesis and dissertation need to be rewritten as a manuscript; they can not be used as is. Often manuscripts developed from theses and dissertations are too long and are not relevant for the journal to which submitted. Strategies for preparing a manuscript from a thesis and dissertation were included in the chapter.

▓ REFERENCES

American Medical Association. (2007). AMA manual of style: A guide for authors and editors (10ᵗʰ ed.). New York: Oxford University Press.

American Psychological Association. (2009). *Publication manual of the American Psychological Association* (6th ed.). Washington, D.C.: Author

Baggs, J. G. (2008). Issues and rules for authos concerning authorship versus acknowledgements, dual publication, self-plagiarism, and salami publishing. [Editorial.] *Research in Nursing and Health, 31*, 295–297. doi: 10.1002/nur.20280

Bradbury-Jones, C. (2007). Enhancing rigour in qualitative health research: Exploring subjectivity through Peshkin's I's. *Journal of Advanced Nursing, 59*(3), 290-298. doi: 10.1111/j.1365-2648.20007.04306.x

Crist, J. D., McEwen, M. M., Herrera, A. P., Kim, S-S., Pasvogel, A., & Hepworth, J. T. (2009). Caregiving burden, acculturation, familism, and Mexican American elders' use of home care services. *Research and Theory for Nursing Practice: An International Journal, 23*(3), 165-179. doi: 10.1891/1541-6577.23.3.165

Demner-Fushman, D., Hauser, S., & Thoma, G. (2005). The role of title, metadata and abstract in identifying clinically relevant journal articles. *Proceedings of the American Medical Informatics Association,* Washington, DC.

Evangelista, L. S., Dracup, K., Doering, L., Moser, D. K., & Kobashigawa, J. (2005). Physical activity patterns in heart transplant women. *Journal of Cardiovascular Nursing, 20*, 334–339.

Hamilton, R., Williams, J. K., Skirton, H., & Bowers, B. J. (2009). Living with genetic test results for hereditary breast and ovarian cancer. *Journal of Nursing Scholarship, 41*, 276–283. doi: 10.1111/j.1547-5069.2009.01279.x

Hays, J. C., Burchett, B. M., Fillenbaum, G. G., & Blazer, D. G. (2004). Is the APOE e4 allele a risk to person-environment fit? *Journal of Applied Gerontology, 23*, 247–265. doi: 10.1177/0733464804267565

Hoit, J. D. (2007). Salami science. [Editorial]. *American Journal of Speech-Language Pathology 16*(2), 94. doi:10.1044/1058-0360(2007/013)

International Committee of Medical Journal Editors. (2008). *Uniform requirements for manuscripts submitted to biomedical journals: Writing and editing for biomedical publication.* Retrieved from http://www.icmje.org/urm_main.html

Johnson, M. E., Dose, A. M., Pipe, T. B., Peterson, W. O., Huschka, M., Gallenberg, M. M.,...Frost, M. H. (2009). Centering prayer for women receiving chemotherapy for recurrent ovarian cancer: A pilot study. *Oncology Nursing Forum, 36*, 421–428.

McIlfatrick, S. (2007). Assessing palliative care needs: views of patients, informal carers and healthcare professionals. *Journal of Advanced Nursing, 57*, 77-86. doi: 10.1111/j.1365-2648.2006.04062.x

Meijers, J. M. M., Janssen, M. A. P., Cummings, G. G., Wallin, L., Estabrooks, C. A., & Halfens, R. Y. G. (2006). Assessing the relationships between contextual factors and research utilization in nursing: Systematic review. *Journal of Advanced Nursing, 55*, 622–635.

Moher, D., Schultz, K.F., & Altman, D.G. (2001). The CONSORT statement: Revised recommendations for improving the quality of reports of parallel-group randomized trials. *Annals of Internal Medicine, 134*(8), 657–662.

U.S. Department of Health and Human Services, National Institutes of Health, National Library of Medicine. (1995). *Full abstracts in MEDLINE.* (NLM Technical Bulletin No. 286). Retrieved from ftp://nlmpubs.nlm.nih.gov/nlminfo/newsletters/techbull/pdf_tb/sepoct95.pdf

Penrose, A. M., & Katz, S. B. (2004). *Writing in the sciences: Exploring conventions of scientific discourse* (2nd ed.). New York: Pearson Longman.

Porter, S. (2007). Validity, trustworthiness and rigour: Reasserting realism in qualitative research. *Journal of Advanced Nursing, 60,* 79–86. doi: 10.1111/j.1365-2648.2007.04360.x

Ryan, F., Coughlan, M., & Cronin, P. (2007). Step-by-step guide to critiquing research. Part 2: qualitative research. *British Journal of Nursing, 16,* 738-744.

Saver, C. (2006). Legal and ethical aspects of publishing. *Association of periOperative Registered Nurses Journal, 84*(4): 571–576. doi:10.1016/S0001-2092(06)63936-7

Steinhauser, K. E., Clipp, E. C., Hays, J. C., Olsen, M., Arnold, R., Christakis, N. A.,...Tulsky J. A. (2006.) Identifying, recruiting, and retaining seriously-ill patients and their caregivers in longitudinal research. *Palliative Medicine, 20,* 745–754. doi: 10.1177/0269216306073112

Tagney, J., & Haines C. (2009). Using evidence-based practice to address gaps in nursing knowledge. *British Journal of Nursing, 18,* 484–489.

U.S. Department of Health and Human Services, National Institutes of Health. (2009). *The Omnibus Appropriations Act of 2009 makes the NIH Public Access Policy permanent* (NIH Notice No. NOT-OD-09-071). Retrieved from http://grants.nih.gov/grants/guide/notice-files/NOT-OD-09-071.html

Wager, E. (2007). Do medical journals provide clear and consistent guidelines for authorship? *MedGenMed: Medscape General Medicine, 9*(3), 16.

6

REVIEW AND EVIDENCE-BASED PRACTICE ARTICLES

Nurses in all clinical settings require the most current and complete evidence of effective approaches to guide their decision making and practice. The evidence should be based on a critical appraisal of studies that answer a specific clinical question or examine best practices and the synthesis of findings from across these studies. The preferential use of such approaches is known as evidence-based practice (EBP). With EBP nurses rely on the review and synthesis of evidence from multiple studies rather than the report of one original research study.

Evidence-based practice though is broader than only the use of research findings to guide clinical decisions. In EBP nurses integrate the research with their own clinical expertise and the patient's preferences and values. EBP is a problem-solving approach to clinical practice and delivery of healthcare, and it is dependent on the nurse's spirit of inquiry and questioning (Melnyk, Fineout-Overholt, Stillwell, & Williamson, 2009). The process begins by identifying a clinical question to which the nurse needs more information to guide practices, searching for evidence to answer that question, critiquing and rating the strength of the evidence (and if appropriate deciding on a change in practice), integrating the evidence with the nurse's clinical expertise and patient preferences, evaluating the outcome of the practice change, and disseminating the EBP results (DiCenso, Guyatt, & Ciliska, 2005; Larrabee, 2009; Melnyk, Fineout-Overholt, Stillwell, & Williamson, 2009; Oermann, 2007).

Methods are now available to nurse-authors for reviewing and integrating individual studies and summarizing the evidence from them to answer a clinical question or explore a topic of interest. These review methods include integrative reviews, systematic reviews, meta-analyses, and metasyntheses. In addition to review papers, nurses also prepare manuscripts on research utilization, which focus on the structures, process, and outcomes of transferring research knowledge and findings into clinical practice. Translating the results of EBP reviews into clinical practice is the final step in research dissemination. Manuscripts on EBP address the effectiveness of new approaches or changes in practice as well as the resources needed for implementation and the process used by nurses in a clinical setting to engage in EBP.

This chapter describes the types of review and EBP articles that are useful for nurses who lack the time or skills to access, appraise, and apply large and accumulating literatures on clinical issues. The chapter also presents guidelines for preparing articles that disseminate the outcomes of those review methods. Only well-designed and conducted reviews should be used as evidence for practice. A detailed description of the methods used by the authors should characterize review articles, such that nurses may evaluate the quality of the review and whether its findings are robust enough for implementation into practice or, if not, what additional research is needed.

TYPES OF REVIEW AND EBP ARTICLES

Integrative Review

An integrative or narrative review provides a summary of empirical and theoretical literature to improve understanding of a particular topic. If comprehensive, this type of review presents the state of the science about the topic. Integrative reviews include both experimental and non-experimental studies (Whittemore & Knafl, 2005). An integrative review tends to be broader in its description and understanding of a topic than a systematic review, which addresses a specific clinical question. In addition to summarizing evidence and presenting the state of the science on a topic, integrative review papers are also written to define concepts and explore theories. Integrative reviews are appropriate for critiquing and reconceptualizing a large or mature body of literature; synthesizing the literature to date on topics with limited or preliminary research; describing the development of a problem and its management; and identifying studies that have flawed designs or implementation (Cook, Mulrow, & Haynes, 1997; Torraco, 2005).

Popay and colleagues identified four elements of an integrated review: (1) a theory of how an intervention works, why, and for whom; (2) a preliminary synthesis of findings of the studies included in the review; (3) an analysis of relationships in the data that might explain differences in the effects across studies; and (4) an evaluation of the rigor and robustness of the synthesis, critical in assessing the strength of the evidence for drawing conclusions and making generalizations to other groups and contexts (Popay et al., 2007). This fourth element is important in determining whether the integrative review can be used for making clinical decisions. While integrative reviews provide a basis for understanding a clinical problem, some may not provide sufficient evidence to guide practice decisions. All EBP reviews of research, including integrative reviews, need to be comprehensive, have an explicit strategy for searching the literature and identifying studies for review, and use a rigorous method for appraising the studies.

Whittemore and Knafl (2005) provided a framework for conducting an integrative review that includes five stages: problem formulation, literature search, data evaluation, data analysis, and presentation of the findings. This framework is useful as a guide for preparing manuscripts of integrative reviews for journals and other types of publications.

Problem Formulation

An integrative review begins with a clear purpose for the review and description of the problem addressed in it. A well-specified purpose and identification of variables of interest guide other stages of the review (Whittemore & Knafl). This same purpose statement can be used in the introduction of an integrative review manuscript to define its scope and explain why the review was done. Clearly articulated purpose statements are helpful to readers and establish the search criteria (Conn, 2009). Exhibit 6.1 is an example of an integrative review paper.

EXHIBIT 6.1

Example of an Integrative Review Article[1]

Pediatric solid organ transplant (SOT) recipients are a unique population of patients experiencing the transition from hospital to home. Management at home following SOT is complex because care includes administration of multiple medications, wound care, central line care, and a time-consuming outpatient schedule for follow-up....

Aim

The aim of this integrative review was to identify factors associated with discharge readiness and propose opportunities for extending research in the field.

Methods

Search Methods

Multiple words were used to search for literature on discharge readiness. The following words were placed in the online indexes individually and in combination with one another: *discharge readiness, discharge, patient discharge education, patient discharge, discharge planning, early patient discharge, pediatric,* and *transition.* The inclusion criteria were: (a) a focus of family and health team factors that influence readiness for hospital discharge, and (b) publication in the English language....

Search Results

A search in CINAHL 1982 to 2008 and MEDLINE 1966 to 2008 was completed. An initial search using the term *discharge* further truncated as *patient discharge education, patient discharge, discharge planning, early patient discharge,* or *transfer* resulted in 8,833 papers. Additional search strategies were employed by combining those results with the following terms, *discharge readiness, transfer, pediatric,* and *transition,* resulting in 432 papers. All abstracts were retrieved and their relevance to the study questions was assessed. Articles were excluded if the focus was on pediatric to adult

Continued

Exhibit 6.1 *Continued*

transition, wound discharge, and long-term care....The studies were evaluated using the Melnyk and Fineout-Overholt (2005) hierarchy of evidence....

Thirty-eight articles were included in the analysis of factors influencing discharge readiness: 14 were pediatric research, 9 were pediatric and adult clinical practice, 4 were obstetrical research, and 11 were adult research articles. The results of the relevant sources obtained during the literature search are summarized in Table 1.

Findings

Support

Support is instrumental to feeling ready to go home in both parents of hospitalized children (Snowdon & Kane, 1995) and family caregivers of adult patients (Artinian, 1993; Congdon, 1994), including feeling comfortable in the home environment (Bent, Keeling, & Routson, 1996). The level of perceived support is different for each parent and may be related to the parent's level of health and available social support (Affleck, Tennen, Rowe, Roscher, & Walker, 1989). The level of support a parent requires may not necessarily correlate with the child's level of illness....

Identification of Individual Parent Needs

Each individual family will have unique and varying stressors that will influence discharge readiness, such as: financial stressors (Snowdon & Kane, 1995), ambivalence before discharge stemming from uncertainty about removing the child from the hospital's professional care (Baker, 1991; Smith & Daughtrey, 2000), adjustment needed to incorporate an infant into the family unit (Baker; Bissell & Long, 2003; Snowdon & Kane), parental competence (Baker), and perceived vulnerability and fear of death (Baker; Bent et al., 1996)....

[1] Selected parts of each section.
From: Lerret, S. (2009). Discharge readiness: An integrative review focusing on discharge following pediatric hospitalization. *Journal for Specialists in Pediatric Nursing, 14*, 247, 250. doi: 10.1111/j.1744–6155.2009.00205.x. Reprinted by permission of John Wiley and Sons, 2010.

In the introduction, the author provides background for readers to understand the problem of the transition from hospital to home for children who have had organs transplants. Management at home is complex considering the child's multiple medications, wound care, central line care, and a schedule for laboratory and clinic follow-up. The author discusses the need to understand the discharge readiness of parents to better prepare them and the child for discharge after an organ transplant and concludes with the aims of the integrative review: to identify factors associated with discharge readiness and propose opportunities for extending research in the field (Lerret, 2009).

Literature Search

An integrative review is a review of research and theoretical literature. It should be comprehensive, especially if used as evidence for practice, because if a review is incomplete and only some studies are considered, the findings may be biased and conclusions may be inaccurate. Multiple bibliographic databases should be searched, as described in chapter 4, combined with other strategies such as ancestry searching (systematically reviewing citations from studies included in the review and from review articles) and hand searching journals, among others (Conn, et al., 2003). The search strategy used for the review should be described clearly for readers including the search terms and how they were combined in the search, the specific databases used, and any additional search strategies employed for locating articles.

Although ideally nurses would review all the relevant literature on a topic or problem and present the literature in the paper, for many reviews this would be a difficult if not impossible task because of the extent of available literature. When authors need to restrict the number of studies included in a review for it to be manageable, the rationale and criteria for deciding which papers to include and exclude in the review should be presented in the manuscript.

In the example of an integrative review article in Exhibit 6.1, the author describes the search strategy she used to explore factors associated with discharge readiness. She includes the databases searched, keywords, and other search strategies used for the review, and she specifies the reasons for articles to be excluded from the review.

Data Evaluation

In this stage of an integrative review, the quality of each of the studies is evaluated. How this is done depends on the types of studies in the review. If only one type of research design was included, then the methodological quality of those studies could be assessed, and scores could be generated to represent different levels of quality. For reviews that include empirical and theoretical articles, different strategies are possible. For example, primary sources might be evaluated based on their methodological quality, informational value, and representativeness of available primary sources; theoretical reports might be assessed using techniques of theory analysis; and multiple instruments might be developed for each type of primary source (Whittemore & Knafl, 2005).

Regardless of the method used for evaluating the studies in the review, the manuscript should describe the method and how it was used to include or exclude papers from the review and evaluate those contained in it. In the sample integrative review paper (Exhibit 6.1), the author evaluated the studies using a hierarchy of evidence and included the level of evidence in the summary table. This can be seen in Table 6.1.

TABLE 6.1

Example of Summary of Included Studies Table

Table 1
Summary of Articles Included in the Integrative Review

Author/Year	Sample	LOE	Conclusion
Summary of Pediatric Research Studies			
Affleck, Tennen, Rowe, Roscher, & Walker(1989)	94 moms of NICU infants	II	Scarce professional resources should be allocated according to the mothers who report needing the most support during the transition home.
Baker (1991)	16 parents of infants <36 weeks	IV	The transition home for parents of premature infants poses unique needs and concerns.
Steele & Sterling (1992)	1, single case study	VI	Patients and their home caregivers are involved in discharge preparation as planners and as learners.
Sheikh, O'Brien, & McCluskey-Fawcett (1993)	34 NICU nurses, 45 mothers of infants	VI	Staff and parents did not agree on topics discussed as part of standard discharge teaching.
Melnyk (1994)	108 mothers	IV	Information alone improves outcomes for families experiencing unplanned childhood hospitalization.
Snowdon & Kane (1995)	16 families	VI	Importance of supporting parental roles in the discharge phase of a child's illness and hospitalization.
Bent, Keeling, & Routson (1996)	20 parents	VI	Suggests that parents are uncertain, stressed, and unprepared for the realities of caring for their children at home.
Kirk (1999)	24 parents, 4 children, and 38 professionals	VI	The care for people with specialized health needs in the community presents challenges for the primary care sector of the health service.
Wesseldine, McCarthy, & Silverman (1999)	160 children	II	Delivering a brief, individual, and simple education and support during a child's stay in hospital decreased readmissions over a 6-month period.
Smith & Daughtrey (2000)	164 surveys, 20 interviews	VI	If discharge is planned and negotiated with parents they experience less anxiety and feelings of being left to cope alone at home.

Continued

TABLE 6.1

Suderman, Deatrich, Johnson, & Sawatzky-Dickson (2000)	20 interviews	VI	Need to recognize the individual needs of parents as learners.
Bissell & Long (2003)	10 parents of infants	VI	Intervention on parent needs positively impact parental experiences.
Domanski, Jackson, Miller, & Jeffrey (2003)	219 admissons	IV	Discharge risk factors for objective illness and treatment criteria were the most reliable predictors of need for social work discharge planning.
Weiss et al (2008)	119 parents of hospitalized children	IV	The "delivery" of discharge teaching by the nurses was the only significant predictor of parental readiness for hospital discharge.
Summary of Obstetric Research Studies			
Bernstein et al. (2002)	55 mothers	VI	Individualized approach ensures quality care and follow-up services.
Weiss, Ryan, Lokken, & Nelson (2004)	1,192 mothers	IV	Patient, provider, and payer factors influence discharge timing.

From: Lerret, S. (2009). Discharge readiness: An integrative review focusing on discharge following pediatric hospitalization. *Journal for Specialists in Pediatric Nursing, 14,* 248. doi: 10.1111/j.1744–6155.2009.00205.x. Reprinted by permission of Wiley Periodicals, Inc. 2010.

Data Analysis

In integrative reviews the data from the primary sources need to be interpreted and synthesized. The method used should be identified prior to beginning the review. Whittemore and Knafl (2005) suggested that research methods used for analyzing mixed-method and qualitative designs are applicable for integrative reviews and allow for comparisons across different types of studies included in the review.

Presentation of Findings

In the final stage, the findings of the review are presented. Conclusions should be supported by evidence from the review. In some manuscripts details about the each of the studies and findings are presented in a table format, but before developing this type of table for a manuscript, authors should check the journal guidelines and review similar articles published in the journal. In the example of an integrative review in Exhibit 6.1, the author presents the results in four subsections, each with a heading. These subsections represent the four major concepts that emerged from the review as influencing discharge readiness: support, identification of individual needs, education, and communication and coordination (Lerret, 2009). The author also includes a table that summarizes studies in the review and their main conclusion (Table 6.1).

Systematic Review and Meta-Analysis

Systematic reviews identify and critically appraise studies to answer a specific clinical or research question. With systematic reviews authors attempt to identify all relevant studies to answer the question, use an explicit and reproducible methodology for searching for studies and selecting them for inclusion in the review, adhere to methodological standards for critically appraising studies, and synthesize findings across them. Systematic reviews appraise multiple studies to answer a clinical question, making them useful for EBP in nursing (DiCenso, Bayley, & Haynes, 2009; Hedges, 2009; Hopp, 2009; Larrabee, 2009; Melnyk & Fineout-Overholt, 2005; Newhouse, 2008; Oermann, Floyd, Galvin, & Roop, 2006). Even though systematic reviews follow an explicit methodology, Sandelowski (2008) noted that they still reflect the perspectives of the authors in terms of the questions established for the review, criteria for studies to include, and how findings are analyzed.

Many systematic reviews include meta-analyses. A meta-analysis extends the critique of the research studies to include statistical analysis of their outcomes. With a meta-analysis statistical techniques are used to integrate the results of studies included in the systematic review. By combining information from all relevant studies, meta-analyses provide more precise estimates of the effectiveness of an intervention or a practice than an individual study (Higgins & Green, 2009). Polit and Beck (2008) suggested that the systematic integration of quantitative evidence through meta-analysis provides more objectivity and precision than a narrative review of the literature (p. 666).

Essential components of a systematic review and meta-analysis are:

- a clearly stated set of objectives and pre-defined criteria for including studies in the review;
- an explicit and reproducible methodology;
- a systematic search with the goal to identify all studies that meet the eligibility criteria;
- an assessment of the validity of the findings of studies included in the review; and
- a systematic presentation and synthesis of the characteristics and findings of the studies (Higgins & Green, 2009).

The key to conducting a systematic review or meta-analysis is use of a protocol. The protocol ensures that the review follows an explicit plan, with the aim of minimizing bias, and specifies the methods to be used. It is a template to guide the review and subsequent updates as new research findings become available.

There are many resources to guide authors in developing these protocols and conducting systematic reviews, with or without meta-analyses, and authors should consult one of those before beginning. A few of these resources, among others, are: the Cochrane Handbook (Higgins & Green, 2009); the Centre for Reviews and Dissemination guidelines (Centre for Reviews and Dissemination, 2009); the Joanna Briggs Institute Reviewers' Manual (The Joanna Briggs Institute, 2008); the Scottish Intercollegiate Guidelines Network (SIGN) guidelines (SIGN, 2009); and materials found at the website of The Evidence for Policy and Practice Information and Coordinating Centre (EPPI-Centre) (EPPI-Centre, 2009).

Systematic reviews begin with a problem and specific questions to be answered and proceed through identifying inclusion criteria for studies, searching for and selecting studies for review, extracting data from the included studies, assessing their quality, synthesizing the findings either quantitatively through techniques such as meta-analysis or using a narrative approach, and describing the results with implications for clinical practice, education, administration, and/ or policy. This process provides a framework for preparing manuscripts of systematic reviews for journals.

Background for Review and Questions

Similar to an integrative review, a systematic review begins with a description of the problem and issues related to the questions being addressed. The background provides the rationale for the review in the context of what is already known. If other reviews have been done related to the question, the background includes a critique of those reviews and why a new one is necessary. The systematic review in Exhibit 6.2 is on administering medications via enteral tubes in adults. In the background the authors identify the importance of using the correct procedure for giving these medications and consequences that can result if the procedure is

EXHIBIT 6.2

Sample Sections from a Systematic Review Article[1]

Objective

The objective of this systematic review was to determine the best available evidence on nursing interventions effective in minimizing the complications associated with the administration of medications via enteral tubes in adults.

Method

An initial limited search of CINAHL and MEDLINE was conducted to identify relevant key words contained in titles and abstracts, and MeSH headings and subject descriptor terms used for each database. An extensive search was then conducted of the following databases using the terms identified and the synonyms used by the respective databases: CINAHL, MEDLINE, The Cochrane Library, Current Contents, EMBASE, Australasian Medical Index, PsychINFO...there was no limit to the year of publication and only studies reported in English were included.

Continued

Exhibit 6.2 *Continued*

Types of Studies

Study designs included were systematic reviews, randomized controlled trials (RCTs) and other research methods such as non-RCTs, longitudinal studies, cohort and case-control studies.

Participants

The review considered studies that included adults (18 years or older) in any setting with any of the following enteral tubes: nasogastric, gastrostomy....

Types of Interventions

The following nursing interventions and considerations related to giving medication via enteral tubes were of interest: (1) nature or form of medication (e.g., liquid/solid ± diluting); (2) verifying tube placement before giving medication; (3) methods used to give medication; (4) methods used to flush tubes; (5) maintenance of tube patency; (6) specific nursing practices for individual types of enteral tubes; and (7) practices to prevent complications.

Outcome Measures

Outcome measures included the incidence of complications, such as mortality, aspiration pneumonia, tube occlusion, enteral feeding implications....

Critical Appraisal

After likely studies for inclusion had been identified by the primary reviewer, each was closely scrutinized for adherence to the inclusion criteria by two independent reviewers. Methodological quality was critically appraised by the reviewers using critical appraisal checklist forms developed by the Joanna Briggs Institute (JBI). The two reviewers then assigned each study a level of evidence using the National Health and Medical Research Council (2000) classifications.

Data Extraction and Analysis

Two reviewers independently carried out data extraction from the included studies using a data extraction instrument developed and used by JBI. A meta-analysis could not be conducted as there were no comparable RCTs. Therefore, data from each study were presented in a narrative summary.

Results

Overall, 5668 records were identified; 5582 were assessed by the primary reviewer as not relevant. Of the remaining 86, 72 were excluded (many were discussion papers). There were 14 studies assessed by two independent reviewers for adherence to the inclusion criteria and then critically appraised for methodological quality; five were excluded. Nine studies were therefore included in the systematic review.…

Tube Occlusion

Two RCTs and four observational studies investigated the outcome of tube occlusion. As part of one double-blinded RCT, tube length and the effect on tube patency were investigated.… Another study, constituting Level IV evidence, investigated the complications associated with enteral nutrition given via nasogastric and nasointestinal polyurethane tubes.… [results continue]

Discussion

There is clearly a paucity of high quality research relating to administering medication through enteral tubes in adults. As the strength of evidence is low, only two studies were RCTs, it cannot be used confidently to justify practice and further research is required.…

Two Level IV studies support the broader literature that the use of solid form medication can result in tube occlusion (Iber, et al., 1996, Pancorbo-Hidalgo, et al., 2001). While three studies considered the number of medications given through nasoenteral tubes and effect on tube occlusion, no conclusions could be drawn because of disparate evidence.… [discussion continues]

[1] Selected parts of each section.
From: Phillips, N. M., & Nay, R. (2008). A systematic review of nursing administration of medication via enteral tubes in adults. *Journal of Clinical Nursing, 17*, 2257–2260, 2263–2264. Reprinted by permission of John Wiley and Sons, 2010.

not carried out effectively (Phillips & Nay, 2008). The authors also establish the rationale for the review—based on limited evidence and conflicting advice in the literature.

Systematic reviews are intended to answer specific questions, often developed using the PICOS framework: Participants, Interventions, Comparisons, Outcomes, and Study designs. The question is then used to develop an objective or multiple objectives for the review. The examples of a systematic review (Exhibit 6.2) and meta-analysis (Exhibit 6.3) illustrate clearly stated and precise objectives for those reviews.

EXHIBIT 6.3

Objectives

The primary objective of this systematic review was to assess the efficacy of prone position ventilation in reducing mortality in adult patients with acute respiratory failure requiring invasive mechanical ventilation. The secondary objectives were to assess the impact of prone position ventilation on oxygenation, ventilator-associated pneumonia (VAP), duration of mechanical ventilation, duration of ICU and hospital stay, adverse effects (such as development of pressure ulcers), and endotracheal (ET) tube complications.

Methods

Identification of Studies

The following databases were searched for reports of RCTs using prone ventilation in adult patients with acute respiratory failure: the Cochrane Central Register of Controlled Trials, MEDLINE, EMBASE, Registry of Current Controlled Trials, Database of Abstracts of Reviews of Effects, NHS Economic Evaluation Database, and the Health Technology Assessment database. The search was performed using the exploded medical subject headings and text words: 'adult respiratory distress syndrome' or.... The search was limited to human studies involving adult patients with no language restriction. In addition, reference lists of all available review articles and primary studies were searched to identify studies that are not found in the computerized searches. The search period was from 1966 to July 2006.

Criteria for Inclusion of Studies

Prospective RCTs comparing prone position ventilation with supine ventilation in patients with acute respiratory failure requiring intubation and mechanical ventilation were included. Studies involving patients with chronic respiratory failure...and nonrandomized trials were excluded.

Types of Participants

Adult patients (>18 years) with acute respiratory failure requiring intubation and mechanical ventilation were included.

Outcome Measures

The primary outcome measure is mortality at the end of study period. Secondary outcomes were changes in oxygenation, incidence of VAP, duration of mechanical ventilation, ICU and hospital stay, complications related to the ET tube, and pressure ulcers.

Quality Assessment of Studies

The quality of the studies included in the analysis was assessed by the description of allocation concealment, the use of intention-to-treat analysis, and Jadad score....

Data Extraction

A standardized data extraction form was designed to extract details on study characteristics and the outcomes of interest.... Data on clinical outcomes including mortality, oxygenation, duration of mechanical ventilation, duration of ICU and hospital stay...and quality of the trials were collected using the data extraction form.

Data Synthesis and Analysis

The outcomes of interest were quantitatively pooled for meta-analysis using a random effects model. The summary meta-analysis for each outcome variable is presented using forest plot graphs.... The literature search, selection of studies, quality assessment, and data extraction were performed independently by 2 authors (R.T. and M.B.). Discrepancies were resolved by consensus.

Results

Description of Studies

A total of 2927 article titles were screened during the search process. Of these articles, only 5 studies [5–7,9,10] met the inclusion criteria. The reasons for exclusion of the rest of the studies are presented in Figure 1. General characteristics and quality assessment of the included studies are presented in Table 1.... The outcome data on mortality, oxygenation, VAP, ICU stay, pressure sores, and ET tube complications were suitable to be pooled in meta-analysis.... The summary meta-analyses of all the variables that were analyzed is presented in Table 3.

Mortality

Of the 5 studies, 4 [5–7,10] included reported data on mortality. None of the individual studies or pooled meta-analysis showed a significant reduction in mortality when prone ventilation was used (OR = 0.98; 95% CI, 0.7–1.3; P =.91) (Table 3 and Figure 2).

Continued

Exhibit 6.3 *Continued*

Oxygenation

Improvement in oxygenation was observed in all the studies included. The improvement in oxygenation with prone ventilation as calculated by weighted mean difference was 21.2 mm Hg (95% CI, 12.4–30.0; P <.0001) (Table 3 and Figure 3). [results continue]

Discussion

This is the first systematic review of the use of prone ventilation in patients with acute respiratory failure. This review allowed performing meta-analysis of the effects of prone ventilation on mortality, oxygenation, duration of ICU stay, VAP, pressure sores, and ET tube complications. The pooled results reveal that prone ventilation significantly improved oxygenation. Among the other variables assessed, mortality, ICU stay, VAP, and ET tube complications were not significantly affected by prone ventilation. [discussion continues]

Conclusions

The results of our meta-analysis, based on a small number of RCTs included, confirm that the use of prone ventilation improves oxygenation in patients with acute respiratory failure. [conclusions continue]

---

[1] Selected parts of each section.
Tiruvoipati, R., Bangash, M., Manktelow, B., & Peek, G. (2008). Efficacy of prone ventilation in adult patients with acute respiratory failure: A meta-analysis. *Journal of Critical Care, 23*, 101–104, 108–109. Reprinted by permission of Elsevier, 2010.

Review Methods

Systematic reviews follow a specific methodology, which is planned in advance and outlined in a protocol. These methods are described in the manuscript, generally in this order:

1. Criteria for studies included in the review, for example, their relationship to the PICOS, years considered, if only English language, and others.
2. Search strategy including the databases that were searched, years included, other limits, search terms, and other search strategies used.
3. Study selection, which is usually done in two stages: an initial screening of titles and abstracts using the inclusion criteria to identify potential studies, followed by screening the full papers (Centre for Reviews and Dissemination, 2009).
4. Data extraction, the process used for collecting information about the study characteristics and findings, for example, forms tailored to the review question.

5. Quality assessment of the individual studies in the review, which is often done with checklists to ensure that studies are appraised using a standardized approach.
6. Data synthesis that includes a description of how the results of individual studies were combined—with a meta-analysis or narrative approach.

This standardized way of presenting the review methods can be seen in the examples in Exhibits 6.2 and 6.3. In conducting a review, authors are likely to adopt a model such as described in the Cochrane Handbook, Centre for Reviews and Dissemination guidelines, Joanna Briggs Institute Reviewers' Manual, or similar source. That model can then be used as the framework for reporting the methods and findings of the review in a manuscript.

Review Results

The results of the review provide details of included and excluded studies with numbers of studies screened, assessed for eligibility, included at each stage, and excluded with the rationale. Authors can develop a flow diagram to show the number of studies remaining at each stage of the review (Figure 6.1).

In presenting the findings of the systematic review or meta-analysis in a manuscript, authors include:

- a report of the study characteristics (e.g., PICOS, sample size);
- citations for each study included in the review (If there are fewer than 50 studies, authors can include them in the reference list with an asterisk; otherwise the references can be submitted as a supplemental document [American Psychological Association, 2009]. Because individual journals may have different guidelines, authors should query the editor);
- results of the analysis of risk of bias in the studies;
- findings of the individual studies (including summary data and meta-analysis results);
- synthesized findings across the studies (for each narrative synthesis and meta-analysis done); and
- results of any secondary analyses (e.g., sensitivity or subgroup analyses).

Tables are useful for presenting the findings, for example, to describe the included studies and their characteristics and to summarize the extracted data. Exhibits 6.2 and 6.3 are typical presentations of the results section. In the systematic review by Phillips and Nay (2008), Exhibit 6.2, the authors use a table to identify the included studies, with the level of evidence specified for each study. The results of meta-analyses are often displayed using forest plots, a graphical representation to illustrate the relative strength of treatment effects. In the meta-analysis used as an example in this chapter (Exhibit 6.3), the authors used six forest plots (on the effects of prone ventilation on mortality, oxygenation, pneumonia, ICU length of stay, pressure ulcers, and endotracheal tube complications) to present their results.

FIGURE 6.1

Flow Diagram to Show Number of Studies Remaining at Each Stage of Systematic Review

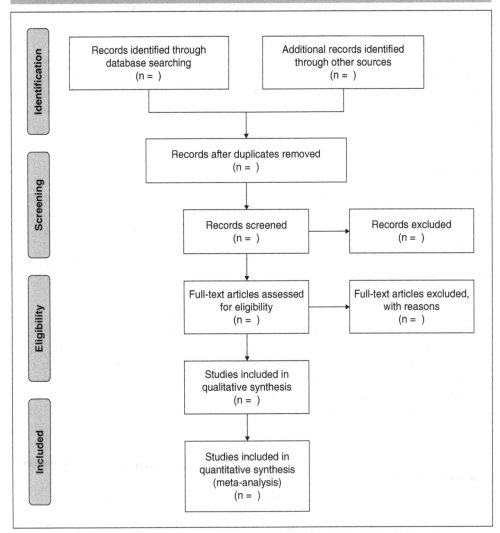

From: Moher, D., Liberati, A., Tetzlaff, J., Altman, D. G., & The PRISMA Group. (2009). Preferred Reporting Items for Systematic Reviews and Meta-Analyses: The PRISMA Statement. *PLoS Med, 6*(6), e1000097. doi:10.1371/journal.pmed1000097. The PRISMA Statement is distributed under the terms of the Creative Commons Attribution License, which permits unrestricted use, distribution, and reproduction in any medium.

Discussion

In the discussion authors summarize the main findings of the study with the strength of the evidence. Considering prior reviews, how do the findings from the systematic review or meta-analysis add to the evidence or raise new questions? The discussion should include the limitations of the review, for example, bias in the studies, difficulties in retrieving studies, and other factors that influence use of the findings in practice. Authors should include a section in the discussion on implications of the findings for clinical practice, education, administration, and/ or policy. Can the findings be used in clinical practice? What are considerations for clinicians prior to adopting the evidence in their own settings? Is more study needed, and if so, what types of questions remain unanswered? The final section is a brief conclusion about the results of the review.

The sample reviews in Exhibits 6.2 and 6.3 demonstrate how the discussion section is written. Authors should be clear as to the meaning of the evidence for clinicians as seen in these examples. In the review on administering medication through enteral tubes, Phillips and Nay (2009) state explicitly that the findings "cannot be used confidently to justify practice" (p. 2264). The meta-analysis in Exhibit 6.3 provided strong evidence confirming "that the use of prone ventilation improves oxygenation in patients with acute severe hypoxemic respiratory failure" (Tiruvoipati, Bangash, Manktelow, & Peek, 2009, p. 109.).

Systematic reviews and meta-analyses are increasingly important in EBP in nursing and other areas of healthcare. They provide strong evidence to guide clinical decisions and are often the basis for developing clinical guidelines (Moher, Liberati, Tetzlaff, Altman, & The PRISMA Group, 2009; Newhouse, 2008). The value of a systematic review, with or without a meta-analysis, depends on "what was done, what was found, and the clarity of reporting" (Moher, et al., p. 1). As with original research papers, their value depends on how well the review is reported.

Metasynthesis

Reviews of qualitative research can also be prepared as manuscripts. Metasynthesis is a broad term of varied approaches to summarizing and integrating findings from qualitative studies (Thorne, Jensen, Kearney, Noblit, & Sandelowski, 2004). The phases of a metasynthesis are similar to other systematic reviews, beginning with a problem and question, identifying types of studies and inclusion criteria, searching for and selecting studies for review, extracting and coding data, and assessing the quality of studies. Polit and Beck (2008) indicated that analytic strategies differ based on the approach used for the qualitative review; readers are advised to check resources on qualitative data analysis for further guidance. The results section of these studies report new interpretations from across studies, with discussion about the strength of the evidence and implications for practice.

Experiential EBP Applications

As nurses implement EBP in their clinical settings, manuscripts can be prepared on these initiatives and their outcomes. Many settings have adopted models of EBP to guide nurses in implementing this process in their clinical practice. An EBP model provides an organized approach to EBP, helps nurses carry out the full process, encourages evaluation, and makes good use of nurses' limited time and resources (Gawlinski & Rutledge, 2008, p. 291). Papers can be prepared on how nurses selected a model, its implementation, outcomes, and implications for other settings. Other potential topics for manuscripts are types of clinical questions asked by nurses that led to a search for evidence, strategies used in clinical settings to facilitate EBP, educating nurses with knowledge and competencies for EBP, methods that worked and were not effective for integrating evidence into the practice setting, and creating a culture of EBP, among many other topics.

A critical need is for nurses to disseminate their evaluations of evidence they implemented in their settings and outcomes of changes in practice. Dissemination of this information is essential to establish the effectiveness of an intervention or approach and determine if it is better than standard practice. Findings of EBP projects implemented in a clinical setting can inform nurses in other settings *if* those outcomes are disseminated.

Research Utilization

Research utilization is the process of transferring the knowledge and findings from an adequate base of research studies into a clinical practice. It is the use of sufficiently rigorous research evidence to guide practice. Studies have identified facilitators and barriers to research utilization, identifying why nurses do not use research based knowledge for making practice decisions. Some of the reasons relate to individual characteristics, such as nurses' lack of ability to read and understand research, and others are organizational factors including the culture of the setting. The organizational culture influences how work gets done, what types of knowledge are valued, and the strategies available in the workplace for nurses to share knowledge with one another (Scott & Pollock, 2008). Estabrooks (2007) called for research to identify individual determinants of research utilization beyond demographic variables and organizational factors that influence research use.

Guidelines for writing research utilization papers depend on the focus and type of manuscript. For example, how to write a manuscript of an original research utilization application in a specific clinical setting should be guided by the principles presented in chapter 5. Strategies for moving research knowledge into practice and action might be developed as manuscripts for clinical specialty journals as discussed in chapter 7. Papers on the development of a theory of research utilization would be guided by concepts in chapter 8 on preparing philosophical and theoretical articles. Other papers on research utilization may be guided by concepts in this chapter.

Synopses That Support Review and EBP Articles

The continued interest in EBP has created the need for review papers that serve as synopses of high quality systematic reviews. Editors of journals with broad clinical readerships seek such synopses in order to disseminate evidence to busy clinicians. The authors prepare streamlined synopses that are rich with headings and bullets to summarize findings, recommendations, and evaluation of the state of the evidence on a specific topic (DiCenso, Bayley, & Haynes, 2009; Oermann, Floyd, Galvin, & Roop, 2006; Oermann, Roop, Nordstrom, Galvin, & Floyd, 2007). An example of such a synopsis of this type is provided in Exhibit 6.4.

EXHIBIT 6.4

Format and Example of a Synopsis of a Systematic Review

Full reference for the systematic review summarized in synopsis:

Fallon, A., Westaway, J., & Moloney, C. (2008). A systematic review of psychometric evidence and expert opinion regarding the assessment of faecal incontinence in older community-dwelling adult. *International Journal of Evidence-Based Healthcare, 6,* 225–259. doi: 10.1111/j.1744–1609.2008.00088.x.

Review question: What is the best practice in assessing fecal incontinence in older community-dwelling adults?

Type of review: Joanna Briggs Institute systematic review with narrative and textual synthesis

Relevance for nursing (brief paragraph establishing the need for the review): Fecal incontinence is a common problem in the care of older people, and its incidence in community settings ranges from 11% to 17%....

Characteristics of evidence: Forty-one papers were included in the review. A thematic synthesis of 25 expert opinion papers was included and 254 conclusions were thematically synthesized into five major themes.... In seven papers, it was recommended that specific assessment tools (i.e., pictorial stool charts, bladder bowel diaries and grading of symptom severity) be used.... [review of evidence continues]

Implications for nursing (few bulleted statements):

- Assessment of fecal incontinence in older adults in the community should be done using a comprehensive assessment plan.
- Continence advisors should have appropriate skills and knowledge in using assessment tools and interpreting their results and in conducting physical examinations.
- Among symptom severity tools, the Vaizey and Wexner scales are the tools of choice but further validation of these is needed.
- For measuring quality of life in people with fecal incontinence, the FIQLS is the tool of choice.

Implications for research (few bulleted statements): There is a need for high quality trials to test the psychometric properties of fecal incontinence assessment tools....

JBI level of evidence: Level I

From: Konno, R. (2009). Review Summaries: Fallon, A., Westaway, J., & Moloney, C. (2008). A systematic review of psychometric evidence and expert opinion regarding the assessment of faecal incontinence in older community-dwelling adult. *Journal of Advanced Nursing, 65,* 773–778. Reprinted by permission of John Wiley & Sons, Inc., 2010.

Authors also might write a synopsis of a single study, providing a brief but detailed summary of a high quality study; an example is provided in Exhibit 6.5. Synopses of single studies are often accompanied by commentaries on the clinical applicability of the findings (DiCenso, Bayley, & Haynes, 2009). The format is similar to an expanded abstract. These are useful as building blocks for research utilization projects, in which nurses are considering how findings of research could be used in practice.

EXHIBIT 6.5

Format and Example of a Synopsis of a Single Study

Full reference for study summarized:

Vandenkerkhof, E., Hall, S., Wilson, R., Gay, A., & Duhn, L. (2009). Evaluation of an innovative communication technology in an acute care setting. *CIN: Computers, Informatics, Nursing, 27,* 254–262. doi: 10.1097/NCN.0b013e3181 a91bf6

Objectives: (1) document perceptions and attitudes of nurses toward use of new communication device (Vocera), (2) compare communication patterns before and after implementation, and (3) document distance traveled before and after implementation

Design: Mixed-method (focus group, pre- and posttest, quasi-experimental)

Subjects: Pre: 11 RNs shadowed for 120 hours; post: 16 RNs shadowed for 150 hours

Setting: 38-bed general surgical unit (H-pattern layout)

Intervention: Vocera personal communication tool

Outcomes: Perceptions and attitudes of RNs, factors that may influence adoption, time for key communication activities (e.g., walking to telephone to answer page). Measured before and 4 weeks after implementation

Main results: Advantages: saves time (97% post implementation), respond promptly to emergency situations. Disadvantages: related to work flow, confidentiality, and training. Attitude associated with behavioral intent before implementation (F = 12, *P* <.01; model adjusted r^2 = 0.25); perceived control associated with behavioral intent post implementation (F = 22, *P* <.01; model adjusted r^2 = 0.45). Time for key communication activities reduced 25%.

Conclusion: Vocera improved communication, other benefits

Commentary: Institutions planning to adopt innovative technology should explore users' attitudes. Ongoing involvement of staff with planning the innovation contributed to its adoption. One strength of the study was the mixed-methods design and collection of information pre and post implementation. However, a limitation was the lack of consistent RNs during pre and posttest.

From: Vandenkerkhof, E., Hall, S., Wilson, R., Gay, A., & Duhn, L. (2009). Evaluation of an innovative communication technology in an acute care setting. *CIN: Computers, Informatics, Nursing, 27,* 254–262. doi: 10.1097/NCN.0b013e3181a91bf6

WRITING REVIEW ARTICLES

This section of the chapter provides additional guidelines for writing all types of review papers. Some journals such as the *Journal of Advanced Nursing* have their own format for preparing different types of reviews, and authors are advised to check those prior to writing the manuscript. Another useful guideline is the PRISMA (Preferred Reporting Items for Systematic reviews and Meta-Analyses) Statement (Moher, et al., 2009). PRISMA, referred to earlier as the QUOROM (QUality Of Reporting Of Meta-analyses) Statement, was developed by an international group of experts including authors of reviews, methodologists, clinicians, medical editors, and a consumer. The PRISMA Statement guides authors in reporting systematic reviews and meta-analyses; it provides a 27-item checklist for reporting these reviews and a flow diagram for identifying the process used and studies included at different phases of the review. There are Microsoft Word templates that can be downloaded for authors' use, including a template for a flow diagram, and other resources that can be accessed at the PRISMA Web site (http://www.prisma-statement.org/).

Title

The title of the paper should include the type of review. This will facilitate searching for specific types of reviews for EBP, research, and other purposes. Authors should use established labels for their reviews because many articles in the nursing literature are titled as "systematic reviews" but lack a critical appraisal of the evidence (Newhouse, 2008, p. 107). The first three examples that follow are the titles of the sample reviews in Exhibits 6.1 to 6.3, and the fourth example is from a metasynthesis:

Discharge Readiness: An **Integrative Review** Focusing on Discharge Following Pediatric Hospitalization

A **Systematic Review** of Nursing Administration of Medication via Enteral Tubes in Adults

Efficacy of Prone Ventilation in Adult Patients with Acute Respiratory Failure: A **Meta-Analysis**

A **Qualitative Metasummary** on Caregiving at End-of-Life.

Abstract

The abstract should specify the background for the review, objective, data sources, review methods, results, and conclusions. For some journals authors also will include a statement on the relevance of the review findings for clinical practice. Two examples of abstracts are in Exhibit 6.6. The structure of the abstract and its length depend on the journal requirements. In the first example, from the systematic review on administration of medication via enteral tubes, the abstract is prepared using a structured format. Some journals use unstructured abstracts written in paragraph form. In that case authors should include at minimum the objective of the review, methods, and major findings, as seen in example 2 in Exhibit 6.6.

EXHIBIT 6.6

Examples of Abstracts From Review Articles

Example 1: Structured Abstract

Title. A systematic review of nursing administration of medication via enteral tubes in adults

Aim. This systematic review aimed to determine the best available evidence regarding the effectiveness of nursing interventions in minimizing the complications associated with administering medication via enteral tubes in adults.

Background. Giving enteral medication is a fairly common nursing intervention entailing several skills: verifying tube position, preparing medication, flushing the tube, and assessing for potential complications. If not carried out effectively harmful consequences may result leading to increased morbidity and even mortality. Until now, what was considered to be best practice in this area was unknown.

Design. Systematic review.

Methods. CINAHL, MEDLINE, The Cochrane Library, Current Contents/All Editions, EMBASE, Australasian Medical Index and PsychINFO databases were searched. Reference lists of included studies were appraised. Two reviewers independently assessed study eligibility for inclusion. There were no comparable randomized-controlled trials; data were presented in a narrative summary.

Results. Identified evidence included using 30 ml of water for irrigation when giving medication or flushing small-diameter nasoenteral tubes may reduce tube occlusion. Using liquid medication should be considered as there may be less tube occlusions than with solid forms....

Conclusion. The evidence was limited. There was a lack of high quality research on many important issues relating to giving enteral medication.

Relevance to clinical practice. Nurses have the primary responsibility for giving medication through enteral tubes and need knowledge of the best available evidence.... There is a need for further studies to strengthen these findings.[1]

Example 2: Unstructured Abstract

Although several variables have been correlated with nursing job satisfaction, the findings are not uniform across studies. Three commonly noted variables from the nursing literature are: autonomy, job stress, and nurse–physician collaboration....A meta-analysis of 31 studies representing a total of 14,567 subjects was performed. Job satisfaction was most strongly correlated with job stress (ES = -.43), followed by nurse–physician collaboration (ES =.37), and autonomy (ES =.30). These findings have implications for improving the work environment to increase nurses' job satisfaction.[2]

[1]From: Phillips, N. M., & Nay, R. (2008). A systematic review of nursing administration of medication via enteral tubes in adults. *Journal of Clinical Nursing, 17,* 2257. Reprinted by permission of John Wiley and Sons, 2010.
[2]From: Zangaro, G. A., & Soeken, K. L. (2007). A meta-analysis of studies of nurses' job satisfaction. *Research in Nursing & Health, 30,* 445. Reprinted by permission of John Wiley and Sons, 2010.

Introduction

The introduction presents the background of the problem and why a review was needed to understand a problem or answer a question. If prior reviews were done, authors should critique those reviews and explain why additional review was indicated. Perhaps published systematic reviews included only one age group, one type of clinical setting, or patients with certain problems. It also may be that prior reviews were inconclusive or that recent research has changed what we know about the topic.

The objectives of the review, or specific questions addressed in it, should be included at the end of the introduction or immediately following it. These should be stated clearly for readers, as seen in the following examples:

- The objective of this systematic review was to determine the best available evidence on nursing interventions effective for minimizing the complications associated with the administration of medications via enteral tubes in adults (Phillips & Nay, 2008, p. 2258).
- What is the effectiveness of interventions to assist caregivers in supporting people with dementia who are living in the community? (Parker, Mills, & Abbey, 2008, p. 137).

Review Methods

The earlier discussion in the chapter on different types of reviews can be used as the framework for writing the methods section of these papers. This part of the manuscript should specify the inclusion criteria for studies, databases searched and dates of coverage, search strategies, process for selecting studies, methods of data extraction and variables for which information was collected, how the quality of individual studies was assessed, and how data were synthesized. Authors should use subheadings to indicate these parts of the methods section. Exhibit 6.2 provides an example of the methods section of a systematic review article showing the specific subheadings used by the authors.

Results

In reporting the results, authors should provide details of studies included and excluded in the review. As indicated earlier, a flow diagram can be used to show the numbers of studies remaining at each stage of the review. In the results section, authors report the characteristics and results of individual studies, often done with tables, and the synthesis of the findings. The results of meta-analyses can be displayed using forest plots, which Hedges (2009) suggested was one of the most convenient ways for nurses to view the results. Exhibits 6.2 and 6.3 provide examples of the results section from a systematic review and meta-analysis.

Discussion

In the discussion section of the manuscript, the main findings of the review are examined considering the strengths and weaknesses of the review methods, quality of the studies included in the review, how bias was controlled and its potential impact on the results, and strength of the evidence for each outcome of the study. The discussion should include an interpretation of the results and whether they are applicable to clinical practice, education, administration, and/or policy. Limitations of the review should be considered when drawing conclusions about the use of the evidence in practice. Reviews are future oriented: they make suggestions for further research and identify new questions that emerged from the synthesis of findings (Conn, 2009). These suggestions should be included in the discussion.

Authors should write a brief conclusion that summarizes the major findings from the review with implications for practice and where additional study is needed. The conclusion may be the final paragraph in the discussion section or a separate section that follows the discussion

▓ SUMMARY

This chapter presented different types of review papers that authors can prepare. An integrative or narrative review provides a summary of empirical and theoretical literature to better understand a particular topic. With an integrative review both experimental and non-experimental studies are included. These are broad reviews to more fully describe and understand the topic in comparison with a systematic review that addresses a specific clinical question. An integrative review progresses through five stages: problem formulation, literature search, data evaluation, data analysis, and presentation of the findings. This framework is useful as a guide for preparing manuscripts of integrative reviews for nursing journals.

Systematic reviews identify and critically appraise studies to answer a specific clinical or research question. With systematic reviews authors attempt to identify all relevant studies to answer the question, use an explicit methodology for searching for studies and selecting them for inclusion in the review, adhere to methodological standards for critically appraising studies, and synthesize findings across studies. For these reasons systematic reviews are useful for EBP.

Many systematic reviews include meta-analyses. A meta-analysis uses statistical techniques to integrate the results of studies included in the review, resulting in a more precise estimate of the effectiveness of an intervention or practice than an individual study.

Essential components of a systematic review and meta-analysis are: a clearly stated set of objectives and pre-defined criteria for including studies in the review, an explicit and reproducible methodology, a systematic search intended to identify all studies that meet the eligibility criteria, an assessment of the validity of the findings of studies included in the review, and a synthesis of the characteristics and findings across studies in the review.

Reviews of qualitative research can also be prepared as manuscripts. Metasynthesis is a broad term of varied approaches to summarizing and integrating findings from qualitative studies. The phases of a metasynthesis are similar to other systematic reviews.

Research utilization articles describe the final stage of research dissemination: translation and evaluation of a sufficient evidence base of knowledge into a specific clinical setting. As nurses implement EBP in their clinical settings, manuscripts can be prepared on these initiatives and their outcomes. Many settings have adopted models of EBP to guide nurses in implementing this process in their clinical practice. Papers can be prepared on how nurses chose a model, its implementation, outcomes, and implications for other settings. Other papers can address research utilization, the process of transferring research based knowledge into practice. A critical need is for nurses to disseminate their evaluations of evidence implemented in their settings and outcomes of changes in practice. Dissemination of this information is essential to establish the effectiveness of an intervention or approach and determine if it is better than standard practice.

REFERENCES

American Psychological Association (APA). (2009). *Publication Manual of the American Psychological Association* (6th ed.). Washington, DC: APA.

Centre for Reviews and Dissemination. (2009). *Systematic Reviews*. Retrieved from http://www.york.ac.uk/inst/crd/pdf/Systematic_Reviews.pdf.

Conn, V. S. (2009). *Western Journal of Nursing Research* welcomes stellar review articles. *Western Journal of Nursing Research, 31*, 3–5 doi: 10.1177/0193945908326378

Conn, V. S., Isaramalai S., Rath S., Jantarakupt P., Wadhawan R., & Dash Y. (2003). Beyond MEDLINE for literature searches. *Journal of Nursing Scholarship, 35*, 177–182.

Cook, D. J., Mulrow, C. D., & Haynes, R. B. (1997). Systematic reviews: Synthesis of best evidence for clinical decisions. *Annals of Internal Medicine, 126*, 376–380.

DiCenso, A., Bayley, L., & Haynes, B. (2009). Accessing pre-appraised evidence: Fine-tuning the 5S model into a 6S model. *Evidence-Based Nursing, 12,* 99–101. doi: 10.1136/ebn.12.4.99-b

DiCenso, A., Guyatt, G., & Ciliska, D. (2005). *Evidence-based nursing: A guide to clinical practice.* St. Louis: Mosby.

Estabrooks, C. A. (2007). Prologue: A program of research in knowledge translation. *Nursing Research, 56*(4), supp 1: S4–S6. doi: 10.1097/01.NNR.0000280637.24644.fd

Gawlinski, A., & Rutledge, D. (2008). Selecting a model for evidence-based practice changes: A practical approach. *AACN Advanced Critical Care, 19,* 291–300. doi: 10.1097/01. AACN.0000330380.41766.63

Hedges, C. (2009). Panning for gold: In search of the meta-analysis. *AACN Advanced Critical Care, 20,* 292–294. doi: 10.1097/NCI.0b013e3181ae4c1f

Higgins, J. P. T., & Green, S. (Eds.). (2009). *Cochrane handbook for systematic reviews of interventions. Version 5.0.2* [updated September 2009]. The Cochrane Collaboration. Retrieved from www.cochrane-handbook.org.

Hopp, L. (2009). The role of systematic reviews in teaching evidence-based practice. *Clinical Nurse Specialist, 23,* 321–322. doi: 10.1097/NUR.0b013e3181be3287

Larrabee, J. H. (2009). *Nurse to nurse evidence-based practice.* New York: The McGraw Hill Companies.

Lerret, S. (2009). Discharge readiness: An integrative review focusing on discharge following pediatric hospitalization. *Journal for Specialists in Pediatric Nursing, 14,* 245–255. doi: 10.1111/j.1744–6155.2009.00205.x

Lowe, N. (2009). Systematic literature reviews. *JOGNN: Journal of Obstetric, Gynecologic & Neonatal Nursing, 38,* 375–376. doi: 10.1111/j.1552–6909.2009.01033.x

Melnyk, B. M., & Fineout-Overholt, E. (2005). *Evidence-based Practice in Nursing & Healthcare.* Philadelphia: Lippincott Williams & Wilkins.

Melnyk, B. M., Fineout-Overholt, E., Stillwell, S. B., & Williamson, K. M. (2009). Igniting a spirit of inquiry: An essential foundation for evidence-based practice. *American Journal of Nursing, 109*(11), 49–52. doi: 10.1097/01.NAJ.0000363354.53883.58

Melnyk, B. M., Fineout-Overholt, E., Stillwell, S. B., & Williamson, K. M. (2010). The seven steps of evidence-based practice. *American Journal of Nursing, 110*(1), 51–53. doi: 10.1097/01.NAJ.0000366056.06605.d2

Moher, D., Liberati, A., Tetzlaff, J., Altman, D. G., & The PRISMA Group. (2009). Preferred Reporting Items for Systematic Reviews and Meta-Analyses: The PRISMA Statement. *PLoS Med, 6*(7), e1000097. doi:10.1371/journal.pmed.1000097

Newhouse, R. (2008). Evidence synthesis: The good, the bad, and the ugly. *Journal of Nursing Administration, 38,* 107–111. doi: 10.1097/01.NNA.0000310729.50913.97

Oermann, M. H. (2007). Internet resources for evidence-based practice in nursing. *Plastic Surgical Nursing, 27*(1), 37–39. doi: 10.1097/01.PSN.0000264160.68623.0a

Oermann, M. H., Floyd, J. A., Galvin, E. A, & Roop, J. C. (2006). Brief reports for disseminating systematic reviews to nurses. *Clinical Nurse Specialist, 20,* 233–238.

Oermann, M. H., Roop, J. C., Nordstrom, C. K., Galvin, E. A., Floyd, J. A. (2007). Effectiveness of an intervention for disseminating Cochrane reviews to nurses. *MEDSURG Nursing: The Journal of Adult Health, 16,* 373–378.

Parker, D., Mills, S., & Abbey, J. (2008). Effectiveness of interventions that assist caregivers to support people with dementia living in the community: A systematic review. *International Journal of Evidence-Based Healthcare, 6,* 137–172. doi: 10.1111/j.1479–6988.2008.00090.x

Phillips, N. M., & Nay, R. (2008). A systematic review of nursing administration of medication via enteral tubes in adults. *Journal of Clinical Nursing, 17,* 2257–2265. doi: 10.1111/j.1365–2702.2008.02407.x

Polit, D. F., & Beck, C. T. (2008). *Nursing research: Generating and assessing evidence for nursing practice* (8th ed.). Philadelphia: Lippincott Williams & Wilkins.

Popay, J., Baldwin, S., Arai, L., Britten, N., Petticrew, M., Rodgers, M., & Sowden, A. (2007). *Methods briefing 22. Narrative synthesis in systematic reviews.* Manchester, UK: University of Manchester, Economic and Social Research Council Research Methods Programme.

Sandelowski, M. (2008). Reading, writing and systematic review. *Journal of Advanced Nursing, 64,* 104–110. doi:10.1111/j.1365–2648.2008.04813.x

Scott, S., & Pollock, C. (2008). The role of nursing unit culture in shaping research utilization behaviors. *Research in Nursing & Health, 31,* 298–309. doi: 10.1002/nur.20264

Scottish Intercollegiate Guidelines Network (SIGN). (2009). *Section 6: Systematic literature review.* Retrieved from http://www.sign.ac.uk/guidelines/fulltext/50/section6.html.

The Evidence for Policy and Practice Information and Coordinating Centre (EPPI-Centre). (2009). *Methods, tools and databases.* Retrieved from http://eppi.ioe.ac.uk/cms/Default. aspx?tabid=88&language=en-US.

The Joanna Briggs Institute. (2008). *Joanna Briggs Institute reviewers' manual: 2008 edition.* Retrieved from http://www.joannabriggs.edu.au/pdf/JBIReviewManual_CiP11449.pdf.

Thorne, S., Jensen, L., Kearney, M. H., Noblit, G., & Sandelowski, M. (2004). Qualitative metasynthesis: Reflections on methodological orientation and ideological agenda. *Qualitative Health Research, 14,* 1342–1365.

Tiruvoipati, R., Bangash, M., Manktelow, B., & Peek, G. (2008). Efficacy of prone ventilation in adult patients with acute respiratory failure: A meta-analysis. *Journal of Critical Care, 23,* 101–110. doi: 10.1016/j.jcrc.2007.09.003

Torraco, R. J. (2005). Writing integrative literature reviews: Guidelines and examples. *Human Resource Development Review, 4,* 356–367. doi: 10.1177/1534484305278283

Vandenkerkhof, E., Hall, S., Wilson, R., Gay, A., & Duhn, L. (2009). Evaluation of an innovative communication technology in an acute care setting. *CIN: Computers, Informatics, Nursing, 27,* 254–262. doi: 10.1097/NCN.0b013e3181a91bf6

Whittemore, R., & Knafl, K. (2005). The integrative review: Updated methodology. *Journal of Advanced Nursing, 52,* 546–553. doi: 10.1111/j.1365-2648.2005.03621.x

Zangaro, G. A., & Soeken, K. L. (2007). A meta-analysis of studies of nurses' job satisfaction. *Research in Nursing & Health, 30,* 445–458. doi: 10.1002/nur.20202

7

CLINICAL PRACTICE ARTICLES

Chapter 7 presents strategies for writing articles about clinical practice. There are many opportunities for preparing these manuscripts: nurses can write about their innovations in practice, unit-based initiatives and projects, updates on clinical topics, new directions in patient care, and research studies and quality improvement projects done in the clinical setting. Lectures and presentations on clinical topics can be adapted into manuscripts for clinical journals, disseminating this new information to readers. Considering the wealth of clinical journals in nursing, these publications provide a venue for nurses to share their work with others.

WRITING FOR CLINICAL JOURNALS

There are many nursing journals that address topics in clinical practice. These articles disseminate new knowledge and skills for patient care, enabling nurses to stay current in clinical practice. With this type of article, nurses in one setting can describe their practice innovations for use and testing by nurses in other settings. They can discuss issues they encountered in patient care and how they resolved those issues, and they can share nursing approaches that worked and ones that did not work, so nurses can build on the experiences of others rather than starting from the beginning. To remain competent, professionals need to continually expand their own knowledge base and skills; clinical practice articles provide a source of information for meeting this need.

Idea for Clinical Article

The process for writing a manuscript on clinical practice begins with an idea, similar to other manuscripts. This idea may come from a patient experience the author had or a clinical situation in which the author was involved, from activities in the clinical setting in which the author participated, and from discussion with nursing staff and other providers. Projects, innovations, and initiatives implemented on the unit and in the clinical setting lend themselves to publication, which is essential to disseminate the work to other nurses for use in their own settings. The idea for a manuscript may evolve from a frustrating experience the author had or an issue in clinical practice that the author eventually resolved. Clinical articles often result from the nurse's own experiences with patients, families, and staff and later reflection on those experiences. Thus, one primary source of ideas for manuscripts for clinical journals is the author's clinical practice and interactions with other nurses and healthcare providers.

Another source of ideas for manuscripts for clinical journals is from lectures and presentations. Educators in academic and clinical settings are continually preparing lectures and other types of presentations, many of which pertain to clinical practice or are intended to keep nurses up-to-date. If the presentation relates to new knowledge and interventions for patient care, a change in practice that will benefit patients across clinical settings, a trend in nursing and healthcare, an issue involving patients and consumers, and so forth, these lectures may be rewritten as manuscripts. Lectures and other types of presentations can be developed into manuscripts for journals that publish papers across clinical practice areas, such as the *American Journal of Nursing*, or journals in specialty areas of practice depending on the topic.

To generate publications, one technique is to write the manuscript first and then develop the lecture or presentation. That strategy encourages nurses to write for publication and use wisely their limited time for writing. Another strategy is to expand conference presentations into manuscripts. Gross and Fonteyn (2008) suggest that conference presentations provide an easy way to write for publication because typically the presentation follows the same order as a manuscript. Course materials that educators develop may be adapted similarly for publications. It is critical, however, that nurses think about a possible manuscript before beginning to develop their lecture or presentation. By planning the paper as the first step, nurses can identify possible journals and conduct the literature review that would be appropriate for that journal and audience.

Ideas for clinical articles also may evolve from research studies, literature reviews, educational experiences, and other activities that lead to new information or a different perspective about nursing practice. When deciding if the idea is worth pursuing for a manuscript for a clinical journal, the author should answer these questions:

- Is the idea new and innovative?
- If the idea is not new, does it provide a different perspective to current practice?
- Is the content relevant to clinical practice, and if so, is it applicable to nursing practice in a specialty area or in general?
- Do nurses *need* this information for their practice and will it improve patient care?
- Will the information be valuable in keeping nurses up-to-date about trends in nursing and healthcare?
- Will the content inform readers about the types of activities and work nurses are doing in other settings and places?

These questions give authors a framework for deciding if the clinical topic is worth pursuing for publication.

Purpose of Article

From this idea the author specifies the purpose of the manuscript. This is an important step because manuscripts for clinical journals can have many different perspectives. What is the goal of the paper? Is it to present new nursing practices and patient care or provide a different perspective to an accepted practice? Will the rationale and related research be emphasized? Is the intent to describe nursing interventions and their effectiveness, to present a clinical guideline and how well it worked with a specific patient population, or to describe an interdisciplinary plan of care? Answering questions such as these enables the author to clarify the purpose of the paper.

Intended Readers

The next step is to identify the intended readers of the manuscript. These readers may be staff nurses, advanced practice nurses, managers, and nurses in other roles. Who will read the article dictates the content included in it.

Manuscripts about clinical practice may be written for a general nursing audience, providing information to help nurses across specialties and settings stay current. Other clinical articles address nurses who practice in a particular specialty area. These articles focus on specific health problems and patient populations or communities. This is an important difference when deciding on the journal for submission because it determines the complexity of the content and types of examples used in the discussion. Clinical articles written for a general nursing audience describe the content more broadly and use more common examples. In planning the content, the author takes into consideration the knowledge and background of the intended readers. This is another reason that selecting the target journal for submission is an early step in the writing process.

In preparing the manuscript, the author also determines the prerequisite knowledge needed by readers to understand the content. This guides the author in deciding on background material to include in the paper for the new information to be clear. For example, in preparing a manuscript on clavicle fractures in children for the journal *Orthopaedic Nursing*, limited background information would be needed about the general care of patients with fractures. However, if the manuscript is written for nurses across specialties as a means of updating them and for general interest, more discussion would be required about common mechanisms of injury, care of patients with fractures, anatomy and function of the clavicle, and other background information.

■ FORMAT OF MANUSCRIPTS ABOUT CLINICAL PRACTICE

The format for writing manuscripts about clinical practice depends on the purpose of the article and journal for submission. Some journals have departments for different types of clinical articles. The author decides prior to beginning the paper if it will be developed for a department in a journal because often these manuscripts have different requirements, e.g., they may be shorter and more focused than the main articles. For example, the *Journal of Nursing Care Quality* disseminates information about patient safety and quality improvement. Manuscripts are limited to a maximum of 18 pages, but papers submitted for publication in one of the departments in the journal are no more than 10 pages including references, tables, and figures. The allowed length is important to know before beginning to write to plan the content.

There is no standard format for writing manuscripts on clinical topics. A manuscript that presents nursing interventions for patients with a particular health problem will be organized differently than one that reviews pharmacology. In contrast to research articles, which follow a standard format, clinical manuscripts vary because of the wide range of topics addressed in them.

Some general guidelines for writing clinical articles follow. However, the author should remember that these guidelines may not pertain to every manuscript depending on its focus.

Title

Every clinical paper needs a title similar to other manuscripts. The purpose of the title is to inform readers what new information will be presented in the paper. Key words that represent the content should be used in the title, and the title should be concise.

Nurses are busy professionals, and with a series of articles to read in a journal and limited time, the title needs to draw the attention of readers. For example, "*No More Surprises*: Screening Patients for Alcohol Abuse" is more of an attention-getter than the title "*Assessment* of Patients for Alcohol Abuse."

Similar to research articles one title may be written, or it may be developed with a subtitle that provides more specific information about the paper. When subtitles are used, the terms that represent the main focus of the article should be placed first in the title. For example:

Single title
Physical and Communication Problems in Feeding Post-stroke Patients with Dysphagia

Title with subtitle
Feeding Post-stroke Patients with Dysphagia: Physical and Communication Problems

Abstract

Not all clinical manuscripts are submitted with an abstract, but when an abstract is required, it should present concisely the content included in the paper and its clinical implications. The abstract is the author's first chance to convince readers that the paper is important to read. Because abstracts are indexed and available in an electronic search, the abstract is critical to guide readers to the paper. Four to five of the most important points, findings, or implications should be integrated in the abstract, using specific terms that others might include in a search (American Psychological Association [APA], 2009).

Abstracts vary in length, ranging from as short as 75 words to 250 words. With some types of papers, though, such as meta-analyses, 300 words might be allowed (American Medical Association [AMA], 2007). How to prepare the abstract for a particular journal and the maximum number of words allowed are described in the author guidelines.

Examples of abstracts for clinical articles are provided in Exhibit 7.1. It can be seen in these examples that the abstracts inform readers about the content in the article and its practical implications.

EXHIBIT 7.1

Sample Abstracts for Clinical Articles

Example 1

Guidelines for the safe administration of drugs through an enteral feeding tube are available, but research shows that often nurses don't adhere to them. This can lead to medication error and tube obstruction, reduced drug effectiveness, and an increased risk of toxicity. This article describes factors to consider before administering a drug through a feeding tube, examines the gap between recommended and common practice, and discusses what the most recent guidelines recommend and why.[1]

Example 2

This article examines the concept of the reproductive life plan and provides information about translating this important idea into practice. The idea of the reproductive life plan was introduced in a report from the Centers for Disease Control and Prevention in 2006, but has thus far received little attention in the nursing literature. Reproductive life plans are important for women and their partners during their childbearing years, for they facilitate discussion about childbearing intentions and choices. Additionally, a dialogue about reproductive life planning may help nurses open a gateway to the use of preconception care as an intervention to improve maternal fetal outcomes. Nurses are ideally prepared and situated to assist women and their partners in learning about and developing reproductive life plans.[2]

Example 3

Two protocols were developed to address risks related to emotional distress in an ongoing, qualitative, community-based study of adolescent dating violence. The first protocol is for use in telephone screening to identify individuals at high risk of adverse emotional reactions. The second protocol guides the interviewer's responses to emotional distress expressed by participants during in-depth research interviews. The study is briefly described, and the process used to develop the protocols is discussed. The process of developing

Continued

Exhibit 7.1 *Continued*

the protocols led the authors to reconsider some previously held assumptions about human subject protections in research on sensitive topics.[3]

---

[1]From Boullata, J. (2009). Drug administration through an enteral feeding tube. *American Journal of Nursing, 109*(10), p. 34.
[2]From Sanders, L. (2009). Reproductive life plans: Initiating the dialogue with women. *MCN: The American Journal of Maternal Child Nursing, 34*, p. 342.
[3]From Draucker, C., Martsolf, D., & Poole, C. (2009). Developing distress protocols for research on sensitive topics. *Archives of Psychiatric Nursing, 23*, p. 343.

Introduction

The first section of the manuscript is the introduction. In the introduction the author presents the purpose of the paper, an overview of the topics in it, the relevance of the content for clinical practice, and the value of the article to nurses.

The first or lead paragraph of the introduction is the most important one because if it is unclear or poorly written, readers will not continue with the article. The lead-in paragraph also needs to capture reader's interest. The author can use the lead-in paragraph to indicate the purpose, topics, and relevance to clinical practice. For example:

> Many patients are unable to report the pain they are experiencing. This places them at risk for pain that is undertreated because of communication problems. This article describes how to assess patient's pain using the basic measures of pain intensity as a framework and following six other steps. The information is important for nurses when caring for patients who are unable to report their pain.

Other types of lead-in paragraphs introduce the topic but focus more on getting the readers' attention. There are three types of opening paragraphs that attempt to get the attention of the readers as their primary purpose: anecdotal opening, placing the reader in the clinical situation, and using statistics.

Anecdotal Openings

Anecdotal openings share a real or simulated clinical experience or present a case scenario that readers can identify with professionally or personally. The opening may describe a patient and health problems, begin with a case scenario, or describe nurses' experiences in caring for patients and their own feelings. Anecdotal openings capture readers' interest by indicating the professional or personal relevance of the information to them as nurses.

The following is an example of an anecdotal opening to an article on adrenal crisis, related physiology, how to differentiate it from other conditions, nursing care and related medical management, and averting future episodes:

> Ms. S, age 52, is brought to the ED with severe abdominal pain, fever, and rapid pulse. She walks slowly and is unsteady. Ms. S has been vomiting for more than

two days, and she has had no appetite for the last week. Her past medical history includes surgery for an adrenal gland tumor. You realize this is not the flu.

This example also shows the contrast in writing style from research articles that tend to be more formal and use an academic style of writing. Often clinical journals prefer a more informal writing style as seen in this example.

Placement in Clinical Situation

A similar type of lead-in paragraph is when the reader is placed in the clinical situation. In this introduction the nurse is involved in the scenario as a realistic participant who needs to make decisions and act in response to the situation. The question for the reader is, "What would you do in this clinical situation?" An example of this type of attention-getter is:

> You have been working in the clinical agency for nearly 10 months. Recently you noticed a colleague having difficulty completing her assignments on time. She is often late for work and asks you to cover for her. Today you notice her moving from one patient to the next without washing her hands.

This example provides the clinical context for the article and engages the reader as a participant in it. Here the reader "becomes" the nurse involved in this dilemma, which the article analyzes and provides options for how the nurse might handle. A personal experience of the nurse, positive or negative, also serves to "connect with readers" who may have had similar experiences and to engage them in the topic.

Use of Statistics

Another attention-getter is through the use of statistics that demonstrate the impact of the information on patient care, the nurse's own practice, or health-care in general. In this type of introduction statistics are presented to show the magnitude of the problem and its implications, signifying the importance of the article. For example:

> The next time you attend a social event, look around the room and consider this: approximately 14 million Americans meet the diagnostic criteria for alcohol abuse or alcoholism.[1] Almost half of all Americans who are 12 years or older currently drink alcohol, and 20.5 percent participate in binge drinking. Among different age groups, the highest prevalence of both heavy and binge drinking is young adults aged 18 to 25 years.[2]

This lead-in paragraph to an article on screening patients for alcohol abuse uses alarming facts to illustrate the magnitude of the problem.

Text

The text or body of the paper following the introduction varies depending on the content. Because clinical manuscripts can address a wide range of topics, from general practice updates to specific interventions for one type of patient problem, there is no one outline that can be used. Some principles, though, guide development of the text for clinical articles:

- Organize the content from simple to complex and from known to unknown.
- Provide background information and scientific rationale so readers can understand the reasons underlying problems, interventions, and outcomes.
- Focus on what nurses need to learn about assessment of patients, significant data to collect, related diagnostic tests, and interpretation of data, considering alternate perspectives and possibilities.
- Focus on what nurses need to learn about patient responses, problems, and diagnoses; interventions; and outcomes. Emphasize related research, evidence and implications for clinical practice.
- Focus on nursing management rather than medical management even though this content also may be included in the paper. The goal is to help nurses assess patients and effectively manage their problems.
- If using a scenario as an attention-getter, relate the content in the paper to the scenario for readers to see how this new information can be used in clinical practice.
- Use examples from clinical practice in the paper to assist readers in applying the new information to patient care. Consider using one scenario throughout the paper as a way of demonstrating how the concepts relate to assessment, diagnoses, interventions, and outcomes. In this way the scenario provides a model of how the new information is actually used in clinical practice.
- Answer questions of "Why?" "What if…" "What are other options and possible decisions?" "How?" Answering these questions promotes the nurses' thinking and clinical judgment about the content.
- When using an acronym, write it out the first time mentioned in the paper, but from that point on use only the acronym for the remainder of the manuscript. For example: "This paper describes the outcomes of a nurse managed clinic for patients with heart failure (HF). Nurse practitioners care for patients with HF both inpatient and in the clinic.
- Use a writing style consistent with the journal. A few clinical journals use "I" and "you" rather than "the nurse." The author should gather information about writing style before beginning the draft.
- Use frequent and specific subheadings that clearly describe the content in that section. The author should review a few articles in the journal for submission because types of subheadings often vary. Some journals use more formal subheadings than do others. This difference can be seen in Table 7.1.

The extent of background information to include is based on the author's professional judgment and an understanding of the reader's needs. When presenting new information not available in nursing textbooks or through other resources, the author includes more background material than would be necessary for a manuscript on a new direction in clinical practice but for a common patient problem known by most readers.

An example of this strategy can be seen in an article on nursing care of patients with renal cell carcinoma (Janotha, 2009). Because this type of carcinoma

TABLE 7.1

Comparison of Subheadings for Clinical Article

Formal	Informal
Venous Thromboembolism	What is VTE?
Pathophysiology	Why VTE Occurs
Incidence of Venous Thromboembolism	How Common is VTE?
Risks Factors of Venous Thromboembolism and Evidence	Assessment of Risk Factors: Be Alert
Nursing Care and Clinical Guidelines	Caring for Your Patient with VTE

VTE: Venous Thromboembolism

is rare, it is unlikely that readers would be familiar with it. The author provides background information about renal cell carcinoma including its incidence and difficulties in diagnosing it. The content includes an explanation of renal cell carcinoma, its etiology, the effects of age on diagnosis and outcomes, the prognosis, and types of treatments. The next section of the paper is entitled "clinical update", and in that part, the author provides follow up information about the case scenario that was used in the introduction.

The content for a clinical paper depends on the topic, journal, and particularly the readers of that journal. The author needs to understand the background of readers because the content should be at an appropriate level for them. A paper on management of hypertension written for a cardiovascular nursing journal would present limited background information because readers of that journal know about this condition and typical treatments. However, that same paper prepared for a general nursing journal would explain the pathophysiology and progression of hypertension, usual treatments, and other basic information for readers to understand the new approaches to managing hypertension discussed in the article. The content, therefore, needs to reflect the emphasis of the journal and background of readers.

The organization of the content is based on the purpose of the manuscript and style of the journal. Authors should organize the content logically, for example, beginning with the background for readers to understand the problem, and then progressing to the care of patients or other focus of the paper. In clinical journals it is important for authors to present the evidence supporting their interventions and identify where further evidence is needed to make decisions about clinical practice.

Conclusion

Every clinical article similar to other papers ends with a conclusion. The conclusion summarizes the information and its value to nurses in their own clinical practice. It also may suggest areas where further work is needed, such as testing of an intervention across settings, but the conclusion should not introduce new information. The conclusion is generally one to two paragraphs in length.

Many of these same principles can be used in writing other types of articles. The author is reminded to follow the format of the journal for submission and gear the paper to intended readers.

WRITING RESEARCH REPORTS FOR CLINICAL JOURNALS

An earlier chapter explained how to write research reports, and while those principles apply to preparing papers on original research studies for clinical journals, there are some additional guidelines to consider when writing these manuscripts. Findings from research need to be disseminated in the clinical nursing literature to reach nurses who can implement them in their own practices and to build the evidence base for nursing. Clinical journals are an effective mechanism for accomplishing these goals. In a descriptive study of 768 articles in clinical specialty journals and 18,901 citations in those articles, Oermann and colleagues (2008) found that nearly a third of those articles were reports of research studies, and 43.2% of the references were to original research studies. These findings are consistent with an earlier study of articles published in maternal/child nursing journals: nearly half (46%) of the 112 articles analyzed were reports of research studies (Oermann, et al., 2007).

Guidelines for Writing

The IMRAD format presented earlier, **I**ntroduction, **M**ethods, **R**esults and **D**iscussion, can be used for a research report intended for a clinical journal. This structure provides a way of organizing the manuscript, and for some clinical journals, these headings can be used with an additional section on clinical implications. In the introduction, the author should identify the clinical problem that led to the study, gap in the research, and why this study was essential to better understand the problem, develop interventions for it, and improve patient outcomes, among other reasons. A good introduction in a clinical journal links the significance of the study to the nurse's own clinical practice. This writing not only sets the stage for the remainder of the manuscript but also captures the reader's interest.

When writing research reports for clinical journals, the literature review is generally less extensive than for a research journal. The review of the literature can be incorporated into the introduction, consistent with the IMRAD format, or presented separately. For example, in a study of policies and practices related to sibling and child visitation in hospital maternity units, the author integrated the literature review in the introduction after identifying why this study was important (Spear, 2009). This research report followed the IMRAD format and had four sections: introduction, method, results, and clinical nursing implications as the discussion section. The final part of the paper was a short conclusion about the research findings and how nurses can use them for examining their own sibling and child visitation policies. The author also developed a table with specific key clinical implications of the study findings. Reviewing research articles in the target clinical journal gives the author a sense of how these manuscripts are developed in terms of the literature review and other parts of the manuscript.

The next section of the manuscript presents the methods that the researcher used to carry out the study. In a research journal, the methods section provides detailed information about the design, subjects, measures, procedures, and data analysis, in that order. Generally, each subsection is labeled similarly. When preparing manuscripts on research studies for clinical journals, the methods section may not as complex or detailed as in research journals. The author should explain what was done, who participated, how they measured and interpreted the results, and how they carried out the study (Oermann, Galvin, Floyd, & Roop, 2006). The principle is to present enough information for clinicians to understand the findings and consider how they might be used in their own clinical setting. Authors should keep in mind as well that clinicians may not have the background to understand the methods and statistical analysis. Instead clinicians want to know how the research findings can guide their practice and work in nursing.

Exhibit 7.2 shows four examples of methods sections published in clinical practice journals. Examples 1 and 2 explain clinical research methods for, respectively, a quantitative study of U.S. nurses' working environments and a qualitative study of population health surveillance activity among public health nurses in one Canadian province. Example 3 describes the method used by nurses to evaluate a scope-of-practice intervention model.

EXHIBIT 7.2

Examples of Methods Section From Articles Published in Clinical Journals

Example 1

Study Design and Sample

The original online survey instrument used in the 2006 survey was based on the AACN healthy work environment standards and on previous research about registered nurses' (RNs) work environments.[8] The 2008 survey used the same questionnaire with only minor modifications (ie, addition of questions to probe results found in the 2006 survey). Once again, convenience sampling was used with AACN members and other constituents invited via e-mail to participate....Frequencies, percentages, standard deviations, and means were determined for each question and cross-tabulated against demographic variables. A total of 5562 RNs responded, with representation from every state and the District of Columbia.[1]

Continued

Exhibit 7.2 *Continued*

Example 2

An interpretive qualitative study design was used to guide data collection and analysis (Draucker, 1999). This inquiry process, which merges the perspectives of the participants, the researcher, and other sources of data in the interpretive process, enabled an in-depth understanding of the everyday practice of public health nurses....

Design and Sample

The study was conducted in the Public Health Service areas of the District Health Authorities (DHAs) in a province in Eastern Canada. At the time of the study, there were approximately 147 public health nurses in the province....

Measures

Ethical approval was obtained from the university's ethics and the DHAs' ethics boards. Potential participants for individual interviews were randomly selected from a roster of nurses who had worked in their positions for at least 3 years. A semi-structured interview guide was used for 90-min face-to-face interviews ($n = 543$). A copy of the audiotaped interview was mailed to each participant. A 30-min follow-up telephone interview was arranged 2–3 weeks later for verification and elaboration of transcript content. Nurses who had participated in the individual interviews and all other public health nurses in the province who met the inclusion criterion were invited to participate in focus group interviews. Five 90-min focus groups were conducted with 31 nurses. The participants discussed emergent themes from the individual interviews, provided feedback, and identified strategies to enhance public health nurses' practice.

Analytic Strategy

Using established procedures for coding and thematic analysis (Lincoln & Guba, 1985; Sandelowski, 1995), the principal investigators and research coordinator independently coded the interviews, identified emergent themes, and arrived at the final coding and thematic structure by consensus.[2]

Example 3

In July 1998, the Section of Public Health Nursing received a federal Nursing Special Project grant, "Public Health Nursing Practice For The 21st Century" to promote population-based public health nursing practice. Part of that grant included a rigorous critique of the Intervention Wheel and synthesis of the evidence relevant to the interventions in the literature. The goal of the critique process was to examine the evidence underlying the interventions and levels of practice. The following questions guided the process: (a) did the 17 interventions encompass the breadth of public health practice;

(b) did the interventions occur at all levels of practice; (c) were there miss-ing interventions, or were there public health nursing activities that could not be classified into the existing interventions; (d) were there overlaps or duplications among the interventions; (e) did the evidence support the origi-nal definitions; and (f) how could these interventions be implemented with excellence. This process incorporated approaches that were refined in the Minnesota Practice Enhancement Project, which included identification of evidence-supported public health nursing practice guidelines (Strohschein, Schaffer, & Lia-Hoagberg, 1999). The entire process was carried out in a series of phases over an 18-month period. Figure 3 outlines the process that was followed, which involved hundreds of public health nurses throughout the nation.[3]

Example 4

Consistent with the scope, three clear questions were identified:

1. How can nurses accurately confirm depressive symptoms in postpartum women?
2. What effective prevention interventions can nurses implement in practice?
3. What effective treatment interventions can nurses implement in practice?

The search strategy was conducted to ensure that all relevant literature was included in the review process. The first structured search looked for the presence of existing evidence-based guidelines that addressed the current scope and could be updated or adapted. Following this review, a systematic literature search was conducted with the assistance of a uni-versity-based librarian. The search methods incorporated several strate-gies including searching in electronic databases (e.g., Medline, PsychLit, Cumulative Index to Nursing and Allied Health, Database of Abstracts of Reviews of Effects, Cochrane Database, Excerpta Medica Database, and Cochrane Collaboration of Controlled Trials) using predefined key words; a structured Web site search; screening the references of retrieved studies and systematic reviews; and hand-searching key journals. On the basis of this search strategy, approximately 450 research articles were retrieved for a critical appraisal.[4]

Note: Selected parts of each section.
[1]From Ulrich, B., Lavandero, R., Hart, K., Woods, D., Leggett, J., Friedman, D., et al. (2009). Critical Care Nurses' work environments 2008: a follow-up report. *Critical Care Nurse, 29*(2), 94.
[2]From Meagher-Stewart, D., Edwards, N., Aston, M., & Young, L. (2009). Population health surveil-lance practice of public health nurses. *Public Health Nursing, 26*, p. 554. Reprinted by permission of John Wiley and Sons, 2010.
[3]From Keller, L.O., Strohschein, S., Lia-Hoagberg, B., & Schaffer, M. A. (2004). Population-based pub-lic health interventions: Practice-based and evidence-supported. Part I. *Public Health Nursing, 21*, p. 459. Reprinted by permission of John Wiley and Sons, 2010.
[4]McQueen, K., & Dennis, C-L. (2007). Development of a postpartum depression best practice guideline: A review of the systematic process. *Journal of Nursing Care Quality, 22*, pp. 200–201. Reprinted by per-mission of Wolters Kluwer Health, 2010.

Another type of method that clinical authors often need to present in a manuscript is their underlying literature search strategy, especially when developing a clinical procedure, document, or innovation. For these projects clinicians search not only the empirical literature but also practice and professional documents from various nursing organizations. For readers to evaluate the value and applicability of the proposal, the search strategy needs to be presented succinctly but convincingly of its comprehensiveness. Example 4 in Exhibit 7.2 provides an illustration of how to describe this type of method in a clinical article.

As with any research paper, the aim of the results section is to present the findings. However, when the readers are clinicians, authors should avoid using complex statistics and for qualitative studies detailed discussions of the theoretical perspective, method, and data analysis. Easy-to-read tables and figures that demonstrate visually the outcomes of the study are valuable to promote understanding of the results (Exhibit 7.3).

EXHIBIT 7.3

Example of Easy-to-Read Tables and Figure

Table 1

Differences in Importance Ratings between Men and Women

Importance Ratings	Men *M (SD)*	Women *M (SD)*	*t*
Able to ask nurse questions	4.13 (.83)	4.12 (.85)	0.07
Having nurse teach me about illness and treatments	4.58 (.81)	4.51 (.89)	0.61
Having nurse teach me self care for discharge	4.56 (.89)	3.91 (.98)	2.51*

*$p = .006$

Table 2

Comparison of Web Sites for Asthma Patient Education

Content Areas	Percent of Web Sites with Content	
	2007 study (N=70)	2009 study (N=145)
Asthma Pathophysiology	72.0	84.4
Asthma Triggers	77.8	92.1
Avoidance of Triggers	67.6	71.2
Action of Long Term Control Medications	62.9	55.6
Action of Quick Relief Rescue Medications	60.4	61.0
Self-care Skills	36.9	52.8
Asthma Action Plan	32.0	41.2

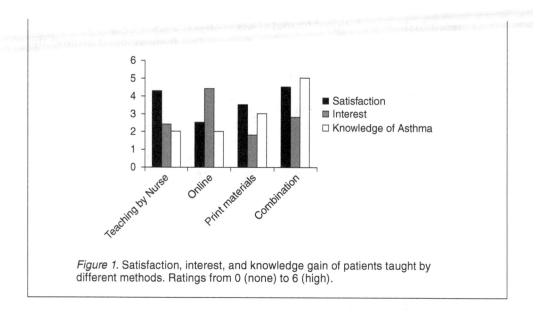

Figure 1. Satisfaction, interest, and knowledge gain of patients taught by different methods. Ratings from 0 (none) to 6 (high).

The discussion section is one of the most important: it allows the author to explain what the findings mean for clinical practice (Oermann, et al., 2006). It is important to be explicit about how the findings can or cannot be used in practice and to identify considerations in implementing the results in one's own setting. For example, a study on the relationship between blood culture contamination rates and workload perceptions done in a children's hospital may not be applicable to adult patients. In the implications authors should guide readers in thinking about how the findings could be used in practice, for example, by describing patient groups, institutions/units or communities, and conditions under which the results are applicable (Becker, 2009; Connelly, 2009).

Writing About Pilot and Evaluation Studies

These same principles apply when preparing a paper on a pilot study or an evaluation of a project or initiative on the unit. These studies may have small samples and may not be as rigorous as other research but nevertheless should be shared with clinicians who are considering similar projects in their own settings. The knowledge gained from evaluations done by nurses of interventions and new initiatives may be important for answering questions about clinical practice. Reports of clinical projects conducted and evaluated in one setting may guide the practice and activities of nurses in another setting.

There are other situations in which the nurse initiated a research study but because of problems in implementation was not able to carry it out as planned. In developing a manuscript about the study, the nurse might view it as a pilot to inform others about its purpose and provide a basis for subsequent research. The nurse also might develop a manuscript on the difficulties encountered in conducting this type of study and possible solutions.

Rather than the conventional format of a research report, manuscripts on pilot studies and evaluations of projects and initiatives can be developed around the problem that led to the study or project, a description of it and the data collected, the findings, and the implications for practice. If changes were subsequently made in practice, then the manuscript also may describe these changes and the evaluation planned to monitor them over time. In manuscripts such as these, the research process may guide authors in deciding on content to include and how to organize it, but they may decide not to use the IMRAD headings.

Some journals do not publish pilot and evaluation studies, and authors should review the journal guidelines and query the editor at the outset. With these studies authors should weigh the conclusions and implications for practice against the sample size and quality of the study, being careful not to overstate them.

▦ WRITING QUALITY IMPROVEMENT REPORTS FOR JOURNALS

Many of the current projects in clinical settings are intended to improve the quality of patient care and can be published in nursing and healthcare journals. In reports about quality improvement studies, nurses can describe problems they examined, interventions they evaluated, and what they learned about their effectiveness. Dissemination of quality improvement (QI) projects is critical to share this information with others who may have similar problems on their units and in their clinical agencies (Oermann, 2009). For nurses and others to use the findings from QI studies, papers need to describe the patient population, clinical or community setting, intervention, and outcomes of the study. Without that information it is unlikely that readers could apply the findings with their own patients.

Yet many published articles on QI studies do not present sufficient information about the project, intervention, process, and outcomes to be implemented elsewhere (Davidoff, Batalden, Stevens, Ogrinc, & Mooney, 2008; Shojania & Grimshaw, 2005). For this reason, guidelines have been developed recently to improve the reporting of QI studies. These guidelines, Standards for QUality Improvement Reporting Excellence (SQUIRE), should be used when preparing manuscripts on QI projects for nursing and healthcare journals (Table 7.2) (Oermann, 2009; Ogrinc, et al., 2008). By using the SQUIRE guidelines, authors can prepare manuscripts that adequately inform readers about the problem that led to the QI project, intervention or initiative developed to solve it, setting in which the project took place, its outcomes, and the local conditions that could influence them (Berwick, 2008).

Although the SQUIRE guidelines provide a format for nurses preparing manuscripts on QI projects, they are only guidelines. Many papers submitted to nursing and healthcare journals will not include each of the items listed, but SQUIRE provides a good framework for authors to follow when preparing a manuscript on a QI project (Oermann, 2009).

TABLE 7.2

SQUIRE Guidelines[1] for Reporting QI Studies in Journals

Section of Paper	Description
Title and abstract	Did you provide clear and accurate information for finding, indexing, and scanning your paper?
1. Title	a. Indicate article is on improvement of quality b. State aim of intervention c. Indicate study method (eg, a qualitative study on call bell responses)
2. Abstract	Summarize key information using journal abstract format
Introduction	Why did you start?
3. Background knowledge	Provide brief summary of current knowledge of problem being addressed in project; include characteristics of setting
4. Local problem	Describe specific local problem addressed in project
5. Intended improvement	a. Describe changes/improvements in processes and outcomes of proposed intervention b. Specify who (eg, champions) and what (events, observations) led to decision to make changes; include why project done now (timing)
6. Study question	State primary and any other questions that QI study was intended to answer
Methods	What did you do?
7. Ethical issues	Indicate ethical concerns of implementing the improvement and study, and how addressed
8. Setting	Specify elements and characteristics of setting most likely to influence change/improvement
9. Planning the intervention	a. Describe intervention in enough detail for others to reproduce it b. Indicate factors that contributed to decision about specific intervention to implement (eg, experiences of nurses with intervention on other units in clinical setting) c. Describe plans for how intervention was to be implemented: what was to be done, how tests of change would be used to modify intervention, and by whom
10. Planning the study of the intervention	a. Outline plans for assessing how well intervention was implemented b. Describe mechanisms by which intervention components were expected to cause changes, and plans for testing if they were effective c. Identify study design (eg, observational, quasi-experimental, experimental) for measuring effects of intervention d. Discuss plans for implementing essential aspects of study design e. Describe aspects of study design that addressed internal validity (integrity of data) and external validity (generalizability)

Continued

TABLE 7.2

Continued

Section of Paper	Description
11. Methods of evaluation	a. Describe instruments and procedures to assess effectiveness of implementation, contributions of intervention components and context factors to effectiveness of intervention, and outcomes b. Report validity and reliability of assessment instruments c. Explain methods to assure data quality and adequacy
12. Analysis	a. Provide details of qualitative and quantitative (statistical) methods b. Align unit of analysis with level at which intervention was implemented, if applicable c. Specify degree of variability expected in implementation, change expected in primary outcome (effect size), and ability of study design (including size) to detect those effects d. Describe analytic methods to demonstrate effects of time as variable (eg, statistical process control)

Results
13. Outcomes
	What did you find?
	a. Nature of setting and improvement intervention:
	  i. Indicate relevant elements of setting (eg, geography, physical resources, organizational culture, history of change efforts), and structures and patterns of care (eg, staffing) that provided context for the intervention
	  ii. Explain actual course of intervention (eg, sequence of steps, events or phases, type and number of participants at key points)
	  iii. Document success in implementing intervention components
	  iv. Describe how and why initial plan evolved and most important lessons learned, particularly effects of internal feedback from tests of change (reflexiveness)
	b. Changes in processes of care and patient outcomes associated with intervention:
	  i. Present data on changes observed in care delivery process
	  ii. Present data on changes observed in patient outcomes (eg, mortality, function, patient/staff satisfaction, service utilization, cost, others)
	  iii. Consider benefits, harms, unexpected results, problems, failures
	  iv. Present evidence on strength of association between observed changes/improvements and intervention components/context factors
	  v. Include summary of missing data for intervention and outcomes

Discussion 14. Summary	What do the findings mean? a. Summarize most important successes and difficulties in implementing intervention and main changes observed b. Highlight study's particular strengths

Continued

TABLE 7.2

Continued

Section of Paper	Description
15. Relation to other evidence	Compare and contrast study results with relevant findings of others
16. Limitations	a. Consider possible sources of confounding, bias, or imprecision in design, measurement, and analysis that might have affected study outcomes b. Explore factors that could affect generalizability, eg, representativeness of participants, effectiveness of implementation, features of local care setting c. Address likelihood that observed gains may weaken over time and describe plans, if any, for monitoring and maintaining improvement d. Review efforts to minimize study limitations e. Assess effect of limitations on interpretation and application of results
17. Interpretation	a. Explore possible reasons for differences between observed and expected outcomes b. Draw inferences consistent with strength of data about causal mechanisms and size of observed changes; pay attention to components of intervention and context factors, and types of settings in which intervention is most likely to be effective c. Suggest steps that might be modified to improve future performance d. Review issues of opportunity cost and actual financial cost of intervention
18. Conclusions	a. Consider practical usefulness of intervention b. Suggest implications for nursing and further QI studies
Other information	Were there other factors relevant to the conduct and interpretation of the study?
19. Funding	List funding sources, if any, and role of funding organization in design, implementation, interpretation, and publication

[1]Guidelines were adapted from Davidoff, F., Batalden, P., Stevens, D., Ogrinc, G., & Mooney, S. for the SQUIRE Development Group. (2008). Publication guidelines for improvement studies in health care: Evolution of the SQUIRE project. *Annals of Internal Medicine, 149,* 670–676.
From Oermann, M. H. (2009). SQUIRE guidelines for reporting improvement studies in healthcare: Implications for nursing publications. *Journal of Nursing Care Quality, 24,* 92–94. Reprinted by permission of Wolters Kluwer Health, 2009.

▨ SUMMARY

Clinical practice articles disseminate new knowledge and skills for patient care, provide information for nurses to stay current in clinical practice, and update them on new technologies and advances in care. With this type of article, nurses in one setting can describe their practice innovations for use and testing by nurses in other settings. They can discuss issues they encountered in patient care and how they resolved those issues, and they can share nursing approaches that worked and ones that did not work.

The process for writing a clinical article begins with an idea. From this idea the author specifies the purpose of the manuscript and then identifies the intended readers. Who will read the article dictates the content included in it. In planning the content, the author takes into consideration the knowledge and background of the intended audience.

There is no standard format for writing clinical articles in contrast to research papers because it depends on the purpose of the manuscript. Some general guidelines for writing clinical articles were presented in the chapter including how to write the title, abstract, introduction and different types of lead-in paragraphs, and body of the paper. Every clinical article ends with a conclusion that summaries the information and its value to nurses in their own clinical practice.

The IMRAD format presented earlier can be used for a research report intended for clinician readers. This structure provides a way of organizing the manuscript, and for some clinical journals, these headings can be used with an additional section on clinical implications.

In the introduction, the author should identify the clinical problem that led to the study, gap in the research, and why this study was essential to better understand the problem, develop interventions for it, and improve patient outcomes, among other reasons. A good introduction links the significance of the study to the nurse's own clinical practice. When writing research reports for clinical journals, the literature review is generally less extensive than for a research journal. The review of the literature can be incorporated into the introduction, consistent with the IMRAD format, or presented separately. In the methods section the author should explain what was done, who participated, how they measured and interpreted the results, and how they carried out the study, keeping in mind that the main readers are clinicians not researchers.

As with any research paper, the aim of the results section is to present the findings. However, when the readers are clinicians, authors should avoid using complex statistics and for qualitative studies detailed discussions of the theoretical perspective, method, and data analysis. Easy-to-read tables and figures that demonstrate visually the outcomes of the study are valuable to promote understanding of the results. The discussion section is one of the most important: it allows the author to explain what the findings mean for clinical practice. It is important to be explicit about how the findings can or cannot be used in practice and to identify considerations in implementing the results in one's own setting. These same principles apply when writing manuscripts about pilot and evaluation studies.

When preparing papers on QI projects, nurses should follow the SQUIRE (Standards for QUality Improvement Reporting Excellence) guidelines. These guidelines provide a format for the manuscript, ensuring that it includes sufficient information about the problem that led to the QI project, intervention or initiative developed to solve it, setting in which the project took place, and its outcomes. Not all items in the guidelines will be included with most manuscripts, but referring to them while planning and outlining the paper will be helpful.

There are many clinical situations in which nurses find themselves that lend to writing for publication. Nurses need to take advantage of these opportunities to disseminate their ideas and innovations to others.

REFERENCES

American Medical Association (AMA). (2007). *AMA manual of style: A guide for authors and editors* (10th ed.). New York: Oxford University Press.

American Psychological Association (APA). (2009). *Publication Manual of the American Psychological Association* (6th ed.). Washington, DC: Author.

Becker, P. T. (2009). Thoughts on the end of the article: The implications for nursing practice. *Research in Nursing & Health, 32*, 241–242. doi: 10.1002/nur.20324

Berwick, D. M. (2008). The science of improvement. *Journal of the American Medical Association, 299*, 1182–1184. doi: 10.1001/jama.299.10.1182

Connelly, L. (2009). The discussion section of a research report. *MEDSURG Nursing, 18*, 300–301.

Davidoff, F., Batalden, P., Stevens, D., Ogrinc, G., & Mooney, S. for SQUIRE development group. Publication guidelines for improvement studies in health care: Evolution of the SQUIRE project. *Annals of Internal Medicine, 149*, 670–676. doi: 10.1136/qshc.2008.029066

Gross, A. M., & Fonteyn, M. E. (2008). Turn your presentation into a published manuscript. *American Journal of Nursing, 108* (10), 85–87. doi: 10.1097/01.NAJ.0000337747.37719.86

Janotha, B. (2009). Symptomatic presentation of renal cell carcinoma in a young adult. *Nurse Practitioner, 34*(6), 9–11. doi: 10.1097/01.NPR.0000352282.89605.7a

Oermann, M. H. (2009). SQUIRE guidelines for reporting improvement studies in healthcare: Implications for nursing publications. *Journal of Nursing Care Quality, 24*, 91–95. doi: 10.1097/01.NCQ.0000347445.04138.74

Oermann, M. H., Blair, D., Kowalewski, K., Wilmes, N., & Nordstrom, C. (2007). Citation analysis of the maternal/child nursing literature. *Pediatric Nursing, 33*, 387–391.

Oermann, M. H., Galvin, E. A, Floyd, J. A., & Roop, J. C. (2006). Presenting research to clinicians: Strategies for writing about research findings. *Nurse Researcher, 13*(4), 66–74.

Oermann, M. H., Nordstrom, C., Wilmes, N. A., Denison, D., Webb, S. A., Featherston, D. E., Kowalewski, K. (2008). Dissemination of research in clinical nursing journals. *Journal of Clinical Nursing, 17*, 149–156. doi: 10.1111/j.1365-2702.2007.01975.x

Ogrinc, G., Mooney, S. E., Estrada, C., Foster, T., Hall, L. W., Huizinga, M. M., Watts, B. (2008). The SQUIRE (Standards for QUality Improvement Reporting Excellence) guidelines for quality improvement reporting: Explanation and elaboration. *Quality and Safety in Health Care, 17*(Suppl 1), i13-i32. doi: 10.1136/qshc.2008.029058

Shojania, K. G., & Grimshaw, J. M. (2005). Evidence-based quality improvement: The state of the science. *Health Affairs, 24*, 138–150. doi: 10.1377/hlthaff.24.1.138

Spear, H. J. (2009). Child visitation policy and practice for maternity units. *MCN, American Journal of Maternal Child Nursing, 34*, 372–377. doi: 10.1097/01.NMC.0000363686.20315.d5

CHAPTERS, BOOKS, AND OTHER FORMS OF WRITING

8

OTHER TYPES OF WRITING

Although research and clinical practice articles are primary formats for nurses to present knowledge to readers, other forms of writing are equally important. Some articles address emerging issues that affect nursing practice, education, or research. These articles may include case reports; descriptions of theory development; commentaries on policies, ethics, or legal aspects of nursing; innovative research methods; historical studies; editorials; and letters to the editor. Nurses also write book reviews and articles for consumer and non-professional audiences. These other types of writing differ in the purposes they are trying to achieve, their format, and often their writing style. Yet all are similar because they address non-trivial topics, provide original insight, and have implications for advancing health and wellbeing.

As with all scientific writing, the first part of any article must convince the reader that it addresses a topic of broad importance. Huth (1999) calls this "passing the 'So what?' test" (p. 10). If the article stands little chance of changing something important for the better, it is probably not worth the author's time to write! For editors and readers, the time and expense of reviewing, publishing, and reading the article would not be justified. The importance of the topic should be made quickly evident in all types of articles, i.e., in the first or second paragraph.

In the first sentence the author should identify a problem or knowledge gap. Then the reader will want to know how the problem is defined, what are its dimensions, and scope. For example, health problems should be described by their incidence, prevalence, and outcomes. At the conclusion of the brief introduction, the reader should understand how the article will address the problem described in an important way.

The paragraphs that follow the introductory paragraphs expand on the background material on the problem. Usually the author summarizes other recent published articles that focus on the problem, describes how much progress has been made in solving the problem, and discusses the background issues that affect the problem. If there is disagreement among published authors, these should be highlighted. The author should identify gaps in the knowledge base in order to provide a rationale for the article. Who needs what in order to accomplish what goal? By the end of the first part of the article, the reader should clearly understand what the rationale for the article is and what the intended objectives are.

The middle part of an article presents the author's original contribution to addressing the problem or issue. When new data are not the focus as in research articles, the original material may include an analysis of secondary material, application of previous material to a new setting, proposal of new dimensions to a problem, refinement of a concept or procedure, report of a new type of case, and other novel material. When presenting such material, authors should be specific and concrete about any new definitions, dimensions, relationships, or flow among the components of the material. Graphics are particularly useful for readers in order to visualize the nature or scope of new material. The author should also describe clearly the settings and circumstances in which the new material was developed or emerged.

The last part of the article should summarize briefly how the aims and objectives of the article were met. The author can be specific about how the original material advances previously published work, as well as what limitations it has. Without over-reaching the logical implications of the original material, the author should reflect on how the contents of the article might be used in patient care settings, educational institutions, research groups, or policy arenas. If additional work would be useful to extend the material, the author should help the reader the see what are the logical next steps. In the sections below, we describe how to approach the rationale and background, original material, and conclusions and implications in specific types of articles.

▪ PROFESSIONAL ISSUES ARTICLES

What about emerging issues in nursing? Information about trends and issues in nursing is becoming increasingly available on the Internet. However, nurses still need publications that analyze issues in terms of why and how they developed, the varied positions that can be taken on them, and multiple strategies for resolving them. Many clinical journals publish this type of paper. Some journals have a department or column on professional issues affecting nurses in that area of clinical practice, societal issues facing patients, and other opinion pieces. The *Online Journal of Issues in Nursing* (OJIN) presents a variety of perspectives on issues in nursing across clinical specialties and settings. The journal recognizes that individuals have differing views on issues and provides a forum for readers to express their opinions and understand others' views (American Nurses Association, 2009).

Professional issues articles begin with a discussion of the issue and why and how it developed. Some articles address information needed to understand the issue itself, increasing nurses' knowledge about it. In these manuscripts the goal is to improve understanding of issues in healthcare and nursing practice, not for nurses to assume a position about an issue. For example, a paper might provide an overview of prenatal testing, an historical perspective, examples of prenatal tests, nursing views, and ethical considerations. Rather than taking a position about prenatal testing, the goal of the author is to present information about the issue and lay a foundation for better understanding related to ethical decisions.

In another approach the author analyzes the issue from different points of view. In this type of article, the issue and the varied perspectives possible are presented for readers with a rationale. For example, a manuscript on whether continuing education should be mandatory or voluntary might present both positions and the rationale for each, leaving the readers to decide on their position. Alternatively, the author might take one point of view and present a rationale to support it. For example, the author might develop a manuscript on why continuing education should be mandatory rather than voluntary.

With issue papers the author includes the assumptions on which thinking is based, the evidence used to guide the analysis of the issue, and how the author developed a position. In preparing these manuscripts, the author is advised to be clear about one's own biases and perspectives so the content reflects an objective analysis of the issue rather than the author's view only.

CASE REPORTS AND HISTORIES

Case reports provide new information by focusing on a single patient, family, community setting, or organization, where in-depth knowledge of the specific case may be informative for understanding larger groups of patients or settings. These manuscripts often begin with why the case was selected and its importance to nursing practice and continue with a description of the case and related care by nurses and other disciplines. For example, Scherr and colleagues (2006) presented a case report on a patient who developed paraplegia following coronary artery bypass surgery. The case highlighted the need for critical care nurses to know spinal cord anatomy, risk factors for spinal cord ischemia, and nursing care of at-risk post-surgical patients.

Although a single case study and its findings cannot be generalized, these articles can be used to describe patient care; illustrate how concepts, theories, and research are used in practice; present issues in a patient's care and strategies for resolving them; and apply new information to a real or hypothetical case. Case reports also can be used for promoting the clinical judgment, decision-making, and critical thinking skills of nurses and nursing students. A case can be presented with multiple decisions possible and different options that the nurse might choose. Consequences of each decision can be examined, followed by the decision the nurse made in the case.

A case report typically includes these content areas:

- Introductory discussion of why this case is significant and how it will help nurses to understand their patients' problems and care. An effective introduction makes it clear why the case is worth reading.
- Description of the case. In this section the author presents relevant data about the case and background information. The case presentation may follow a chronological sequence or may represent one particular phase of the health problem.
- Nursing care planned and implemented for the patient, family, or community; evaluation of its effectiveness; and implications for nursing practice. The

author might include in this section changes in practice suggested as a result
of this case.

- Alternate decisions possible in the case and consequences of each. This is an
important section if the case is designed to promote nurses' clinical judgment
and critical thinking skills. The author might also include in this section how
nurses might approach the patient's care from different perspectives.
- Ethical considerations. Cases may be used to present ethical issues in a patient's
care and strategies for resolving ethical dilemmas.
- Conclusions with implications for clinical practice or research. The manuscript should conclude with a discussion of the implications of this case for the
nurse's own practice and what it means to the care of other patients. If systematic research is needed to generalize to populations, the author should specify
research questions (American Psychological Association, 2009).

Publications in nursing, medicine, and other healthcare disciplines must protect the rights of individuals to privacy, as discussed in chapter 5. Except in rare
cases, patient names, initials, and case numbers should be omitted from published case reports. The Uniform Requirements suggest that identifying information about patients should not be published unless it is essential for scientific
purposes, the patient or legally authorized representative give written informed
consent for publication in print and on the Internet, and the patient or legally
authorized representative be allowed to review the manuscript before giving
informed consent for the information to be published (International Committee
of Medical Journal Editors [ICMJE], 2008). When informed consent is obtained,
it should be indicated in the published article. Only essential details should be
provided (American Medical Association [AMA], 2007).

The author is cautioned to query the editor if interested in a case report, as
some journals do not publish case reports as articles. For these journals there
may be a department for which the case would be appropriate. As an example,
the *Journal of Obstetric, Gynecologic, and Neonatal Nursing* (Wiley Interscience,
2009) has a category for manuscripts that are case reports, i.e., reviews of cases
that present new information for nursing and inter-professional care.

PHILOSOPHICAL AND THEORETICAL ARTICLES

Other topical articles may be philosophical in nature or deal with theory development or testing. The format used to develop these manuscripts should fit the
goals of the paper, the philosophical theory used for its development or the position taken, or the structure of the theory or framework.

Manuscripts of this type might discuss the development of nursing theory,
present the results of the testing of concepts and theories in a defined population,
analyze an existing theory and propose an extension of it or an alternative theory, identify a flaw in a theory, or compare different theories. Varied philosophical perspectives can be analyzed and compared. In general, these papers should
include a review of the literature that serves as the foundation for the author's
thinking and perspective. The authors should discuss the internal consistency

and external validity of the theory, and implications for nursing research and further development of the theory. In writing philosophical and theoretical manuscripts, the author is careful to present and order ideas so they are logical and sequenced appropriately. It is important to present a sound argument to support ideas and defend them using theory and research.

As an example, Covell (2009) developed a middle-range theory of how nursing knowledge is stored in healthcare organizations. She began the paper by describing the philosophical background on intellectual capital, including human, relational, and structural capital. Next, she presented the methods she used to search the business and health-related literatures and to synthesize, re-define, and analyze previous work on intellectual capital for a new setting. Based on published evidence in support of the emergent theory, she described the implications for organizational and patient outcomes in healthcare settings. In this way the content and its organization reflected concepts of theory development in nursing.

Some journals in nursing are devoted to nursing science and theory development. For example, the primary purposes of *Advances in Nursing Science* (ANS—Lippincott Williams & Williams, 2009) are to contribute to the development of nursing science and to promote the application of theories and research findings to nursing practice. Articles deal with theory development, concept analysis, development of extensions or alternative theory to existing theories, practical application of research and theory, and other areas related to nursing science (ANS, 2009). *Nursing Science Quarterly* (NSQ—Sage Publications, 2009a) also publishes manuscripts focusing on nursing theory development, nursing theory-based practice, and quantitative and qualitative research related to existing nursing frameworks (NSQ, 2009).

POLICY ARTICLES

Nurses shape organizational and public policies in such a way that affects nursing practice, education, and research. Articles are needed that describe the circumstances in which the need emerged for new or revised policies, how the structure and processes of new policies developed, and the outcomes of policy review and evaluation. Authors should clearly describe how data were gathered to understand the problem. What stakeholders were consulted? How were resources coordinated? What decisions were implemented? What did the evaluation plan entail? The general purpose, scope, timeline, and responsibilities of the policy should be summarized with enough specificity that the reader can evaluate its applicability to one's own setting and circumstances.

Policy-related articles may be appropriate for several kinds of journals. Some journals, such as *Policy, Politics and Nursing Practice* (Sage Publications, 2009b), are dedicated to publishing a broad range of articles that describe the impact of public policy, legislation, and regulation on nursing practice and, conversely, of nurses on health policy.

Authors may also find that editors of specialty journals are interested in articles on relevant policies for education or practice, especially when new general policies from oversight groups appear. For example, following the publication of general guidelines on substance abuse among nursing students from the AACN, Monroe (2009) described a prototype for implementing such a policy in a university setting. The article, published in the *Journal of Nursing Education*, provided readers with a thorough example of applying professional standards in an educational setting. Similarly, in a clinical journal focused on urologic nursing, Spencer (2009) summarized available clinical and government policy regarding the management of urinary incontinence and described implications for translation of research into practice guidelines.

ETHICS ARTICLES

Although many types of articles written by nurses will feature a brief discussion of the ethical implications of a topic, authors may also organize an article to focus specifically on organizational or patient care-related ethical issues. A journal such as *Nursing Ethics* features a broad range of such articles. Recent ones have focused on the ethics of resuscitation and genetics, cross-cultural studies, how ethics are represented in the nursing curriculum, and professional codes of conduct. Specialty journals and organizations also publish articles that focus on ethical practice related to specific kinds of care. Recent examples of ethics articles include a case study of a patient's refusal of emergency care for religious reasons (Pasci, 2008), a concept analysis of the development and attributes of ethical sensitivity among professional nurses (Weaver, Morse, & Mitcham, 2008), and the ethical obligations of teaching spiritual care to nursing students in a public university (Lantz, 2007).

The organization of an ethics paper will be dictated by the type of information being presented. All of the articles noted above begin with a description of the background of the ethical dilemma or concern and what is at stake in a thorough investigation of it. The middle section includes the specifics of the original cases or data, laid out in a logical framework that makes clear what the author has found. The articles conclude with a synthesis or analysis of what was learned in such a way that readers take away new insights into ethical development or practice.

Some ethics articles may be similar to a research article, with introduction, methods, results, and discussion sections. For example, de Casterle and colleagues (de Casterle, Izumi, Godfrey & Denhaerynck, 2009) introduced their ethics article by documenting a gap in past research on barriers to ethical action in clinical settings: the research failed to consider the ethics of daily decision-making in nursing care. Then, in the methods section, they described a meta-analysis of nine studies of nurses' ethical behavior at the bedside, all of which used the identical test for ethical behavior based on one theory of moral development. Results showed that nurses employed nursing conventions rather than patient characteristics to guide ethical decisions. The authors concluded with a discussion of conformist nursing practice and next steps in promoting ethical development.

ARTICLES ON LEGAL ISSUES

Nursing practice, education, and research is constrained and empowered by legislation and regulation. Therefore, articles on legal issues are of critical interest in generalist nursing and specialty journals. For example, the *Journal of Nursing Law* (Springer, 2009) publishes analyses of legislation related to nursing practice, education, and administration, with emphasis on emerging trends and influences.

Articles on legal issues are structured according to the material to be presented. A nurse lactation consultant collaborated with a law student to write an article comparing breastfeeding legislation in states with high and low breastfeeding rates (Chertok & Hoover, 2009). Their brief introduction included background literature on the nutritional value of human milk for infants and the variability of breastfeeding behavior and activism across the U.S. The extensive middle section first contrasted legal language of the right to breastfeed with language decriminalizing breastfeeding as an indecent act. Next, the authors described specific examples of laws regarding breastfeeding during jury duty and in the workplace. A detailed table compared breastfeeding rates in five regions of the U.S. and legislation in their constituent states. A brief conclusion noted time trends in legislative activity on breastfeeding and a call to action among legislators, healthcare providers, and consumers to provide societal support for this healthy activity.

Legal implications for professional practice are also important areas for articles by nurses. These topics include the nurse's role in informed consent, high risk nursing specialties, and issues involving professional liability insurance (*Journal of Nursing Law*, 2009).

ARTICLES ON RESEARCH METHODS

Nurses often identify concepts from grounded theory studies or clinical practice for which valid and reliable assessment tools are not available. When developing and testing original tools and scales, authors must use a rigorous research protocol. When they draft a report of such studies, the results should be presented using the IMRAD format described in chapter 5. Even when refining tests of validity and reliability of scales in new demographic populations or when using a subset of the original questionnaire items, authors should use a research manuscript format for presenting the findings.

However, some methodological innovations can be presented using nonresearch formats. Authors might describe the need for a translation of a specific survey tool into the language of a high risk group of patients, what translation and back-translation procedures were employed, where the new tool was pilot tested, and what kind of next steps would demonstrate reliability. Another author might have developed ethical and effective strategies either for recruiting subjects who are often under-represented in research studies or for retaining patients in high stress circumstances over time for longitudinal studies. These manuscripts should include the background on the lack of a suitable methodological strategy, the original contribution of the authors to filling the need, and implications for how to apply it in the practice of research or practice.

▨ HISTORY OF NURSING ARTICLES

Articles on the history of nursing are found throughout scientific publications. A search of the *Cumulative Index of Nursing and Allied Health Literature (CINAHL)* database yielded 147 citations alone to articles with titles that included "Florence Nightingale" published widely between 2000 and 2009. *Nursing History Review* is one peer-reviewed, scholarly journal that focuses on the history of nursing, healthcare, health policy and society, as well as a department for book reviews (American Association for the History of Nursing [AAHN], 2009a). Articles on history of nursing appear in the *Bulletin of the History of Medicine* (Johns Hopkins University, 2009) and the *Journal of the History of Medicine and Allied Sciences* (Oxford University Press, 2009). Some specialty journals also publish articles on the history of nursing. For example, *Public Health Nursing* has a department for history manuscripts that concern "any aspect of the development of public health nursing or the role of nurses in the evolution of population-based care in any country, including original historical research, critical analyses of past events or trends, and oral histories or biographies" (Wiley Interscience, 2009b, p.3).

The structure and formatting of scientific articles on the history of nursing are subject to the same principles as those for all research studies, as described in Chapter 5. The primary source data for nursing history articles includes diaries, journals, correspondence, organizational records, photographs, manuscripts, audio-visual records of oral histories, and other original material (AAHN, 2009b). Data from such sources requires the author to introduce the material with a description of the import of the knowledge gap that will be addressed by the article. The manuscript should also describe, analyze, and synthesize the data succinctly for the reader. The author should make clear to the reader how the particular historical record presented in the article will contribute to nurses' understanding of their professional identity, patients' perspectives, or evidence-based decision-making (Borsay, 2009). Regardless of the order of presentation, all articles on the history of nursing address the significance, approach, and meaning of the research.

▨ EDITORIALS

Some journals have editorials that are written only by the editor, but with other publications nurses may be asked to write a guest editorial. Preparing an editorial for a journal requires a different type of writing than used for other manuscripts. Editorials are short essays that represent the official opinion of the publication or an invited guest editor (AMA, 2007). Often editorials are issue oriented, related to the theme of articles in the journal. For example, if the theme of the journal is genetic counseling, the editorial may focus on related ethical considerations.

An editorial also may be a critical review of an original paper in the journal or a summary of new developments in the field. Editorials that comment on papers in the journal may provide an alternative view of the issue or even a different interpretation of the data. New findings may have been presented recently that readers should be aware of when they read the article; editorials are a way of providing these other perspectives. An editorial also might emphasize the practice implications of articles in the journal.

Editorials are usually short, so the first task of the author is to plan the content within a limited number of words. In comparison to manuscripts that generally range from 15 to 18 pages of text, editorials may be only 3 to 6 typed pages.

Many editorials can be written using the following format: statement of the problem, issue or opinion; possible solutions and approaches; supporting evidence for each; and the author's conclusion based on this evidence. In some situations the author may indicate that there is the lack of evidence to support a decision or an action and more study is needed.

LETTERS TO THE EDITOR

Letters to the editor are an essential component of holding authors accountable for what they write (AMA, 2007). Comments, questions, and criticism of previously published articles stimulate public debate that can be healthy for the common good. Letters to the editor usually comment on a recently published article and are sometimes accompanied by a brief response from the author, which is solicited by the editor. Letters to the editor engage a large audience, are often monitored by opinion leaders, and provide new information to the audience of the publication.

While anyone can write a letter to the editor, not everyone can get it published. Journals, newspapers, and other types of publications receive many letters, only some of which they publish. Letters may be written to the journal's editor to provide an alternate perspective to an earlier article; they may be sent to a newspaper to explain a topic to the public or present a viewpoint about an issue.

Not every journal publishes letters to the editor, so the author should first check the information for authors page or scan copies of the journal. If commenting on an article published earlier in the journal, the author should make this clear in the beginning of the letter. The letter should focus on a scientific, clinical, or ethical implication of the original article and avoid personal attack on the author (AMA, 2007). The writing style and format are similar to editorials. Because most journals limit the length of letters to the editor, the author should keep this in mind and prepare a letter that is short and to the point.

Authors also can send letters to newspapers, magazines, and other types of publications. Carroll (1999) presented six tips for writing these letters: (1) be concise, (2) present only one topic, (3) clearly state the viewpoint, (4) state opinions directly, (5) if responding to comments made by others, do not use stereotypes for describing them, and (6) be accurate.

REVIEWS OF BOOKS AND OTHER MEDIA

Nurses might write book or media reviews for journals describing what the work is about and addressing its quality. This is a good opportunity for nurses with limited writing experience. Book reviews are typically short pieces similar in length to editorials, and authors need to communicate their ideas clearly and succinctly.

The purpose of the review is to inform readers about the quality of the book and its content so they can decide whether to purchase it. Authors should provide a substantive overview of the contents of the work, followed by a comparison to other similar products. For instance, a new instructional film or textbook may emphasize topics that were secondary or absent in older works. Praise or criticism should be supported with evidence from the work. Rather than saying the book is "too basic for experienced nurses and they should not buy it," the author can cite examples from the book that demonstrates the depth of content and then conclude that the "book is most useful to new graduates."

Guidelines for writing a book review are:

- Identify the purpose of the book. This is generally stated in the preface and introduction. Then assess if the book achieves this purpose.
- Describe the types of readers for whom the book would be valuable, for instance, students as a course text, in-service educators, nurse practitioners, staff nurses, and so forth. In most situations books are appropriate for more than one audience, and these should all be included in the review. For example, if the author is a nurse practitioner, a book may seem too basic for one's own practice, but if reviewed from the perspective of new graduates or staff nurses, it may be at the appropriate level.
- Assess if the content is up-to-date and reflects research findings if available.
- Review how the book is designed. Are there sufficient headings and sub-headings? Are there visuals to support the content? For textbooks, are strategies included to promote learning, such as, chapter objectives and learning activities?
- Review the references. Are they current? If older references are included in the chapters, are they classic in the field? Does the book have references from other fields?
- Include the book price, its value, and if it is unique (Hill, 1997).

WRITING FOR CONSUMERS AND NON-PROFESSIONAL AUDIENCES

Another type of writing is for consumers and non-professional audiences. Nurses have the background and education for writing health articles for the public, and they need to take the initiative to prepare articles of this nature.

Consumer magazines are a major source of health education for the public, and these publications allow nurses to share their expertise with readers (Penrose & Katz, 2004). Examples include general news magazines, specialty magazines that target demographic interest groups (health and fitness, parents), company publications, and newspapers.

With this type of writing, the author needs to be clear about who reads the publication so the content and writing can be geared to them. Examples can be used that are relevant to the readers' knowledge level and needs. A manuscript on how to choose a primary care provider would have different examples if written for a magazine read by parents of young children compared with one geared to older readers.

Before starting to write, the author should be clear about what is important to the readers and how the readers might apply the information provided in the article. What does the author hope the reader will do with the information? Finally, it is important for the author to write the article in such a way that relates to the direct experience of the readers. Be as specific and concrete as possible about the problems faced by the reader, the supporting evidence for its scope and impact, and any recommendations that are included in the article.

The format and content of articles for popular audiences differ from articles written for scientific or professional readers. The author should avoid using technical terms and develop the manuscript at a level that readers without any healthcare background can understand. Any terminology should be defined clearly. The author should use her expertise to provide an analysis of any complex issues using simple but accurate wording, using pictures wherever allowed by the publishers. Comparisons can often help the reader to understand important differences. For instance, instead of describing the symptoms of only the H1N1 virus, the author could compare and contrast them with symptoms of other viral diseases. Other effective writing strategies for popular audiences include storytelling, examples, and graphics.

The author can begin by writing health pieces for newsletters and local newspapers. This provides experience in gearing the writing to a non-professional audience and deciding what information is most important to communicate to the public. In general, the conventions for writing for popular audiences are not as formulaic as for professional audiences. Therefore, the nurse-author can improvise and be creative, to the benefit of the readers.

SUMMARY

What about issues in nursing? These papers analyze issues, why and how they developed, varied positions that can be taken, and multiple strategies for resolving them.

Other topics may be philosophical in nature or deal with theory development or testing. In writing philosophical and theoretical manuscripts, the author is careful with how ideas are presented and ordered so they are logical and sequenced appropriately. It is important to present a sound argument to support ideas and defend them using theory and research.

Nurse-authors may also write articles on public and organizational policies developed by nurses or that affect their role, ethical challenges that they confront, legal and regulatory precedents with implications for patient care and professional practice, and methodological innovations for research studies. History of nursing articles use primary source material to inform current readers about the roots of their professional identity, perspective of patients, and evidence-based practice. Case reports provide new information on nursing practice and the care of patients with particular health problems through the presentation of an actual case.

With some journals nurses may be asked to write the editorial. Editorials may be issue oriented, summarize new developments in the field, or critically review an original paper in the journal. Nurses also might write book reviews describing what the book is about and addressing its quality, letters to the editor, and articles for consumers and non-professional audiences.

There are many situations in which nurses find themselves that lend to writing for publication. Nurses need to take advantage of these opportunities so their ideas are communicated to and used by others.

▦ REFERENCES

American Association for the History of Nursing. (2009a). Guidelines for contributors. *Nursing History Review.* Retrieved from http://www.aahn.org/guidelines.html

American Association for the History of Nursing. (2009b). Guidelines for contributors. *Nursing History Review.* Retrieved from http://www.aahn.org/methodology.html

American Medical Association. (2007). AMA manual of style: A guide for authors and editors (10th ed.). New York: Oxford University Press.

American Nurses Association. (2009). About OJIN. *Online Journal of Issues in Nursing.* Retrieved from http://www.nursingworld.org/MainMenuCategories/ANAMarketplace/ ANAPeriodicals/OJIN/FunctionalMenu/AboutOJIN.aspx

American Psychological Association. (2009). *Publication manual of the American Psychological Association* (6th ed.). Washington, D.C.: Author.

Borsay, A. (2009). Nursing history: An irrelevance for nursing practice? *Nursing History Review 17,* 14–27. doi: 10.1891/1062–8061.17.14

Carroll, P. (1999). Getting heard: Writing opinion pieces for the newspaper. *Nurse Author & Editor, 9*(3), 4, 7–8.

Covell, C.L. (2008). The middle-range theory of nursing intellectual capital. *Journal of Advanced Nursing, 63*(1), 94–103. doi: 10.1111/j.1365–2648.2008.04626.x

de Casterle, B.D., Izumi, S., Godfrey, N.S. & Denhaerynck, K. (2008). Nurses' responses to ethical dilemmas in nursing practice: Meta-analysis. *Journal of Advanced Nursing, 63*(6), 540–9. doi: 10.1111/j.1365–2648.2008.04702.x

Hill, K. (1997). Book reviewing: Keeping the audience in mind. *Nurse Author & Editor, 7*(1), 4, 7–8.

Huth, E.J. (1999). *Writing and Publishing in Medicine* (3rd ed.). Baltimore: Williams & Wilkins.

International Committee of Medical Journal Editors. (2008). *Uniform requirements for manuscripts submitted to biomedical journals: Writing and editing for biomedical publication.* Retrieved from http://www.icmje.org/urm_main.html

Johns Hopkins University. (2009). *Project MUSE: Journal of the History of Medicine.* Retrieved from http://muse.jhu.edu/journals/bhm/

Lippincott Williams & Wilkins. (2009). Instructions for Authors. *Advances in Nursing Science.* Retrieved from http://edmgr.ovid.com/ans/accounts/ifauth.html

Lantz, C.M. (2007). Teaching spiritual care in a public institution: Legal implications, standards of practice, and ethical obligations. *Journal of Nursing Education, 46*(1), 33–8.

Monroe, T. (2009). Educational innovations. Addressing substance abuse among nursing students: Development of a prototype alternative-to-dismissal policy. *Journal of Nursing Education, 48*(5), 272–8. doi:10.9999/01484834–20090416-06

Oxford University Press. (2009). *Journal of the History of Medicine and Allied Sciences.* Retrieved from http://jhmas.oxfordjournals.org/

Pacsi, A.L. (2008). Case study: An ethical dilemma involving a dying patient. *Journal of the New York State Nurses Association, 39*(1), 4–7.

Sage Publications. (2009a). About the journal. *Nursing Science Quarterly.* Retrieved from http://www.sagepub.com/journalsProdDesc.nav?prodId=Journal200789

Sage Publications. (2009b). About this journal. *Policy, Politics, and Nursing Practice.* Retrieved from http://www.sagepub.com/journalsProdDesc.nav?prodId=Journal201332

Scherr, K., Urquhart, G., Eichorst, C. & Bulbuc, C. (2006). Paraplegia after coronary artery bypass graft surgery: Case report of a rare event. *Critical Care Nurse, 26*(5): 34–6, 38–40, 42–5.

Spencer, J. (2009). Summary of current policy to address urinary incontinence. *Urologic Nursing, 29*(3), 149–54.

Springer Publishing Corporation. (2009). Author guidelines. *Journal of Nursing Law.* Retrieved from http://www.springerpub.com/journal.aspx?jid=1073–7472

Weaver, K., Morse, J. & Mitcham, C. (2008). Ethical sensitivity in professional practice: Concept analysis. *Journal of Advanced Nursing, 62*(5), 607–18. doi: 10.1111/j.1365–2648. 2008.04625.x

Wiley Interscience. (2009a). Guidelines for authors. *Journal of Obstetric, Gynecologic, and Neonatal Nursing.* Retrieved from http://www.wiley.com/bw/submit.asp?ref=0884–2175&site=1

Wiley Interscience. (2009b). Author guidelines. *Public Health Nursing.* Retrieved from http://www.wiley.com/bw/journal.asp?ref=0737–1209&site=1

9

BOOKS AND BOOK CHAPTERS

Writing a book or book chapter is different from an article because the author has more opportunity to provide background information and discuss related content, with more pages allowed, than in a manuscript for a journal. While a journal manuscript may be 15 to 18 double spaced pages, a chapter may be 30 to 50 pages depending on the book length. Books also provide an opportunity for the author to develop strategies that guide readers in learning the content such as including bulleted lists that emphasize the key points, case scenarios that demonstrate how the content applies to clinical practice, learning activities and questions for discussion at the end of each chapter, and so forth.

Whereas articles generally focus on one topic, books address multiple but related content areas. A book designed for use in an undergraduate maternity course contains the range of topics needed by students at that level to understand maternity nursing and gain knowledge and skills for safe and competent practice. Even a book with a more specific focus such as case management will contain the content areas needed to understand and implement case management in varied clinical settings.

One consideration for faculty members is that books and book chapters are not peer reviewed and often carry less weight in tenure and promotion decisions than publications in refereed journals. Although the publisher may have experts review the book proposal or prospectus, specific chapters, and sometimes the finished book manuscript, this review is generally done to identify missing content, suggest changes in organization, recommend a different emphasis among chapters, and assess other areas important to the publisher. These expert reviewers do not conduct a peer review of the rigor of the content. Lang (2010) indicated that academic institutions may not accept book chapters and books as evidence of scholarly achievement: first authored, original research papers published in peer-reviewed journals are the standard. New and tenure-track faculty members need to understand the types of dissemination important in these decisions in their school.

WRITING A BOOK

Nurses with experience writing journal articles will have a sense of the time commitment in writing a manuscript and following the paper through to publication.

Yet, a journal manuscript compared with a book takes a short time. A major consideration before embarking on a book is this time commitment: books without contributed chapters can easily take one year or more to complete. Experienced authors will have an idea of how to approach a large writing project such as a book, their writing style and process established, and contacts with other experts who might contribute chapters to the book if it is an edited work. Nevertheless, writing a book requires an extensive time commitment that authors should weigh against their other responsibilities.

Some questions potential book authors should answer for themselves when deciding if they want to write a book are:

- Is there a clear need for the book, and who might read it?
- What content would be in the book?
- Is there sufficient content for a book length manuscript, which might be 450 pages or more? When considering that a journal article is often restricted to about 18 manuscript pages, the magnitude of writing a book becomes clear.
- Would the book be developed from chapters contributed by other authors or written by an author or coauthors?
- Are coauthors and contributors available, and what are their writing styles and habits, e.g., with submitting manuscripts on time?
- Are there administrative and other resources available to assist with contacting contributors, managing their submissions, and handling other details?
- If approached by a publisher to serve as an editor of a book, what resources and assistance will be provided by the publisher, for example, contacting potential chapter authors, consulting with them on their individual chapters, communicating with them, monitoring their progress, reviewing drafts, and editing the final versions of the chapters?
- Is time available in one's own work schedule and considering personal circumstances to write the book?
- What are the benefits personally and professionally for writing the book?
- What is the quality of the publisher?

Types of Books

There are different types of books that nurses might write. These include textbooks for students, which may be written for particular courses; resource books for nurses in clinical practice, teaching, administration, and other roles; handbooks and manuals, which present abbreviated versions of content and are practical such as a handbook on health assessment and manual on clinical nursing skills; case studies usually in a specific clinical area, such as critical care; and edited books that contain chapters written by different authors and are coordinated by an editor or editors. Some nurses also write novels, short stories, essays, and poetry for the general public.

Authored Versus Contributed Book

If thinking about writing a book, an early consideration is whether the author or coauthors will write all of the chapters themselves or if the book will be a contributed text. An authored book is one in which the author or coauthors assume full responsibility for the content of the text, writing each chapter in it, the front matter (beginning pages), and other parts of the book, and complete all of the related activities required for its publication. In a contributed book, in contrast, authors or coauthors write individual chapters under the guidance of an editor who assembles those chapters into a book. With a contributed text, the heading of each chapter includes the authors' names and sometimes credentials; their affiliations are listed usually in a contributors' page in the front matter. The editor's name, or names of multiple editors, is on the title page, and the book's cover would indicate the editor, but not the contributors.

A contributed book allows the editor to invite experts to prepare chapters in their area of specialization. The editor may not have a background in those topics, which are important for the book to meet reader needs. Editing a book requires less time than writing all of the chapters, but the editor is responsible for ensuring accuracy of content, a similar format for presenting the content across chapters, transition between chapters, and that the chapters as a whole contain the relevant information for the aims of the book. Issues with a contributed book are the different writing styles of chapter authors, varying levels of details and specificity with how authors develop their content, authors not adhering to the format for chapters, and authors not submitting their chapters on time, according to the due dates set by the editor. With some books, contributors are paid an honorarium, but with others, they are not compensated financially.

Initial Contact With Publisher

The idea for a book may be initiated by the author, often as a result of the author's inability to find a book for teaching a course or to meet a professional or personal need. Existing books in an area of specialization may be out-of-date or not available because of current advances in the field of practice. In those situations the author will approach different publishers to find one interested in publishing the work.

Alternately, authors with known expertise may be asked by a publisher to write a book. In this instance the publisher may not have a book in that content area to market to faculty for courses and for other readers. The publisher may be aware of the nurse's work based on journal articles and other publications or from suggestions of nurses and authors. Usually the acquisitions editor contacts the author to inquire about the author's interest.

Publishers include commercial firms that publish books in nursing, medicine, allied health, and other fields; organizations such as the American Nurses Association; and university presses. Commercial scholarly publishers such as Springer and Elsevier publish books for profit in nursing and other fields. Some commercial publishers focus on clinical nursing books and textbooks for undergraduate nursing students while others publish more specialized books with smaller markets. It is important for authors to explore publishers that have experience marketing to the audience of the book being considered. Some of the publishers have more experience with nursing books than do others, and authors should have this information at hand when deciding on which publisher to contact about their ideas.

Professional organizations such as the American Nurses Association have book publishing divisions. Often these books meet specific needs of the members of the organization and are marketed primarily to that group.

University presses are another type of publisher but do not commonly publish nursing books. They tend to publish books in the arts and humanities that have a regional focus and that are of interest to a wider audience than nurses or nursing students.

Large commercial publishers of fiction and nonfiction books for the general public are not likely to be interested in books aimed at nurses or nursing students. If a nurse is thinking about writing a novel or series of short stories, those publishers might be interested. Some authors also publish their own work, but some of the issues are a lack of technical assistance through the publication process, need for a printer, and how to advertise and market the book, among others. With self publishing the author absorbs all of the costs.

Prospectus

Whether the author approaches the publisher with an idea or is contacted by the acquisitions editor or another representative of the publisher, the process begins with a literature search and completion of a prospectus. The prospectus is the proposal or plan for the book, outlining its goals and how the author envisions the development of content.

Publishers have their own formats for preparing the prospectus, which generally include the following information:

- Purpose of the book and why it is needed
- List of chapters in the book and content of each
- Features of the book
- Contributors, if any, and chapters they will prepare
- Intended readers including the level of nursing students if it is a textbook
- Courses the book could be used in and other market considerations
- Competition including a review of every competing book on the market and statement as to why the proposed book would be better
- Timetable for its completion
- Size of the book including total number of pages, and
- Sample chapter.

Exhibit 9.1 is an example of a prospectus that authors would complete for a book.

Authors should contact a publisher first, and if there is interest in the proposal, then prepare a prospectus for that publisher. It is risky to begin writing the manuscript without a publisher in case none can be found. It may be that the market is too small, or there are too many books on the same content. While the topic may be important to the author, there may be minimal interest in it from the publisher's point of view. In other cases the publisher may be interested only if the focus changes considerably. For these reasons the author is advised to contact publishers before beginning to write.

EXHIBIT 9.1

Example of Book Prospectus

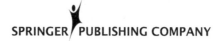

SPRINGER PUBLISHING COMPANY

11 W. 42nd Street
New York, NY 10036–8002
Tel: 212–431–4370
Fax: 212–941–7842
www.springerpub.com

Book Proposal Guidelines
Type your response in the area below each question.

Editorial Information

What is the tentative title of your book?

Who will be the authors and/or editors? Please provide a current CV or resume for each primary author/editor.

Will some chapters be contributed by others? If yes, please list those whom you plan to invite: include name, credentials, and affiliation for each within the table of contents.

Provide a description of the book's contents (3–4 paragraphs). Include what the book will contribute to the literature; its main themes and objectives; its distinctiveness in comparison to current competitor titles; and what pedagogical features it will include (e.g., if a textbook, will it include objectives, review questions, case studies, etc.).

What are the Key Features of this book? (Please provide a list of why people will buy this book in list format.)

Who is your book's intended audience? (Please list specific education, specialty, or practice areas and/or professional associations, as appropriate.)

If this is a textbook, please indicate whether it is intended for the undergraduate or graduate-level audience. Include a list of programs and course titles where the book should be considered for adoption. If enrollment numbers per program or course are available, please include them.

Table of Contents (Please provide an annotated list of sections and chapters, including authors per chapter, with degrees and affiliation for each.)

How long will the manuscript be? (Please include an estimate of the number of manuscript pages, illustrations, and photographs.)

What is your estimated completion date for the manuscript?

Continued

Exhibit 9.1 *Continued*

Marketing and Sales Information

Please list what you think are the Key Sales Features and Benefits. (List the kind of information that should be highlighted, for example, on the book's back cover as well in print and web advertisements for the book.)

Professional Associations to consider for marketing:

Journals that should receive copies for book review purposes:

What books provide the most direct competition to your book? (Your list should include author's last name, title of book, publisher and year of publication, price, length in pages, any special features such as DVD, Instructor's Resource Guide. Please note how your book is different or better.)

Reprinted by permission of Springer Publishing Company, 2009.

Responsibilities of Author and Publisher

The prospectus is then submitted to the publisher who reviews it and, if interested, sends the author a contract. The review of the prospectus may take from a few weeks to months depending on the publisher. It is likely that the prospectus will be sent to external reviewers for feedback as to whether the book should be published and suggested changes in content or focus.

The contract is a legal document outlining the responsibilities of the author, or editor if a contributed book, and the publisher. The author is responsible for preparing the book and submitting it on time. The publisher is responsible for getting the book into production, copyediting the manuscript, designing the book, carrying out other details to produce it, and marketing it. Details of the book such as its focus, due date, number of manuscript pages, and royalties are included commonly in book contracts; some of the details can be negotiated while others cannot. The contract will include information about transfer of copyright similar to a journal article. Authors should read the contract carefully and consult with experts if unsure about some aspect of it.

Once the contract is signed, publishers will provide authors with detailed information about how to prepare and submit the book manuscript. This information will include guidelines on the overall format of the book and individual chapters; details on the format of the pages such as size of the margins and spacing; use and preparation of displays, boxes, tables, figures, and illustrations; numbering and placement of those in the text; abbreviations and other style considerations; responsibilities for permissions; and format for submission of the final manuscript. The manuscript is likely to be submitted electronically and as a hard copy.

Authors are generally responsible for preparation of figures and any artwork included in their book. Similar to journals these need to be in a format ready for production, i.e., camera-ready. If the author intends on including multiple illustrations or artwork in the book, it would be good to discuss this with the publisher prior to signing the contract because the author may need assistance in developing them.

Authors who serve as editors of contributed books have added responsibilities to define the content and length of each chapter for contributors, develop schedules for submission, and make sure that contributors adhere to them. With some books contributed chapters may be peer reviewed to provide feedback on the quality of the content and its comprehensiveness; contributors would need to consent to revise their chapters based on that feedback. With a contributed book it is important that format and writing style are consistent across chapters. This may require rewriting by the editor.

Some publishers send the completed book manuscript for external review to identify omissions of content and possible redundancies. With journal manuscripts, authors typically do not receive copyedited pages to review but instead are sent the page proofs, with copyedits already included, to check prior to publication. The proofs are the pages as they will appear in the publication. For book manuscripts, however, authors receive the edited versions and page proofs to review. With contributed books, individual chapter authors may be asked to review the edited versions of their chapters and page proofs, or the editor may do this for all of the chapters in the book.

The publisher's responsibilities include copyediting the manuscript, designing the book, moving it through production, and marketing it. Authors may have different contacts with the publisher during this process, beginning with the acquisition editor who contacted the author about writing the book, reviewed the prospectus, and provided feedback on the book's contents. Once the contract has been signed, the author may interact with other editors such as the managing editor who will guide the author or editor in preparing the manuscript, answer questions, and ensure the book is ready for production.

When the book manuscript has been submitted, the publisher is responsible for copyediting it, developing the manuscript pages into proofs of the pages, and completing other details. Authors will review the edited pages, which include changes suggested by the copyeditor to improve understanding of the text, correct grammatical errors, and modify the text to adhere to the publisher's style. Except for style, other changes need to be read carefully and approved by the author: copyeditors will not have expertise in the content and may suggest revisions that change the intent of the text. Copyeditors also will include queries for the author to answer. While changes can be made in this phase of production, once the copyedited pages become page proofs, few corrections can be made. Exhibit 9.2 provides an example of a copyedited page, with the editing done using the track changes feature in Microsoft Word. Exhibit 9.3 shows the subsequent proof of that same page.

The other major responsibility of the publisher is marketing the book. At some point in the production phase, the author will be asked to complete a marketing questionnaire that provides detailed information to guide the publisher with these activities. An example of a marketing questionnaire is provided in Exhibit 9.4.

EXHIBIT 9.2

Sample Copyedited Page

Copyedited Page

<LRH>**Part I** Basic Concepts ~~of Evaluation and Measurement~~

<RRH>**Chapter 1** Assessment and the Educational Process

<CN>~~Chapter~~ 1

<CT>Assessment and the Educational Process

<tct>In all areas of nursing education and practice, the process of assessment is ~~an~~ important ~~process~~ for obtaining information ~~to make decisions~~ about student learning, to judge performance ~~and~~ determine competence to practice, and arrive at other decisions about students and nurses. Assessment is integral to monitoring the quality of educational and health care programs. By evaluating outcomes achieved by students, graduates, and patients, the effectiveness of programs can be measured and decisions can be made about needed improvements.

<p>Assessment provides a means of ensuring accountability for the quality of education and services provided. Nurses, like other health professionals, are accountable to their patients and society in general for meeting ~~their~~ patients' health needs. Along the same line, nurse educators are accountable for the quality of teaching provided to learners, outcomes achieved, and overall effectiveness of programs that prepare graduates to meet the health needs of society. Educational institutions also are accountable to their governing bodies and society in terms of educating graduates for present and future roles.

Process of Writing Books

The purpose of the book guides the depth and complexity of the content. Similar to other types of manuscripts, the author needs to keep the goals of the book and readers in mind when preparing the text. A book written for prelicensure nursing students will be more explanatory and may include multiple displays, tables, and summaries to guide their learning about the content than that same book written for readers who have a background in the content. Authors are experts in the content they are communicating to others but need to think about readers as novices and plan how best to explain the ideas to them.

Table 9.1 lists the typical parts of a book in their order. The content of the book was outlined in the prospectus, and the author can start by developing a more detailed outline for each of the chapters. This should be done before beginning to write because the author may identify gaps in or overlapping content once the chapters are planned in more detail. For contributed texts, editors should provide guidelines for writing each chapter, including the use of displays, boxes, learning activities for readers, and other strategies, and the topics to be included.

EXHIBIT 9.3

Proof of the Page

1

Assessment and the Educational Process

In all areas of nursing education and practice, the process of assessment is important for obtaining information about student learning, to judge performance and determine competence to practice, and to arrive at other decisions about students and nurses. Assessment is integral to monitoring the quality of educational and health care programs. By evaluating outcomes achieved by students, graduates, and patients, the effectiveness of programs can be measured and decisions can be made about needed improvements.

Assessment provides a means of ensuring accountability for the quality of education and services provided. Nurses, like other health professionals, are accountable to their patients and society in general for meeting patients' health needs. Along the same lines, nurse educators are accountable for the quality of teaching provided to learners, outcomes achieved, and overall effectiveness of programs that prepare graduates to meet the health needs of society. Educational institutions also are accountable to their governing bodies and society in terms of educating graduates for present and future roles. Through assessment, nursing faculty members and other health professionals can collect information for evaluating the quality of their teaching and programs as well as documenting outcomes for others to review. All educators,

From: Oermann, M. H., & Gaberson, K. (2009). *Evaluation and testing in nursing education* (3ʳᵈ ed.). New York: Springer Publishing Company, p. 3. Reprinted by permission of Springer Publishing Company, 2009.

EXHIBIT 9.4

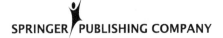

SPRINGER PUBLISHING COMPANY

11 W. 42nd Street
New York, NY 10036–8002
Tel: 212–431–4370
Fax: 212–941–7842
www.springerpub.com

Marketing & Sales Author Questionnaire

Type or paste text in the gray areas below each question; each gray field will automatically expand to accommodate your response. Please return this form to: marketing@springerpub.com

General Information

Date:

Title:

Subtitle:

Publication Date:

Author's or Editor's name(s), degree(s) and affiliation(s) as it should appear in promotional material (List all authors/editors appearing on the book's cover).

Corresponding author's mailing address, telephone, fax, and e-mail:

Description of Book's Contents Your answers to the following three questions will be used as a starting point for the printed and web-based promotional material we prepare, as well as for the copy that appears on the back cover of your book. Write descriptions that sell the book to its intended audience.

1. Please describe the major focus and intent of the book. List the major ideas, points of view, and research findings and practical applications.
2. What are the most important sales features? List in descending order of importance in bullet-point format.
3. What books provide the most direct competition for your book? (Please also include a brief description of what makes your book different or better.)

Author(s)	Title	Publisher

1.

How is your book different?

2.

How is your book different/better?

3.

How is your book different/better?

4.

How is your book different/better?

5.

How is your book different/better?

Marketing & Sales

4. A major portion of our promotional efforts are direct mail flyers, other printed material, and email campaigns. Please list the groups of professionals to whom we should send mail.

5. Do you have a mailing list or an e-mail list of colleagues or other professionals who can be used for the promotion?

   ☐ Yes (if "yes" please send us a copy via mail or e-mail) ☐ No

6. List the professional associations whose membership lists may be useful for us to consider when sending direct mail promotion; if you hold current or past positions within these associations, e.g., book review editor, current president, past president, or board member, please also provide us with this information.

7. If your book is primarily a textbook, please provide a list the titles of sample course titles for which the book might be adopted.

8. If possible, please provide names, snail-mail, and e-mail addresses of 10 colleagues whose influence over course adoptions would merit their receiving information about your newly published book (attach as a separate page).

9. Please list the professional meetings (both major and minor) where your book should be displayed. If you are a presenter, please also provide us with the dates and locations of the events, and a contact name and information with whom we can work to coordinate the display and sale of your book.

   Name of Meeting   Next Meeting Date   I Will Attend/Contact

10. Special Sales: In addition to individual professionals and students, we may be able to sell your book in quantity through non-traditional venues,

Continued

Exhibit 9.4   *Continued*

such as to workshops, training programs, societies, government agencies, manufacturing or pharmaceutical companies. If these or other special sales opportunities might be viable, please list them below.

11. Web site Addresses: Please list all of the website addresses (URLs) for websites you maintain or contribute to, as well as URLs of videos, blogs, or any other online content. (We would like to link to these as "related content: from your springerpub.com book page.)

Review Copies

12. List the journals that should receive copies for book review purposes. (We customarily send books to the major journals in the field; please list other specialty journals relevant to the book's content.)
13. If there is an alumni publication or employer newsletter that should receive a review copy or other announcement for the book, please list the publication or newsletter title(s) and provide contact information:

Endorsements

14. If your book contains a foreword written as an endorsement for the book, please provide a quote or quotes that you think would be appropriate for promotional purposes:
15. Please provide a list (including contact information) of ideas for people who could provide marketing endorsements for the book. We will contact these individuals, offer to send them page proofs for use in writing their endorsement and ask their permission to quote their endorsement in promotional materials.

Reprinted by permission of Springer Publishing Company, 2009.

Authors should receive the prospectus and outlines of their chapter and others in the book to better understand how their chapter fits into the book as a whole. It also is important in a contributed book for the editor to develop a realistic timetable for chapter authors to follow, requirements of each chapter, and information about the writing style (Chambers, Wakley, Nineham, Moxon, & Topham, 2006).

The process for writing a book is no different than other manuscripts except for the length of the project and the need to stay on a strict time frame. When writing a book, the author must keep to deadlines and persevere or the book will never be completed. Techniques discussed in other chapters on preparing to write, organizing the writing project, and working with groups are important when writing a book. The author needs to view the writing project as a series of smaller "assignments" each with their own due dates for completion (Oermann, 1999). For large writing projects deadlines must be met because lost

TABLE 9.1

Typical Book Contents Submitted by Author

Part	Content
Front Matter	Title page with the book title and authors' names, credentials, and affiliations. There may be a half-title page (prepared by the publisher) with the book title only that precedes the title page.
	Copyright page including the copyright date, International Standard Book Number (ISBN), edition, and other publication data.
	Dedication.
	Contributors (author names, credentials, and affiliations).
	Table of contents.
	Foreword (statement by an expert, not the author or editor, about the book and its relevance).
	Preface (discussion by the author or editor about the content of the book often with a summary of each chapter, how the book can be used, and intended readers). In some books the preface serves as an introduction.
	Acknowledgements (this page might be earlier in the front matter following the dedication).
Text	Chapters of the book. They may be grouped into sections or parts, each with its own title. References are included at the end of each chapter. Displays, boxes, tables, figures, and other illustrations follow and are labeled with the chapter number and number representing the order in which each one was cited in the chapter.
Back Matter	Appendices.
	Glossary if relevant (definition of terms in the book).
	Bibliography (may be included in addition to the references with each chapter).
	Index (prepared when the book is completed). Although authors can index the text themselves, it is usually done by the publisher or indexer.

time is difficult if not impossible to make up. Exhibit 9.5 provides tips for completing chapters, books, and other writing projects that extend over a period of time.

WRITING A BOOK CHAPTER

The process of writing a book chapter is the same as journal articles although with chapters the author typically has more pages allowed; chapters might be from 30 to 50 manuscript pages depending on the book length and other chapters in it. With these additional pages, authors have an opportunity to explain their

EXHIBIT 9.5

Tips for Completing Books

Work on one chapter at a time

Develop an outline of topics to be covered in the chapter

Divide the topics into smaller, manageable parts

Treat each part as a separate writing project and assign a realistic due date to each part

Keep a running list of related activities that need to be completed for each chapter in the book; assign due dates to these

Keep the due dates in a prominent place

Finish a chapter in its entirety before beginning the next one

Find your prime time for writing and use it for *writing the book*

Use other times of day for completing related activities, such as, writing for permissions and checking references

Be persistent—complete on time each separate project that you identified for completing the book

Adapted from Oermann, M. H. (1999). Extensive writing projects: Tips for completing them on time. *Nurse Author & Editor, 9*(1), 8–10.

topics more thoroughly and develop the content in more depth. This is essential for chapters in textbooks, which are primary sources of information for learning about a topic. Because chapters in a book meet a particular goal, chapter authors are guided by the editor as to content to include, format of the chapter, displays and other materials to include, and other requirements. Chapter authors need to be committed to preparing the chapter as specified and meeting the editor's due dates.

Although chapters are not considered as evidence of scholarship in some schools of nursing, depending on the tenure and promotion criteria, writing a chapter in a leading book may be advantageous to the nurse's career. Writing a chapter is a way of getting one's name known (Fraser, 2008). It also provides a way of becoming immersed in a content area and developing expertise in it. Lang (2010) suggested too that the chapter author can continue the association with the editor and other contributors if the book is revised over the years.

SUMMARY

Writing a book requires time and commitment: while experienced authors know how to write and may have contacts with experts who could contribute chapters to the book, nevertheless, preparing a book takes time. An early consideration is whether the author or coauthors will write all of the chapters themselves or if the book will be a contributed text. In a contributed book, authors or coauthors write individual chapters under the guidance of an editor who assembles those chapters into a book.

The idea for a book may be initiated by the author, often the result of the author's inability to find a book for teaching a course or to meet a professional or personal need. Or, authors with known expertise may be asked by a publisher to write a book. Usually the acquisitions editor contacts the author to inquire about the author's interest. Publishers include commercial firms that publish books in nursing, medicine, allied health, and other fields; organizations such as the American Nurses Association; and university presses.

Whether the author approaches the publisher with an idea or is contacted by the publisher to write a book, the process begins with a literature search and completion of a prospectus. The prospectus is the proposal for the book outlining its goals and how the author envisions the development of content. Typical content in the prospectus was discussed in the chapter. The prospectus is then sent to the publisher who reviews it and if interested, sends the author a contract. The contract is a legal document outlining the responsibilities of the author, or editor if a contributed book, and the publisher.

The author is responsible for preparing the book according to the format of the publisher and submitting it on time. Editors of contributed books have added responsibilities to define the content and length of each chapter for contributors, develop schedules for submission, and make sure that contributors adhere to them. The publisher is responsible for getting the book into production, copy-editing the manuscript, designing the book, carrying out other details to produce it, and marketing it.

The process for writing a book is no different than other manuscripts except for the length of the project and the need to stay on a strict time frame. When writing a book, the author must keep to deadlines and persevere or the book will never be completed.

▦ REFERENCES

Chambers, R., Wakley, G., Nineham, G., Moxon, & Topham, M. (2006). *How to succeed in writing a book.* Oxford: Radcliffe Publishing.

Fraser, J. (2008). *How to publish in biomedicine: 500 tips for success.* Oxford: Radcliffe Publishing.

Lang, T. A. (2010). *How to write, publish, & present in the health sciences: A guide for clinicians and laboratory researchers.* Philadelphia: American College of Physicians.

Oermann, M. H. (1999). Extensive writing projects: Tips for completing them on time. *Nurse Author & Editor, 9*(1), 8–10.

THE WRITING PROCESS

10

WRITING PROCESS

At this point in the process of writing, the author has identified the type of manuscript, the purpose of the paper, potential journals, and the audience to which the paper will be geared. The author has obtained author guidelines from the target journal, has conducted or updated the literature review, has completed other preparations for writing, and is now ready to begin writing the manuscript.

Writing for publication involves an iterative process of both forward motion and retreat (Murray & Moore, 2006). The forward motion of engagement in writing is the creative and energized time when thoughts and words are flowing onto the page or computer screen. But good writing also includes a time of retreat, when the author takes a step back from the newly created article to review, revise, refine, and enhance the material (Murray & Moore). Both kinds of involvement with one's written work are important to produce the article that will meet the author's goals.

Chapter 10 focuses first on preliminary questions to ask before starting to write and on organizing the content into an outline. Next, the chapter describes how to write the first draft of the manuscript. Finally, the chapter describes the steps in revising the content and organization of the paper and then revising the writing structure and style. Some principles are provided for improving how the paper is written, although the chapter does not address all aspects of prose structure and style that are important in writing for publication.

PREPARING TO WRITE

Writing for publication requires careful planning, organization, and personal strategies to keep on target until the paper is completed. It cannot be done haphazardly. With an outline, even if brief, and materials assembled, the author can move quickly into writing the first draft. The author should plan on revising the first draft a number of times until satisfied with the final copy.

Before beginning the outline, the author completes other preparations to facilitate the writing process and eliminate unnecessary distractions. These preparations include reviewing the author guidelines for the journal to clarify the format and other requirements; gathering materials about the project, innovation, or practices described in the manuscript; and assembling analyses of data and other information about the research project. These preliminary activities are important to allow authors to focus on their writing once they begin rather than on time consuming, and sometimes distracting, tasks such as finding evidence needed to support ideas, locating statistical analyses of data, and checking references. The goal is to assemble all materials prior to writing the first draft.

The literature review should be available if references need to be checked during the writing phase. No writer, even an experienced one, can rely on memory to cite a reference in a manuscript. Authors even in high quality journals make too many errors in their reference lists. This can be avoided by carefully checking each reference when preparing the manuscript.

This is not the time to learn a new word processing or reference management program or how to develop tables, and so forth. When the author begins to write, all other necessary activities of this nature should have been done so the author is able to concentrate on preparing the first draft.

Review Purpose and Audience

Before writing the first draft, the author should spend time planning how to approach the topic. Reviewing the purpose of the manuscript is the first step in this planning. It is often helpful to record the purpose on a note card that is visible as a way of keeping the manuscript focused on this main point. The author should be able to track the main point from the beginning of the manuscript to the end.

The author should then think about the intended readers. What is their level of knowledge and expertise? Why is the article important to them? The intended readers, combined with the purpose of the manuscript, guide the author in writing the first draft. If the primary audience is nurses in the same specialty field or a related one, authors are essentially writing for their peers and therefore are able to use technical and highly specialized language in the writing. Examples from nursing practice and case studies that focus on nursing care would be easily understood by readers and therefore appropriate for inclusion in the manuscript.

The primary audience of other journals, though, may be readers from different disciplines. *The Joint Commission Journal on Quality Improvement* (Joint Commission Resources, 2009) is a journal that provides information on measuring, assessing, and improving the performance of healthcare organizations. When writing for this journal, authors would avoid using terms and examples unique to nursing and instead would write for understanding by any professional involved in measuring and improving performance.

Review Writing Style of Journal

In writing the manuscript, the author needs to use a writing style consistent with the journal. Journal editors will not send a manuscript for peer review if it does not conform to the conventional writing style of the journal. Journal readers will find it easiest to absorb the information in the article if the author has used a form of writing that readers expect. Before beginning the process of writing, it is helpful to read paragraphs from several articles published in the journal to become familiar with its conventional style.

Formal Writing Style

There are different ways of categorizing writing style. One way is to classify styles of writing as formal or informal. A formal style is expected in scientific and scholarly journals. Authors using a formal style may refer to themselves in the third person, as "the researchers" or "the authors". Many sentences may be constructed in the passive voice. An example of a clearly written introductory paragraph in the formal writing style follows:

> Genes are the basic physical and functional units of heredity, units that carry information from one generation to the next. The configuration of an individual person's genes (i.e. one's genotype) has been implicated in the natural history of physical illness and cognitive impairment. Genotype, which is present at birth, may express itself in illness and impairment only very late in life (Snowdon, 2001). Elders and their families who are concerned about a family history of specific health problems, or individual susceptibility to cognitive problems, may increasingly face the decision of whether to test for a specific gene profile. Unfortunately, most of the research to date examines whether clinical outcomes are worse in the presence of a specific gene. There is little research concerning implications of genotype for broader, non-clinical dimensions of quality of life. This article addresses the degree to which the presence of a widely discussed gene, APOE ε4, is associated with poor quality of life. (Hays, Burchett, Fillenbaum, & Blazer, 2004, p.247.)

Informal Writing Style

An informal writing style may use more active voice sentences. Typically, with a more informal style, personal pronouns such as "I" and "we" are used as subjects of sentences.

Similarly, informal writing style often uses the personal pronoun "you" to engage the reader in the topic and personalize the information. In the following example of an informal writing style, the personal pronoun "you" is used:

> *You* can help the patient break down his overall stress into separate concerns that can be addressed one at a time. *You* can also refer the patient to the nurse practitioner if needed.

Develop an Outline

An outline is a general plan of the content to be included in the manuscript and its organization (Davidhizar & Dowd, 2007). Outlines enable the author to specify content areas to include in the manuscript and decide how to organize these topics logically so the information is clear to readers. If the journal prescribes a basic structure for the type of article being drafted, the author can use the headings of that structure to frame the outline.

Some authors prefer not to develop an outline, but even experienced authors may drift in their writing and find near the end of a manuscript that certain content areas were omitted or that the organization was unclear. It is easier and quicker to revise an outline than a draft of an entire paper, so the time devoted to outlining is worth it in the long run.

The author should view the outline as a working document; the outline is not a final product but instead is a tool to aid writing the first draft. Some authors find it helpful before writing the draft to review the outline a few days after its initial development to assess if changes are needed and to add details to the content.

Advantages of Outlines

Oermann (2000) identified five advantages of outlining before starting to write the first draft. An outline:

- Provides a way of planning content to include in the manuscript and deciding how to organize it
- Suggests headings and subheadings that might be used with the manuscript
- Allows the author to focus on the content when writing the draft rather than how to organize it
- Keeps the author on target
- Assists the author in developing an argument to support a position in the manuscript.

Types of Outlines

Outlines may be formal or informal. A formal outline uses a standard format such as Roman numerals or decimals. Authors can prepare an outline themselves with Roman numerals or decimals, or can use the outline mode in the word processing program. For instance, Microsoft Word's outline view automatically formats the outline and assigns numbers. When changes are made in the level of the outline, the content is automatically renumbered. For some authors, though, it is easier to develop an outline themselves rather than use word processing software for this purpose.

Outlines can also take the form of matrices, spiderwebs, charts, or other graphics (Gallaudet University, 2009). Authors may try several formats to stimulate thinking and idea generation. There is no right or wrong type of outline. The best outline is the one that fits the material, encompasses a comprehensive scope for the manuscript, and constrains the authors from wandering away from its focus.

Outlines can grow and develop from many sources. Some authors jot notes as they read through the background literature and following conversations with colleagues; others keep diaries or record their thoughts digitally. These notes can then be transferred to sticky-notes or note cards for development or reorganization into an outline. Outlines for an article may be generated from interim material used for other purposes. Murray and Moore (2006) suggest that procedure guides, lectures notes, learning resource packets, and other material prepared for uses other than writing an article lend themselves naturally to an outline format.

How much detail to include in the outline depends on the author and what style best facilitates writing the manuscript. There is not one correct way to develop an outline. Every author should develop a style of outlining that best meets the need. For some authors, developing a detailed and formal outline is essential to stay on target and not have to think about how to structure the content. For these people outlining saves valuable time later when writing the first draft. For others, a brief list of topics to be covered in order in the manuscript is sufficient to guide writing. Regardless of the format, it can be valuable to use the same type of outlining for each writing project.

Examples of outlines are in Exhibits 10.1 and 10.2. Exhibit 10.1 shows an outline and subsequent text developed from that outline. Exhibit 10.2 is a sample outline for a research manuscript.

EXHIBIT 10.1

Sample Formal Outline and Article

Outline for Article: "Using Grand Rounds for Staff Development"

I. Grand rounds
  A. Types
    1. Observation and interview of patient or several patients on unit
    2. Web cast of grand rounds conducted elsewhere
    3. Multimedia program of grand rounds
  B. Uses
    1. Observe patient with specific condition
    2. Discuss assessment and analysis of data
    3. Propose interventions
    4. Examine issues in care
    5. Collaborate with others
    6. Keep nurses up-to-date
II. Delivery of grand rounds
  A. On Web
  B. Public access television
  A. Via intranet, independent study
  B. Videotape

Article: "Using Grand Rounds for Staff Development"

Grand rounds involve the observation and often interview of a patient or several patients in the clinical setting, a Web cast of grand rounds conducted elsewhere, or a multimedia program of the grand rounds. Grand rounds provide an opportunity for new graduates and experienced nurses to observe a patient with a specific condition, discuss assessment and interpretation of data, and propose interventions and changes in the plan of care. Rounds are valuable for examining issues facing patients, families, and communities, and exposing nurses and other providers to clinical

Continued

Exhibit 10.1 *Continued*

situations they may not have encountered in their own practices. Grand rounds may involve nursing staff only or be interdisciplinary.

Grand rounds that are offered on the Web or on public access television can be used to bring new information to nurses worldwide. For example, Public Health Grand Rounds is a series of Webcasts that present case studies on public health issues (North Carolina Institute for Public Health, 2009). Rounds delivered using this methodology can educate nurses across settings and geographic areas. Grand rounds can be done live in the classroom and delivered via the intranet. They can be videotaped and completed by nurses as independent study. Grand rounds are valuable for highlighting nurses' clinical expertise and promoting best practices (Iacono, 2008).

Techniques for Outlining

Before beginning the outline, the author should review quickly the materials gathered, making a list of relevant topics and notes on how the material might be grouped into topics and in what order. This gives the author a general sense of how the content will be organized.

If unsure how to organize the content, the author might record key content areas on separate index cards. This can be done as the author is reviewing the materials in preparation for beginning the manuscript. Each index card should have a major content area listed on it; these content areas represent the main topics to be covered in the manuscript. The author can then arrange the cards in a logical order, rearranging as needed until comfortable with the organization. Subtopics can be recorded with the relevant content area and then organized logically. This technique allows the author to easily change the outline until it represents the best order in the author's judgment.

Some authors may prefer to outline their ideas in a picture or map. A concept map is a graphic or pictorial arrangement of key concepts and their interrelationships. Concept maps facilitate and record the author's thinking that underlies the understanding of their topic (Hay, 2008). Mapping concepts visually helps authors connect key ideas together and organize them logically.

The shape of the related concepts is entirely dependent on the author's understanding, similar to the way an architect would draft or design plans for a building (Hay, 2008). After the ideas are written down, the author can order the ideas to guide their logical presentation in the article. The authors can use different shapes (circles, triangles, squares) connected or combined by different types of lines to depict different types of information and their interrelationship. The logical order of the information can flow from left to right or top to bottom. The author's ideas may lend themselves to a scene, e.g., an iceburg or forest, where elements of the picture are labeled. The important idea is for authors to get as much of the content of their ideas onto paper to gain perspective on its best organizational structure.

EXHIBIT 10.2

Outline for Research Manuscript

Introduction

  Extensive research on defining and measuring healthcare quality
  Limited attention to consumers' perspectives of quality care
  Purposes
    Identify importance to consumers of indicators of quality healthcare and nursing care
    Examine relationships of health status and demographic variables to consumer views

Methods

  Exploratory design
  239 consumers, convenience sample
  How selected (waiting rooms of clinics and neighborhoods)
  Instruments
    Quality Healthcare Questionnaire
    SF-36

Results

  Indicators of quality healthcare most important to consumers (Table 1)
  Indicators of quality nursing care most important to consumers (same table)
  Differences based on race/ethnicity, income, and educational level (Table 2)
  Correlations of indicator ratings and health status (SF-36) (Table 3)

Discussion

  Consistency of findings with other studies
  Important implications for teaching patients in clinics
  Limitations of design and sampling
  Next steps in research agenda

When the outline is complete, it should clearly show the main topic or content area. Identifying the main idea prominently helps keep the writing focused on the purpose of the manuscript. This is especially important when writing the first draft because the main point should be highlighted early in the introduction to the paper.

WRITING THE FIRST DRAFT

Each author develops a *way* of writing—what works best for them. With a well thought-out outline and materials available that might be needed during the writing, the author is ready to begin the draft. The draft can rarely be written all at one time. Instead the author should find the best time for writing and work on the draft over the next few weeks. The author should be careful not to extend the time for writing the draft for too long a period. When this happens, it is difficult to keep track of ideas and remain motivated about the writing project.

In preparing the first draft, the author should write as quickly as possible to get the ideas on paper. This forward momentum is intended to instill confidence and a feeling of productivity (Murray & Moore, 2006). There will be time in the future to be concerned about grammar, spelling, punctuation, and writing style. These will be revised later. The author may not feel ready to write, but it is important to begin (Murray & Moore). The goal with the first draft is to get the ideas on paper, using the outline for organizing them.

With the outline or concept map the author should be able to start at the beginning of the manuscript with the main idea and write through each section to the end. Content can be re-ordered if needed by modifying the outline. Some authors, though, do not write each section of the manuscript in order. With experience authors develop their own styles of writing and techniques for completing writing projects.

Drafting a Title and Abstract

A first draft of the title and abstract should accompany the first draft. The author may use these elements along with the outline to keep the draft focused as it is being written or may craft a title and abstract once the first draft is complete. Since the title conveys the purpose of the paper and the abstract includes the main ideas in each section of it, writing these first may help the author clarify the main points to be conveyed in the paper. As the first draft is revised and refined, it is likely that the title and abstract will also undergo some change.

Managing Reference Citations in the First Draft

The references used in the body of the first draft should conform to the format requirements of the target journal. Most journals use either name-year or citation sequence system.

In the name-year system, such as with the American Psychological Association (APA) (APA, 2009) reference format, the author's name and date of publication are cited in the paper. References are then organized alphabetically on the reference list. For example, a paper by Hays, Davis, and Miranda (2006) used the name-year format in their introduction, as follows:

> Environmental quality is one of 10 Leading Health Indicators of *Healthy People 2010* (U.S. Department of Health and Human Services, 2000).

In the citation-sequence system, references in the reference list are numbered in the order they first appear in the text instead of the author and date. If the example above had appeared in a journal requiring citation-sequence references, it would appear as:

Environmental quality is one of 10 Leading Health Indicators of *Healthy People 2010*.[1]

In the reference list at the end of the paper, number 1 refers to the reference to *Healthy People 2010* published in 2000. Only the number, though, is listed in the text of the paper.

Even if the target journal uses the citation-sequence system, the author's last name and date of the publication should be recorded in the drafts of the manuscript. The references can be numbered later. If numbers are assigned prior to the final copy, they will need to be changed every time content is shifted and a reference is added or deleted. To make it easier to correct the reference format with the final manuscript, the author can insert a symbol before each citation in the text and can use the "find" function in the word processing program. With this function the author can move quickly through the document to find the references and then replace them with a number.

If using a bibliographic management program, references are marked in the text and then converted to the proper reference format later. The author should learn how to use this software before writing the first draft.

Even though this is the first draft, authors should be careful about how they cite references to avoid errors. Sometimes in an effort to quickly write the first draft and get ideas expressed, authors make notations about references as a way of remembering to include them in the manuscript but later forget to check them for accuracy.

Producing the Draft

The medium for preparing the first draft depends on author preference. Most authors compose the draft directly on the computer although some people may prefer to write on paper first, then type it into an electronic file or have someone else type it. Regardless of the process used, each draft should be numbered and dated. This allows the author to refer back to earlier drafts. One easy way to number and date the drafts is by inserting this information in a header or footer; this is shown in Exhibit 10.3. Another way is to label the electronic file name with this information.

If writing alone and working from the beginning section to the end, pages can be numbered sequentially. However, some authors write sections in a different order from how they will eventually appear and in these instances, a system should be devised for numbering pages within each section. Otherwise the author may be faced with a situation in which pages were printed off from the computer for review, but it is unclear as to their order. If there are coauthors who are submitting drafts of sections to the primary author, a system should be devised for noting the name of the contributor, numbering and dating the draft, and numbering the pages of the contributed section.

Line Numbering and Exhibiting Revisions of Drafts

When writing in a group, and exchanging sections of the manuscript for critique, it is helpful to number the lines. The lines can be numbered automatically by the

EXHIBIT 10.3

Labeling Drafts

[Teaching Portfolio, 1ˢᵗ draft, 1/12/10]

Documenting the quality of teaching in the classroom, in clinical practice, and in the learning and simulation laboratories through student evaluations of teaching alone negates other sources of information about the teacher and the context within which the teaching has occurred. Teaching portfolios provide a solution to this issue because they allow faculty to compile materials that more fully represent the scope and quality of their instruction and supervision of students.

[Teaching Portfolio, 2ⁿᵈ draft, 3/5/10]

Teaching portfolios are being used more widely for documenting teaching effectiveness in nursing education programs. Promotion, tenure, reappointment, and merit decisions are based on an assessment of the quality of teaching, research, service, and clinical practice depending on the mission and purposes of the nursing program. Teaching portfolios allow faculty to compile materials that more fully represent the scope and quality of their instruction and supervision of students.

word processing program, which enables coauthors to communicate more easily where changes are needed. For example,

    245 The physical environment is a core element in the practice models of public
    246 health nursing pioneers such as Florence Nightingale (1960) and Lillian Wald
    247 (1915), in currant community health nursing assessment and intervention
    248 frameworks (Anderson & McFarlane, 2000), and in the standards mandated by
    249 professional nursing organizations (American Nurses Association, 1999)....

With line numbering an author can indicate that "current" in line 247 is misspelled.

Other word processing functions that can be used to show revisions of drafts are through annotations, inserting comments, and marking the revisions with different colors while editing. Manuscripts can then be sent electronically to coauthors indicating the queries and suggesting revisions in the draft with one of these techniques.

▩ PREPARING TO REVISE

After a period of active work on the first draft, the writing process includes a period of retreat from writing (Murray & Moore, 2006). There are three reasons to step back from the work accomplished. The first reason is to rest and relax. Even though writing can be exhilarating, authors may over time experience stress and frustration as part of the creative process. Stepping back from the first draft can be an antidote to those negative feelings. The second reason to retreat from writing is to seek the comments and views of others. In the pre-submission phase when the article is emerging, the perspectives of other like-minded colleagues serve as proxies for the eventual readers of the article. Chapter 3 discusses in more detail the structure and processes of writing in a group context. The third reason to retreat from active writing is to prepare for the active phase of revising the draft. A period of deliberate preparation to revise can make this phase more efficient and productive (Murray & Moore).

Putting the First Draft Aside

During the retreat phase of writing, Murray and Moore (2006) suggest practical guidelines for getting the most out of their retreat from writing:

- Make a complete break from your writing. Print out a copy of what has been written, read it through, and then store it out of sight with other resources being used to write.
- Schedule a start time for your revision. Plotting out the next writing phase on the calendar ensures that the break from writing will not entail some underlying anxiety about when the project will be re-engaged. Don't let too much time elapse before the next writing period. Negotiate with professional colleagues and personal contacts to identify the dedicated space on the calendar.
- Develop a prioritized to-do list for the draft revision. Decide what the most important or easiest steps will be to get back into active writing mode. Writing down the next steps ensures that the break from writing will not entail more anxiety about remembering what priorities were in the author's mind.
- Be active in an environment away from writing space. Select a non-sedentary activity that is at least moderately enjoyable to engage muscles not used in writing. Avoid taking a break that entails simply other desk-work.

Getting Feedback From Others

If the break from writing comes after the author completes the entire first draft of the manuscript, it can be sent to coauthors to read. Circulating the article to coauthors can also be delayed until after the author has revised the draft for content and organization, as described below. Colleagues who are experts in the content or the method described in the manuscript can also serve as reviewers of the content and organization of the paper. Feedback from collaborators, experts, and readers who represent a constituency for the final draft is an essential ingredient for the writing process.

As the author approaches the phase of writing when feedback from others is appropriate, the author may experience resistance to proceeding. The following observations may assist writers to overcome barriers to seeking feedback from others:

1. Feedback can only improve one's writing if the author requests it, but getting feedback does not entail losing control of one's writing.

2. Feedback can protect against unreliable or invalid information only if the author opens oneself to review by trusted others.
3. Feedback should be timed to arrive before the author is committed to a final product.
4. Feedback requests of others should be specific, i.e., to identify missing parts of the whole, to focus on a particular section, to serve as devil's advocate by saying "yes, but...", or to check grammar and punctuation.
5. Feedback requests should be contextualized, e.g., the author should communicate to those asked for feedback about what stage of writing the author is in, the reasons that the article was written, and whether the draft is responding to earlier feedback or not previously seen.
6. Feedback should be approached with calmness and objectivity (Murray & Moore, 2006).

Review by Coauthors

When to send the draft to coauthors is a decision of the first author or whoever is responsible for organizing the preparation of the manuscript. Usually, coauthors are asked to critique a second or subsequent draft of the manuscript rather than the first draft. The first draft may not contain the essential content, and the lead author may find in revising the draft that a reorganization of the content is warranted. However, it is best for coauthors to read an early draft after the content has been revised for accuracy and structure by the lead author. Coauthors have a variety of strengths and expertise such that comments from each may be focused on separate parts of the emerging article.

Drafts should be numbered, dated, and labeled with the co-author's name as a means of tracking revisions of the manuscript. If contributors are reading drafts of individual sections of the paper, this should be noted. As the lead author receives suggestions for revisions, these can be made in subsequent drafts. All versions of the manuscript should be kept by the lead author or individual organizing preparation of the paper in case authors need to refer later to them. The "reviewing toolbar" of word processing programs is useful for tracking changes and comments by coauthors in a digital format.

The final version of the paper must be read and approved by each co-author to meet the requirements for authorship as described in earlier chapters. A record of which coauthors have drafted or provided critical revisions of each draft is crucial for required documentation authorizing that authorship criteria have been met during the writing process.

Review by Colleagues

The author might ask colleagues who are not coauthors to review and critique the manuscript. Often colleagues can identify missing content, problems with the organization of the content, and areas in which the presentation of the information is unclear. Ideally, colleagues asked to critique the manuscript, at this point in the revision process, have some understanding of the content. The goal of this revision is to improve the content and its organization. The author can then acknowledge these individuals in the manuscript as long as they give written approval.

Anticipating the Revision Phase

During the period of rest from writing, the author may think of new ideas or possible improvements for the first draft. To provide a record of any thoughts related to the topic or written draft, the author should keep notepads or digital recorders handy for recording them. It is not important to evaluate the usefulness of these thoughts during this time. If they are stored securely for retrieval during the revision phase, the author is free to allow the mind and body to take a needed break from the active writing process.

▧ REVISING THE FIRST DRAFT

With the essential elements of the article arranged on the page into a preliminary logical order and with a period of retreat from the article, the author is ready to begin revising the first draft. The author should begin to revise based on the list of priorities developed at the end of the first phase of writing and any notes taken during the period of retreat. Some of the priorities may have changed, and ideas jotted down may be dismissed. However, these early changes allow the author to gain momentum for revising the draft.

   Authors will revise the content, organization, grammar and punctuation, and writing style of the first draft. Some authors may revise content and organization first, until they are satisfied that all elements are in their logical place, and then focus on elements of style and accuracy. Other authors will choose to proceed from first paragraph to last paragraph, revising all elements as they go. Still others will work from the "inside outwards", focusing first on the original material in the center of the article and then moving to "set up" that material well in the introduction and background section and "wrap up" the contributed material with the final section of the article. However, the following elements must be addressed before a final draft is complete.

Number of Drafts

There is no set number on how many drafts to write until satisfied with the finished product. Some authors need to revise their drafts more than others. In the first few drafts, authors should continue to focus on expressing the content clearly and thoroughly. Only when satisfied with the content should the author begin to revise grammar, punctuation, spelling, and writing style. The author should avoid trying to write a finished manuscript as a first draft and instead should focus on including the essential content. The key in writing the first and early drafts is to get the content on paper and organize it effectively. During the revising phase, the author engages in an iterative and interactive cycle of changes. Each article will emerge from its own pattern, and the author will develop increasingly comfortable patterns of writing, resting, seeking advice, incorporating the advice of others and authorial evaluations, resting, and so forth.

There comes a time, however, when the author needs to stop modifying the content, or the drafting phase will never end. "Perfection is the ideal, but an obstacle to done" (Williams, 2009, p.5).

Revising for Content and Organization

In revising the content and its organization, the authors become their own peer reviewer and editor. It is important to allow oneself to be receptive to criticism of own work; the author should view the draft as a "work in progress" that needs to be revised rather than as a finished product. Change is a key ingredient for growth and development, as an author and as a professional. If convinced of the perfection of a draft of the article, the author may be unwilling to make changes that are essential to improve it. Authors must always keep in mind that the ultimate goal of the article is to communicate to the readers, whose needs guide all changes and improvements.

The principles described earlier for preparing each section of the manuscript may be used as a framework for revising the first and later drafts in terms of content and organization. Exhibit 10.4 provides a list of questions the author can use to revise the paper.

Review Title

If the author developed a working title, this can be reviewed first. The title should capture the purpose of the manuscript and, for research manuscripts, should indicate the objective of the study, which may have shifted in focus over multiple drafts.

EXHIBIT 10.4

Revising Content and Organization: Questions to Ask

Title

Does the title communicate the purpose of the manuscript?
Is the title informative?
Is it accurate?
Is the title too long? If so, what words can be omitted?

Abstract

Does the abstract summarize the most important content in the paper?
Does the abstract of a research manuscript describe the background, purpose, methods, results, and conclusions of the study, within the length allowed?

Text

Is the purpose of the paper clear and introduced early in the discussion?

Does the introduction explain why the content is important to readers and how it will improve their knowledge or skill?

Can the main concepts expressed in the purpose be traced from the introduction to the end of the text?

Is important literature reviewed and synthesized?

Is the literature review relevant for the goals of the paper and journal?

Is the original contribution of the paper fully described?

Is the literature current?

Is any content missing?

Is there any content that is repetitive in the text?

What content can be omitted from the paper?

Is the content accurate?

Is the content sequenced clearly and logically?

Is it clear how the content may be used in the nurse's own work and setting?

References

Are all references essential?

Have any important references been omitted?

Are the references consistent with the citations in the paper?

Tables and Figures

Do tables and figures display specific data that supplement and support the text?

Are they consistent with the text?

Is each table and figure essential?

Headings and Subheadings

Are the headings and subheadings effective in organizing the content of the manuscript?

Are they substantive, informing readers of the content that follows?

Do they provide transition from one topic to the next?

Are the correct levels of headings and subheadings used to reflect the importance of the content area?

Are there at least two headings or subheadings grouped sequentially at each level employed in the paper?

Continued

Exhibit 10.4 *Continued*

Additional Questions for Research Manuscripts

Are the purposes of the study, research questions, and/or hypotheses stated clearly for readers?

Are the gaps in knowledge and limitations of prior studies emphasized to provide support for the current study?

Does the methods section adequately describe the study design, subjects, measures, procedures, and data analysis?

Does the results section present the findings of the study, addressing the original purposes of the research?

Are the main findings presented first?

Are the findings presented without discussion, which is provided in the subsequent section of the paper?

Are the results described accurately and precisely?

Are statistics reported correctly, using conventional format?

Does the discussion section interpret the results and explain what the findings mean in terms of the purpose of the study and how they advance previous studies?

Are inconsistencies with prior research addressed?

Are implications of the study discussed?

Regardless of when the title is prepared, following the final revision of the article, the author should critique the title to determine if revisions are needed in it.

Review Abstract

In reviewing the abstract the author examines if it adequately summarizes the purpose of the current draft and indicates the most important content within the length allowed by the journal. For research manuscripts the abstract should describe the key elements of the body of the article as ultimately developed.

Review Text

After critiquing the title and abstract, the author is then ready to review the text. First, the author should re-read the body of the article to determine if content is missing. It is helpful to read the draft as a whole without interruption. Sometimes identifying missing elements requires the fresh eyes of a coauthor or colleague. It may be that the outline was missing a section of content or in writing the paper, the author failed to elaborate sufficiently about a particular topic related to the central idea. The author may have made claims about the background issues that omit evidence from the literature. These gaps should be filled by appropriate references. Or, the author may have stated that there is one or more objectives for the article but neglected to describe the background for each of the concepts or population groups noted in the objectives. It is helpful to identify all of the nouns in the research questions or hypotheses or in each of the objectives to make certain that each has been addressed thoroughly in the article.

Second, the text should be reviewed to eliminate repetitive content and to assess if any content can be omitted considering the purpose of the paper. In writing the first draft authors often repeat ideas in different sections of the manuscript and frequently include more content than essential. Repetition should be avoided, and information not immediately relevant to the topic should be deleted. It is better to prepare a shorter manuscript that is focused than a longer one with content not essential to the goals of the paper. It may be that entire sections or paragraphs of the manuscript may be eliminated; in these instances the author should save the deleted content in a separate file in case it is needed later.

Because the author has devoted much time and effort to writing the first draft, it is sometimes difficult to delete content. The author, however, should be willing to make these changes to improve the manuscript and avoid having the material become distracting to the editor or peer reviewers during the submission process.

Third, once the author has revised the content of the draft, the next step is to assess its organization or structure. Although an outline was used for writing the draft, the content in the outline may not have been structured clearly, or the author may have strayed from the outline in writing the draft. The author also may find that the broad organization of content is consistent with the outline and is clear, but the content within each section of the paper needs reorganization. For research papers using the IMRAD format, the broad content areas are predetermined, but how the content is organized within each of these sections should be evaluated.

Some authors find that making a 'reverse outline' from the first draft can diagnose problems with the structure and organization of the article (Duke Writing Center, 2009). This strategy involves taking the first draft as the starting point and listing on a fresh piece of paper the concept or premise that is addressed in *each* of the paragraphs of the article. By examining the actual structure and organization of the ideas in the paper in this way, the author is frequently able to see where ideas were introduced too late or out of logical order for the reader.

Fourth, the accuracy of the paper should be reviewed. For research papers it is particularly important to check the accuracy of the data reported in the manuscript, statistical results, and conclusions reached from the findings. Each statement in the draft should be reread for accuracy and whether it is supported adequately by the discussion.

Fifth, the end of the manuscript should bring the ideas to a closing, summarizing the main points covered in the paper. The author should check that the manuscript does not end in mid-air without concluding remarks. New concepts should not be introduced at the end, and the author should be able to trace the development of the main points of the paper from the beginning through the end. A few sentences are usually sufficient to summarize the conclusions from the article and to prioritize the next steps based on its implications for practice, teaching, administration, and future research.

Review References

The author should remember that the literature review in a paper provides the background information for readers but is not intended to be an exhaustive review of every article on a topic. In reviewing the references, the author should ask whether they are essential to support the goals of the paper and consistent with the intended journal and readers. Unnecessary references should be omitted. When citing support for a statement, key references should be used rather than a long list of citations.

Review Tables and Figures

Consistent with eliminating unnecessary content and insuring accuracy, the author should review each table and figure to determine if it is essential to the paper and its content matches what is described in the text. Some tables may be omitted because they duplicate the content in the text. Sometimes new tables should be developed to replace material that became unwieldy as the text was revised. Tables and figures should supplement the text not duplicate it. This is a good time for the author to recheck numerical data in the table for accuracy and consistency with the information reported in the text.

Review Headings and Subheadings

Headings and subheadings emphasize for readers the content covered in each section of the manuscript. They give structure to the overall paper, provide transition from one topic to the next, inform readers of the content that follows, and suggest the importance of each subject area. By dividing the manuscript into sections, headings also make the paper more attractive visually (American Medical Association [AMA], 2007). The revision of the paper provides an opportunity for the author to add headings and subheadings to the manuscript if not done already or to review those written.

Headings and subheadings are often identified by using the outline developed for the manuscript but should conform to the best organizational structure for the final draft. Headings of the same "level" represent topics of equal importance (APA, 2009). For example, research papers following the IMRAD format include four predetermined Level 1 headings that are of equal importance (Introduction, Methods, Results, Discussion). The author may choose to insert subheadings within these general areas or may be required by convention to do so, as with the Level 2 subheadings of Methods (Design, Sample, Intervention, Measures, and Analysis). For non-research papers, the author should select headings and subheadings to organize the content and indicate for readers the topics that follow. The target journal prescribes the levels of headings and their formatting, and the author is advised to review sample articles in the journal to determine the levels typically included in its publications.

There is no correct number of headings to use in an article. Because headings are meant to subdivide material into multiple parts, there should be at least two headings at each level used. If two or more are not needed, then no headings at that level should be used.

Headings and subheadings can be short sentences, phrases, single words, or questions. Headings should not contain a single abbreviation, an abbreviation with its first explanation, a citing of figures or tables, or references (AMA, 2007). Exhibits 10.5 and 10.6 present two documents, the first without headings and the second with them. This table shows how headings improve readability and make the organization clearer for readers.

EXHIBIT 10.5

Sample Document Without Headings

An evidence-based approach to teaching in nursing begins with educators reflecting on their own teaching practices and questioning if there is a better way of helping staff learn. This is the crucial step because without raising questions, we continue to teach as it has "always been done."

Questions raised about educational practices lead to the second phase—searching the literature for research studies that might answer those questions, critically appraising those studies, and synthesizing the evidence. This requires ability to search databases for relevant studies, some background in research methodology to critique studies and make sense of the research evidence, and an understanding of strategies for rating the strength of the evidence.

The two databases most familiar to nurse educators are MEDLINE, the National Library of Medicine's bibliographic database covering nursing and other healthcare fields, and the Cumulative Index to Nursing and Allied Health Literature (CINAHL), the database covering nursing and allied health literature. These two databases are a good starting point for a search because educational studies in nursing and other health fields are indexed in them. For evidence to answer educational questions, though, the search might be extended to include the Education Resources Information Center (ERIC) and PsycINFO databases.

The third phase of adopting an evidence-based approach to teaching involves making a decision as to whether those findings are ready for implementation, based on the evidence, and if appropriate for own setting. Educators need to determine if the findings are relevant to *their* needs and environments.

Adapted from: Oermann, M. H. (2007). Approaches to gathering evidence for educational practices in nursing. *Journal of Continuing Education in Nursing, 38,* 251–252. Reprinted by permission of Slack Incorporated, 2009.

EXHIBIT 10.6

Sample Document With Headings

Question Educational Practices

An evidence-based approach to teaching in nursing begins with educators reflecting on their own teaching practices and questioning if there is a better way of helping staff learn. This is the crucial step because without raising questions, we continue to teach as it has "always been done."

Search for Evidence

Questions raised about educational practices lead to the second phase—searching the literature for research studies that might answer those questions, critically appraising those studies, and synthesizing the evidence. This requires ability to search databases for relevant studies, some background in research methodology to critique studies and make sense of the research evidence, and an understanding of strategies for rating the strength of the evidence.

The two databases most familiar to nurse educators are MEDLINE, the National Library of Medicine's bibliographic database covering nursing and other healthcare fields, and the Cumulative Index to Nursing and Allied Health Literature (CINAHL), the database covering nursing and allied health literature. These two databases are a good starting point for a search because educational studies in nursing and other health fields are indexed in them. For evidence to answer educational questions, though, the search might be extended to include the Education Resources Information Center (ERIC) and PsycINFO databases.

Decide on Relevance of Evidence

The third phase of adopting an evidence-based approach to teaching involves making a decision as to whether those findings are ready for implementation, based on the evidence, and if appropriate for own setting. Educators need to determine if the findings are relevant to *their* needs and environments.

Adapted from: Oermann, M. H. (2007). Approaches to gathering evidence for educational practices in nursing. *Journal of Continuing Education in Nursing, 38,* 251–252. Reprinted by permission of Slack Incorporated, 2009.

Guidelines for preparing the headings and subheadings are:

1. Develop substantive headings that inform readers of the content in the section that follows.
2. Write headings and subheadings as short sentences, phrases, single words, or questions.

3. Do not use a heading for the introduction because the first part of the manuscript is assumed to be the introductory section (APA, 2009).
4. Avoid having only one subsection in a section, similar to principles for outlining (AMA, 2007).
5. Follow the style manual or author guidelines for how to level the headings, how to position them in the manuscript, and other details for typing them.
6. Abbreviations should not be used in headings even if expanded earlier in the manuscript. Instead, the author should write out the term or phrase.
7. Subheadings within a section should have parallel grammatical structure.

Revising for Style

Publication of the manuscript depends more on the substantive content than on writing style, but poorly written papers may influence the critique by peer reviewers and the editor and ultimately the acceptance decision. If similar papers are under review, the one that is well written will more than likely be accepted. Poor writing structure and style also may result in the manuscript requiring extensive revisions prior to acceptance for publication. It is important, therefore, that the author carefully edit the manuscript so it is well written.

Writers do not intend to write without clarity and grace. Some bad writing occurs because the author does not understand the topic and adds words to mask the knowledge deficiency (Williams, 2009). Some writing is grammatically accurate but sounds jerky because authors write slowly and painstakingly to avoid breaking supposed rules of writing. Some writing is awkward because it represents a first attempt to mimic the style of a new and unfamiliar genre such as scientific writing. Whatever the reason for poor writing style, authors can improve their writing with attention and practice.

The following section provides a framework for revising the style of any draft of an article. The author revises for style only after being satisfied that the necessary content is in place and organized appropriately in major sections of the article. In other words, the content of the draft should be complete and accurate. Revising for style should be accomplished by focusing first on paragraphs and then on sentences and words (Figure 10.1). This system enables the author to edit broad elements of the paper first, then more specific ones. Otherwise, changes may be made in words, phrases, and sentences that need to be modified again when the paragraph is edited.

The discussion that follows is not intended to be an exhaustive list of points to consider when editing the draft to improve the writing. The discussion highlights

FIGURE 10.1

Scheme for Revising Writing Structure and Style

Check paragraphs ⟶ Check sentences ⟶ Check phrases ⟶ Check words some of the aspects the author checks when editing the writing structure and style.

In these revisions, the author should continue to keep earlier versions of the paper for referral later if needed. If the author is making one's own revisions, the manuscript may be modified easily on the computer. Alternately, some authors prefer to print hard copies and revise the prose on the hard copy so as not to be distracted by word processing. If revisions are made first on the hard copy, the author might use proofreading marks to indicate changes. Appendix 2 includes a list of proofreading marks and an example of their use in revising a draft.

Revising Paragraphs

One way to begin revising a first draft is to edit the paragraphs. In editing the paragraphs, the author should check the: (1) coherence, (2) length, (3) structure, and (4) transitions between paragraphs.

Coherence

Coherent paragraphs share a common theme and include all aspects of that theme and none from different themes. The subjects of all of the sentences in the paragraph are related to each other (Williams, 2009). At least one of those sentences—usually the first or the last sentence—explains to the reader the paragraph's basic claim. Sentences in coherent paragraphs "add up, the way all the pieces in a puzzle add up to the picture on the box" (Williams, 2009, p.60).

Length of Paragraphs

Long paragraphs often can be divided into two smaller ones by identifying breaks in the flow of ideas or how details might be grouped together into separate thematic paragraphs. For example, a lengthy paragraph on different addiction models might be divided into separate paragraphs, each describing one of the models. The initial paragraph in the sequence could specify the models discussed, listing them in the same order as explained in the paragraphs that follow. As a rule of thumb, paragraphs that extend beyond a single double-spaced page are too long and should be divided (APA, 2009).

Structure

In editing the paragraph structure, the author is concerned with the sequence of ideas. As noted earlier, the beginning sentence often explains the basic premise of the paragraph. The author should then confirm that there is a clear sequence of ideas developed from sentence to sentence through the paragraph. Authors can make their sentences flow more graceful by selecting subjects for each sentence that are related conceptually. Later in this chapter we will discuss ways to construct sentences in which the subjects are thematically related.

Authors can also use *metadiscourse* to guide the reader through the unfolding ideas in a paragraph. Metadiscourse includes all of the elements of writing that point not to the content of the article but rather to the writing itself, the readers, or the authors (Williams, 2009). For example, when constructing a paragraph, the author can alert the reader that a series of sub-themes will be presented in the writing by using terms noting seriation, e.g, "first," "second," "finally," to guide the reader through the paragraph. In a paragraph that begins, "There are two major principles in evaluating a burn wound," the reader expects the paragraph to cover these two principles, with a sentence that begin "First…" followed eventually by a sentence that begins with "Second…." These words do not concern the topic of the paragraph, which is the evaluation of burns. Rather, the words are used to inform the reader about how the writing of the paragraph is constructed, i.e., metadiscourse.

Transitions Between Paragraphs

To develop ideas in the paper, paragraphs need to be linked to one another. When the reader completes one paragraph and begins the following one, there should be a sense of moving to a new idea or different points about the topic. The first sentence of the new paragraph introduces the next theme to be discussed in the article and often echoes the preceding paragraph. Readers should be able to track the main idea from the beginning of the paper to the end by following the content from one paragraph to the next. Readers should not be disappointed to find a paragraph with a new theme that follows illogically from the preceding paragraph's theme.

To edit the transitions between paragraphs, the author should read the last sentence of a paragraph and first sentence of the next paragraph. The example in Exhibit 10.7 shows how paragraphs are connected so there is a transition between them and how ideas are developed by reading a sequence of paragraphs.

EXHIBIT 10.7

Sample Paragraphing with Transitions

Evaluation fulfills two major roles: formative and summative. Formative evaluation judges students' progress in meeting the objectives and developing competencies for practice. It occurs throughout the instructional process and provides feedback for determining where further learning is needed.

Considering that formative evaluation is diagnostic, it typically is not graded. Teachers should remember that the purpose of formative evaluation is to determine where further learning is needed.

Summative evaluation, on the other hand, is end-of-instruction evaluation designed to determine what the student has learned in the classroom, an online course, or clinical practice. Summative evaluation judges the quality of the student's achievement in the course, not the progress of the learner in meeting the objectives.

Adapted from: Oermann, M. H., & Gaberson, K. (2009). *Evaluation and testing in nursing education* (3rd ed.). New York: Springer, pp. 10–11.

Revising Sentences

Once the paragraphs in each section of the article are thematically coherent and flow logically from one to the next, the author focuses on improving each sentence within a paragraph. Below are several recommended strategies for constructing sentences that readers will find easy to understand.

Cohesion

Even when all of the sentences in a paragraph are focused on a single theme, sentences may need revision to insure that they link together as pairs, i.e., to insure cohesion. Williams (2009) makes two recommendations for constructing sentences that link together as puzzle pieces. First, authors should "begin sentences with information familiar to your readers" (p. 59), using a key word from the previous sentence or a word logically related to the topic of the previous sentence. Second, authors should "end sentences with information readers cannot predict" (p. 59), allowing readers to read each sentence from the familiar to the new, from easy to hard. Readers find material easy when the new sentence uses a word or two from the previous sentence.

For example, an article on environmental health (Hays, Davis & Miranda, 2006) included a paragraph that began by describing environmental health "mandates" and "action suggestions" developed by the American Nurses Association and the Institute on Medicine. The sentence that followed this description linked backwards to easily recognizable material before introducing new information, as follows: "In this context of **mandate** and **action**, two professional schools at Duke University collaborated to integrate environmental health science into the entry-level nursing curriculum" (p. 443).

Characters and Action

Put the main character and its action up front. "Begin your sentences with elements that are relatively short: a short introductory phrase and clause, followed by a short concrete subject, followed by a verb expressing a specific action" (Williams, 2009, p. 69). The early short phrase or clause frames the subject for the reader, who wants to know quickly the subject of the sentence and what the subject did to what or whom. These basic elements can be followed for several lines of additional details about the topic. The sentence above uses the short introductory phrase, "In this context of mandate and action." The two professional schools are the active agents. The action verb is "collaborated." The remainder of the sentence provided extensive information about where, what and who (the University, the scientific focus, the degree program.)

Active Versus Passive Voice

Write as many sentences as possible in the active voice, which is preferred by editors for brevity and clarity (Penrose & Katz, 2004; APA, 2009). The active voice states who or what the person is doing; the passive voice suggests that the subject is being acted upon. The active voice keeps readers' interest better than the passive voice (Williams, 2009). Here is an example of passive and active voices:

Passive voice: The clinical guidelines were developed by the interdisciplinary team.

Active voice: The interdisciplinary team developed the clinical guidelines.

Although the active voice is preferred, the passive voice may be more appropriate if the author does not know or the reader does not need to know who is responsible for the action.

Use of the First Person as Subject

Use first person pronouns sparingly to indicate actions that are unique to the writers (Williams, 2009). In the introduction to the article, the authors might state: "In this paper we will explain (or address, present, review)...." In the concluding sections, the authors might summarize as: "In this paper, we have developed (or argued)...." This is a second type of metadiscourse that helps the reader understand the content and follow its logic by using words that refer to the authors rather than to the content of the manuscript.

When referring to actions of a research team that includes others besides the writers, authors should use the third person plural. For example, state that the "Researchers recruited diabetic patients...." or "Interviewers implemented screening procedures..." rather than saying, "We recruited..." or "We implemented...."

Length of Sentences

Authors naturally vary the length of their sentences, and most fall between 15–30 words. Short sentences suggest urgency or certainty (Williams, 2009). Long sentences require particular attention to assure balance and rhythm.

Balanced Sentences

Construct sentences so that they are internally balanced using coordinating words, punctuation, transitional words, or parallel word forms. Coordinating words such as *and, or, nor, but* and *yet* contribute to internal balance between parts of a sentence. Punctuation such as semicolons between two or more related independent phrases indicate that these are generally balanced in importance. When transitional words are used, such as *although* or *since*, the sentence communicates to the reader the continuity of thought across a balanced sentence structure (APA, 2009). Parallel construction of verbs and nouns throughout the sentence also balances a sentence. Authors should check that parallel structure is used in sentences that contain a sequence of phrases or words.

In the following example, there is an unbalanced use of gerunds (ending in "–ing") and infinitives (beginning with "to") as direct objects; these are revised to use gerunds throughout the sentence.

Original: Benefits of simulations are learn*ing* how to use equipment, develop*ing* ability to perform a procedure, and *to practice* complex technological skills in a laboratory environment rather than with actual patients.

Revised for parallel structure: Benefits of simulations are learn*ing* how to use equipment, develop*ing* ability to perform a procedure, and *practicing* complex technological skills in a laboratory environment rather than with actual patients.

Sentences That Compare Elements

To avoid ambiguous and illogical comparisons, identify both elements in the comparison and use parallel construction for each element.

Ambiguous: "Previous research suggests that residents of public housing units are more disabled." (The reader is left wondering, more disabled than whom?)

Illogical: "Previous research suggests that residents of public housing units were more disabled than single-family dwellings." (Dwellings are not disabled; people are disabled.)

Correct: "Previous research suggests that residents of public housing units were more disabled than residents of single-family houses."

Mechanics of Sentence Construction

In this stage of revision, the author also ensures that each sentence is grammatically correct. One common problem with sentence mechanics includes *subject-verb agreement*. The sentence's subject must match in number to the form of the sentence's verb(s). Subject-verb pairs must be consistently singular or plural. Two common problems occur when using intervening words or nouns of foreign origin. For example,

The *number* (singular) of applicants to second degree nursing programs *rises* (singular) during periods of unemployment.

The *data* (plural) *show* (plural) a positive trend.

Another common problem is with *pronouns*. A pronoun must match in number and gender (masculine, feminine, neuter) the noun to which it refers earlier in the sentence. Pronouns used with present participles must be in the possessive form. Authors should check the antecedents of pronouns and when using pronouns make it clear to what word they are referring. For example:

Jones and Smith reported that patients learned effectively with videotapes. *They* were satisfied with the quality of the instruction.

In the second sentence it is not clear to whom "they" refers—is it Jones and Smith or the patients who were satisfied with the quality of the instruction? Ambiguity often results when sentences begin with "it" and "this," requiring readers to refer to the prior sentence. Authors are advised to check each pronoun for clarity.

A third common problem is with *modifiers and adverbs*. Authors should place each modifying phrase and adverb as close as possible to the word it modifies in the sentence and be certain that the sentence contains the word that an existing modifier is intended to describe. They also should check for misplaced modifiers. Often this problem can be avoided if the modifying word, phrase, or clause is placed close to the word it is modifying. In the first example, the modifier is misplaced; the patient has congestive heart failure not the nurse.

Original: The patient was transferred to the home health nurse with congestive heart failure.

Revision: The patient *with congestive heart failure* was transferred to the home health nurse.

Lastly, authors need to check that the *punctuation* is correct. Style manuals such as the APA (2009) and AMA (2007) include extensive instructions regarding punctuation of sentences in scientific writing. Two of the most commonly misused elements in sentence construction are the comma and the semicolon.

The semicolon is used in only two circumstances. First, use a semicolon to separate two independent clauses (that could otherwise stand alone as separate sentences) but which are thematically related and are not joined by a conjunction such as *and* or *but*. Second, use a semicolon to separate a series of three or more elements, any of which already contain commas.

The comma is more common but has related uses. Its first usage is to separate two independent clauses that are joined by a conjunction. A second usage is to separate a series of three or more elements that do not already contain commas. A third usage is to separate from the main part of the sentence any nonessential or nonrestrictive clause (one whose omission would leave intact the meaning of that sentence [APA, 2009]). Other uses are to separate the year in a date, the year in a reference citation, and groups of three digits in most numbers. Commas should NOT be used to separate essential clauses (whose omission would change the meaning of the sentence) or between two parts of a compound predicate (which could not stand alone as separate sentences).

Revising Words

When revising sentences, the author likely made numerous changes in the words used to describe ideas and connect sentences. The focus of this last phase of revising the manuscript is to examine the words used in each sentence, to insure that they convey the correct meaning and that the writing is clear, concise, and accurate. For some authors, reading the manuscript out loud helps identify where revisions are needed. Following are some recommended strategies for choosing words that readers will find easy to absorb.

Concision

Publishing is expensive, and the author should write as concisely as possible. Use of many words is not required to demonstrate a topic's importance. Authors should select only necessary and accurate words to express their ideas and eliminate all others.

Williams (2009) lists six types of words that should be deleted:

1. Words that mean little or nothing, e.g., *really, certain, various*
2. Words that repeat the meaning of other words, e.g., *each and every*
3. Words implied by other words, e.g., *basic fundamentals, large in size*
4. Phrases that could be expressed in a word, e.g., *if* rather than *in the event that*

5. Words in the affirmative that could replace a negative, *different* versus *not the same*
6. Useless adjectives and adverbs, e.g., *abstract idea, tried as much as possible*.

We applied these principles of concision to the following example:

Less concise: *In order to* evaluate neck masses, a thorough and complete examination of the head and neck region should be performed by the nurse practitioner *using a systematic process*.

"In order to" is an unnecessary phrase that can be omitted while still preserving the meaning of the sentence. Similarly, examinations are done systematically so the phrase "using a systematic process" is not needed. By eliminating unnecessary words in this sentence it reads:

More concise: To evaluate neck masses, the nurse practitioner should perform an examination of the head and neck regions.

Precision

The value of journal space also underlies the need to choose the most precise and complete information available to inform the reader. Sizes and amounts can be described in more and less precise ways. In general, "approximations weaken statements" in the scientific literature (APA, 2009, p.68).

Less precise: There was a *large* increase in the number of patients admitted to home care with the initiation of case management.

"Large" in this sentence is vague; it would be better to present the actual increase in numbers of patients admitted to home care within a particular time period.

More precise: Case management increased home care admissions by 35% over one year.

Words have precise meanings that communicate the same common understanding to all readers. Sometimes the meaning of simple words can confound the writer and confuse the reader as much or more than long unfamiliar words. Authors should check their manuscripts for some of the most common imprecise word usages. For example:

- among (for a group of three or more objects) versus between (for two objects):

  The work to be done was divided *among* the three nurse managers.

  The work to be done was divided *between* the nurse manager and the clinical coordinator.

- effect (noun) versus affect (verb):

  The *effects* of the intervention were decreased pain and improved coping.

  Patients were *affected* positively by the intervention, reporting decreased pain and improved coping.

- normal and abnormal; positive and negative (the findings and results of tests and examinations are normal, abnormal, positive, or negative, not the tests and examinations themselves):

  Incorrect: The physical examination given by the nurse practitioner was normal.

  Correct: The *findings* from the physical examination given by the nurse practitioner were normal.

▪ which (relative pronoun used to introduce a nonessential clause) versus that (relative pronoun used to introduce a necessary clause):

The patient should have a complete assessment, *which* is described in this article, when admitted to the hospital.

The author should check *that* the statistics are reported correctly.

Words to Avoid

There are a number of guidelines for word choice that will help readers engage with the text.

▪ Avoid abstract words. Authors may be tempted to use abstract words to make their writing seem more formal. This can be a mistake. Penrose and Rose (2004) note that abstract language often exhibits "false objectivity created by an inflated and vacuous style" (p.222). Abstract words are often verbs that have been turned into nouns, called *nominalizations* (Williams, 2009). Examples of nominalized verbs are: investigation, expansion, intention, decision, and many others. Use of nominalizations obscures both the actor and action taken.

Instead of using abstract nominalized words as the subject or object of a sentence, authors should ask two questions: (1) what is the underlying action verb? and (2) who is doing the action? Next, the author should construct a new sentence in which the actor serves as the subject and the previous nominalized verb serves as a true verb. Clearer and more concrete words (and sentences) emerge from this strategy. For example:

Abstract: A review of falls investigations in nursing homes was completed.

Concrete: We reviewed how investigators have studied falls in nursing homes.

Abstract: Understanding how nutrition problems impact overall health and mortality in late life has been limited by a lack of population-based samples and longitudinal designs.

Concrete: Researchers usually study late life nutrition using convenience samples and cross-sectional studies, which limits understanding of its impact on health and mortality.

▪ Avoid jargon, colloquialisms, and abbreviated terms such as "temp" and "lab." Jargon represents technical shorthand that is immediately understood by a limited group of people and, as such, will be exclusive of and grating to larger communities of discourse (APA, 2009). Jargon and other shorthand terminology can be used in the drafts of the paper as a way of capturing the ideas for the manuscript, but they need to be rewritten during the revision.

Original: The nurse *prepped* the patient for surgery after checking *lab* values.

Revised: The nurse *prepared* the patient for surgery after checking *laboratory* values.

▪ Avoid words that imply a bias for or against any group of persons. Historically, such groups have been distinguished by gender, sexual orientation, racial and ethnic identify, disability, and age (APA, 2009). The following guidelines may assist authors in revising specific words to avoid bias.

▪ Be as specific as possible about relevant characteristics. Instead of *elders,* refer to *persons 65–83 years of age.*

- Avoid labels and impersonal terminology. Instead of *depressives* or *diabetics* refer to *people with depressive disorder* or *patients with diabetes*.
- Acknowledge participation by using action verbs. Instead of "The survey was administered to students", state that "Students completed the survey" (APA, 2009, p.73).
- Use the plural form of nouns and verbs. For example:

  Original: The nurse begins health teaching when *she* completes the initial assessment of learning needs.

  Revised: Nurses begin health teaching when *they* complete the initial assessment of learning needs.

  Original: The patient should have an opportunity to choose *his* own treatment.

  Revised: Patients should have the opportunity to choose *their* own treatments.

- Select non-specific forms of words to avoid assumption of an unknown characteristic, for example, using committee chair or chairperson rather than chairman.

Mechanics of Word Choice

Rules and conventional uses of English grammar and scientific writing are myriad and complex. It is not possible to describe the universe of such conventions here. Three frequent stumbling blocks are described below because they are prevalent in formal writing.

- Check verb tense so it is consistent throughout the paper and the correct verb tense is used. The correct verb tense is needed so readers know when the action occurred. For instance, in the first statement below, the use of past tense indicates to the readers that the study was completed earlier and is presented for historical purposes.

  In 2005 Jones completed the first study that evaluated the effects of using a smartphone for teaching patients in clinics.

If the study by Jones remains important, the author might revise the sentence using the present perfect tense and delete the date:

  Jones has completed a study on evaluating the effects of using the computer for teaching patients in clinics.

In referring to current studies, present tense may be used:

  Smith reports that computers are effective for teaching patients in clinics.

- Check for spelling errors. The spell-checking function in word processing programs identifies misspelled words although medical and specialized terms often need to be checked by the author. The author also should be alert to words that are spelled correctly but misused in the sentence, for instance, principle versus principal. Only careful reading by the author, not the word processing program, will locate these errors.
- Check capitalization of proper nouns, names of organization and institutions, and others. Exhibit 10.8 is a checklist for authors to use in revising their drafts

EXHIBIT 10.8

Checklist for Revising Writing Structure and Style

Paragraphs

Ideas sequenced clearly through manuscript as a whole and in each section

Paragraphs focus on one topic and present details about it

Clear sequence of ideas developed within and between paragraphs, using sequencing terms as needed

Clear transitions between paragraphs

First sentence of paragraph introduces subject and provides transition from preceding paragraph

Paragraphs appropriate length

Sentences

Sentences clearly written and convey intended meaning

Characters and their actions are apparent in sentences

Sentences appropriate length

Variety in types of sentences and how they begin

Clear transitions between sentences within paragraphs

Subjects and verbs agree in each sentence

Comparisons specify all elements

First person used sparingly

Sentences are balanced by use of punctuation and coordinating, transitional, or parallel words

Words

Words express intended meaning and used correctly

Clear antecedents for pronouns

Information provided with maximum possible precision

No misplaced modifiers

Excessive and unnecessary words omitted

Stereotypes, abstractions, nominalizations, jargon, and abbreviated terms avoided

Active voice used

Throughout the manuscript

Grammar: Correct?

Punctuation: Correct?

Capitalization: Correct?

Spelling: Correct?

for writing structure and style. As mentioned earlier in the chapter, this discussion is not exhaustive of principles to consider in improving writing but highlights some important ones for the author to follow.

Revising for Scientific Style

Publications in nursing and healthcare often include abbreviations, symbols, measures, and other labels for presenting specialized content. Similar to formats for references, journalistic style is particular and dictated by the editor and publishers. This information may be provided in the journal guidelines, but usually the author refers to a style manual such as the *AMA Manual of Style: A Guide for Authors and Editors* (AMA, 2007) or the *Publication Manual of the American Psychological Association* (APA, 2009). In the revision of the manuscript, the author verifies the proper use of abbreviations, nomenclature, units of measure, numbers and percentages, and statistics. Exhibit 10.9 summarizes these principles in the form of a checklist for the author to use.

EXHIBIT 10.9

Checklist for Scientific Style

Abbreviations

Expanded first time cited in text followed by initials in parentheses
No abbreviations in title or abstract
No author-invented abbreviations

Nomenclature

Standard nomenclature used

Units of Measure

SI used for measurements except for temperature, blood pressure, and time

Numbers and Percentages

Figures used for numbers 10 and above
Figures used for statistics, fractions, decimals, and percentages
Words used for numbers below 10 except when grouped with numbers 10
    and above in same sentence
Words used for common fractions
Words used if sentence, title, or heading begins with number
Percentage used when specific number not included

Statistics

Statistical analysis and interpretations correct
Data in text consistent with tables and figures

Complete information reported with each statistic
Accepted abbreviations and symbols used
Statistics typed correctly

Abbreviations

An abbreviation is a shortened form of a word, such as U.S. for United States. An acronym is a word formed from the initial letters of words in a phrase, such as CINAHL, which stands for Cumulative Index to Nursing and Allied Health Literature. An acronym is pronounced as a word. An initialism is a name formed from the initials of an organization such as ANA for American Nurses Association (AMA, 1998). For the purposes of writing a manuscript, the author can think about these together, all representing a type of abbreviation in writing.

Most journals discourage abbreviations in manuscripts because abbreviations commonly used in one specialty in nursing may not be understood by readers with different clinical backgrounds and experiences. The exceptions though are standard and approved abbreviations, such as those found in a style manual, and when words are repeated throughout a manuscript, for example, using CINAHL rather than Cumulative Index to Nursing and Allied Health Literature.

When abbreviations are used, the author writes out the words the first time cited in the manuscript followed by the initials in parentheses. From that point on, the initials can be used alone. For instance,

> Length of stay (LOS) decreased from 4.0 to 2.5 days after implementation of the critical pathway. With improved medication management, LOS decreased by an additional 1.2 days.

Abbreviations, though, should not be used in the title or abstract (APA, 2009). The reader should understand words and phrases in the title and abstract without referring to the text. This is important particularly in bibliographic databases that contain abstracts of articles; the abstract should be clear to individuals searching the database.

In the first draft it is best to write out the words and avoid using abbreviations, then to add these during the revision. Otherwise, content might be reorganized altering the first time the abbreviation is used in the manuscript. It also allows the author to keep a draft without abbreviations in case this information is needed later.

Nomenclature

For clinical papers the author may need to refer to specific diseases, diagnostic tests, terminology, medications, and names for other entities. Nomenclature is the formulation of names to represent these entities. For example, the author might describe care of a patient with stage IV cancer, indicate that the patient had a grade 4 systolic murmur, report an Apgar score of 9 at 1 minute, and include the PO2 value in a manuscript. Some symbols may be used without expanding them the first time cited in the paper, such as PO2, while others should be written out the first time, such as positive end-expiratory pressure (PEEP). For medications, authors should use the nonproprietary (generic) name that is the official name of the drug (AMA, 2007). Authors are not expected to remember these rules and instead should write out the terms in the first draft, then in the revision refer to the style manual for how to correctly cite them in the paper.

Units of Measure

The International System of Units (SI) is considered the universal measurement standard, providing uniformity in expressing measurements (AMA, 2009). It is a refinement of the metric system. Non-SI units used in papers are measurements for temperature, blood pressure, and time. The requirements for metric style are well established, so authors should be careful to check the style manual to be consistent with it.

Numbers and Percentages

There are a number of style requirements when reporting numbers and percentages. A few are summarized here, but again the author is advised to check a style manual.

1. In general, use figures for numbers 10 and above, e.g., 30 years old, 10 cm wide, 15% of the group, and 207 participants.
2. Use words for numbers less than 10, e.g., Subjects completed five instruments.
3. However, for numbers below 10 that are grouped with numbers 10 and above in the same sentence or paragraph, use figures. For example:

    In 4 of the 27 patients, acute pain was reported.

    The children ranged in age from 2 to 11 years.

4. Use figures for statistics, fractions, decimals, and percentages, e.g., $P=.04$, 5½ days, 0.25, and less than 8%.
5. Use words for common fractions, e.g., one-fourth.
6. If a sentence, title, or heading begins with a number, use words to represent the number, e.g., Twenty-four of the patients were discharged within five days of admission.

Percent means by the hundred; the word *percent* and symbol % are used with a specific number (AMA, 2007). Percentage is used when a number is not included. For example:

Eighty percent of the nurses had high levels of job satisfaction.

Pain was reported by 25% of the patients.

Of the 120 patients, 62 (51.7%) had improved scores on the posttest.

Anxiety was reported by a small percentage of the nursing students.

Statistics

Reporting statistics in research papers was described in Chapter 6. In the revision of the paper, the author should check carefully that the statistical analysis is correct, the data in the text are consistent with the tables and figures, and complete information is included when reporting the statistics. What constitutes complete information depends on the statistic reported, and the author should consult a style manual or statistics book for direction.

In reporting statistics, accepted abbreviations and symbols must be used. Common ones are listed in Appendix 1. Many statistical abbreviations, such as SD for standard deviation, are not expanded the first time cited in the text. Others, though, such as ANOVA may be written out at the first mention in the text with the abbreviation in parentheses, depending on the style manual. The author should follow the guidelines specified in the style manual.

In checking the statistics, the author should:

1. Review the original statistical analysis to confirm that the statistics reported in the manuscript and interpretations are correct.
2. Compare the data and statistics reported in the text with the tables and figures.
3. Refer to the style manual or statistics book to ensure that complete information is presented with each statistic reported, the appropriate abbreviations and symbols are used, and they are typed properly.
4. Use the statistical term not the symbol when referring to a statistic in the narrative. For example, instead of "The M score was 125," the text should read, "The mean score was 125."
5. Use an uppercase and italicized N for the number of subjects in the total sample, e.g., $N = 206$. A lowercase n also in italics represents the number of subjects in a portion of the total sample, e.g., Group 1 included managers ($n = 32$) and staff ($n = 16$).

SUMMARY

Before beginning the first draft, the author completes preparations to facilitate the writing process and eliminate unnecessary distractions. These preparations include reviewing the author guidelines for the journal to clarify the format and other requirements; gathering materials about the project, innovation, or practices described in the manuscript, and assembling analyses of data and other information about the research project. The goal is to assemble all materials before writing the first draft.

After reviewing the purpose of the manuscript and intended audience, the author writes an outline, which is a general plan of the content to be included in the manuscript and its organization. Outlines may be formal, such as one developed using Roman numerals, or informal such as topics listed in order.

Using the outline, the author writes the first draft. The important principle here is to get the ideas on paper. This is not the time to be concerned about grammar, spelling, punctuation, and writing style—these are revised later. The goal with the first draft is to present the content following the format of the outline and in a logical order.

Between the first draft and subsequent revisions, the author plans a period of retreat from writing. In anticipation of retreating, the author re-reads the first draft, jots down any priorities for revision that come to mind, and schedules a firm time to begin the revision. Then, it is important to take a complete break from the manuscript, away from the desk, doing something physically active. If a first draft is circulated to colleagues or coauthors, the author should alert them to the stage of writing that has been achieved and what would be a helpful contribution from them. Any thoughts that occur to the author during the retreat period could be jotted on a notepad for later consideration.

The initial revisions of the draft focus on the content and how it is organized, not on grammar, punctuation, spelling, and writing style. There is no set number of revisions to make until satisfied with the content, although writing at least three drafts is likely.

If the author developed a working title, this can be reviewed first. In reviewing the abstract, the author examines if it adequately summarizes the purpose of the paper, indicating the most important content within the length allowed by the journal. For research manuscripts, the abstract should describe the study purpose and background, methods, findings, and conclusions.

In reviewing the main body of the paper, the author begins by reading the introductory section. The key is to assess if the introduction explains the content covered in the paper and its importance to readers. After critiquing the introduction, the author then is ready to review the rest of the text. The author should reread the draft to determine if content is missing, if content can be omitted, and if there is repetitive content; to assess the organization or structure of the paper; and to determine the accuracy of the content. Unnecessary references should be deleted at this stage, and each table and figure should be reviewed to determine if it is essential to the paper.

Headings and subheadings emphasize the content covered in each section of the manuscript. They indicate the organization of the manuscript, provide transition from one topic to the next, inform readers of the content that follows, and suggest the importance of each subject area. In the revision stage, the author has the opportunity to add headings and subheadings to the manuscript.

After the first draft is revised, the author continues revising the drafts until satisfied with the content and its organization. Usually, coauthors are asked to critique a second or subsequent draft of the manuscript rather than the first draft. The final version of the paper must be read and approved by each co-author to meet the requirements for authorship.

Publication of the manuscript depends more on the substantive content than on writing style, but poorly written papers may influence the critique by peer reviewers and the editor and, ultimately, the acceptance decision. Therefore, the author must carefully edit the manuscript so that it is well written. The author can begin by editing paragraphs, then move to revising sentences, phrases, and words. This system enables the author to edit broad elements of the paper first, and then move to specifics. In the revision of the manuscript, the author verifies the proper use of abbreviations, nomenclature, units of measure, numbers and percentages, and statistics.

The chapter discusses some of the aspects of writing for the author to check when editing the writing structure and style. It also emphasizes the importance of authors being cautious to give proper credit to their sources.

REFERENCES

American Medical Association (AMA). (2007). *AMA manual of style: A guide for authors and editors* (10th ed.). New York: Oxford University Press.

American Psychological Association (APA). (2009). *Publication manual of the American Psychological Association* (6th ed.). Washington DC: Author.

Davidhizar, R., & Dowd, S.B. (2007). The successful nurse scholar as interdisciplinary collaborator and leader. *Nurse Author & Editor 17,* 4.

Duke Writing Center. (2009, December 8). Reverse outlining [Handout]. Retrieved from uwp. duke.edu/wstudio/resources/handouts/WS%20Handouts/reverse_outline.pdf

Gallaudet University. (2009). *Mapping.* Retrieved from http://aaweb.gallaudet.edu/CLAST/Tutorial_and_Instructional_Programs/English_Works/Reading_%28ESL%29/Reading_and_Mapping_Strategies/Mapping.html

Hay, D. B. (2008). Developing dialogical concept mapping as e-learning technology. *British Journal of Educational Technology, 39*(6), 1057–1060.

Hays, J. C., Burchett, B. M., Fillenbaum, G. G., & Blazer, D. G. (2004). Is the APOE e4 allele a risk to person-environment fit? *Journal of Applied Gerontology, 23*(3), 247–265.

Hays, J. C., Davis, J. A., & Miranda, M. L. (2006). Incorporating a built environment module into an accelerated second-degree community health nursing course. *Public Health Nursing, 23,* 442–452.

Joint Commission Resources. (2009). *The Joint Commission Journal on Quality Improvement.* Retrieved from http://www.jcrinc.com/26813/newsletters/32/

Murray, R., & Moore, S. (2006). *The handbook of academic writing: A fresh approach.* New York: McGraw Hill.

Oermann, M. H. (2000). Refining outlining skills: Part 1: The topic or sentence method. *Nurse Author & Editor, 10*(2), 4, 7–8.

Williams, J. M. (2009). *Style: The basics of clarity and grace* (3rd ed.). New York: Pearson Longman.

11

REFERENCES

Most papers written for publication in nursing include references. The references in the manuscript document the literature reviewed by the author in preparation of the paper and provide support for the ideas in it. Chapter 4 discussed how to conduct and write a literature review for a manuscript. It described purposes of a literature review, bibliographic databases useful for literature reviews in nursing, selecting databases to use, search strategies, analyzing and synthesizing the literature, and writing the literature review. The outcome of chapter 4 was to develop skill in conducting literature reviews for writing papers in nursing.

In this chapter the focus is on citing the references in the manuscript and preparing the reference list. Journals have different reference formats, and the author must prepare the references according to the journal guidelines. Examples are provided of how to cite references in the text and on the reference list using the name-year system and citation-sequence system. The author will need to consult a style manual for more information about preparing different types of references using each of these systems.

REFERENCE STYLES

Journals differ in the styles they use for citations and references. Two of the reference styles used widely in nursing and healthcare journals are the name-year system and citation-sequence system. The name-year system, such as found in this book, uses the author surname and year of publication. The American Psychological Association (APA) publication style is based on this system.

The other reference format is the citation-sequence system. This reference style is included in the Uniform Requirements for Manuscripts Submitted to Biomedical Journals, adopted by many journals (International Committee of Medical Journal Editors [ICMJE], 2008). When submitting a manuscript to a journal that uses the Uniform Requirements, authors would follow those guidelines for preparing the manuscript including the references. Other journals use a similar style for citing and organizing references, such as the American Medical Association (AMA) style. There are many adaptations of both of these systems by journals: in preparing the citations in the text and the references, the author needs to follow carefully the information for authors' page or the style manual that the journal has adopted.

Citations are how the work is documented in the text. The citation informs the readers that the statement or idea in the text was developed by the author(s) cited. In some reference styles the citations are documented by author surname and year of publication, allowing readers to find the complete reference on the alphabetized list at the end of the manuscript. Other formats call for the citations to be noted by a number that corresponds to a publication on the reference list.

The reference list, at the end of the manuscript, provides the documentation of the publications reviewed by the author in preparation of the paper and the means for readers to retrieve them for their own work. A reference list cites the resources actually used in preparing the manuscript whereas a bibliography includes other publications and information related to the content of the paper. The bibliography provides additional readings about the topic not cited in the manuscript. Most journals require reference lists not bibliographies, although the author might prepare a bibliography for other types of writing projects.

References are placed at the end of the paper following the text and before the tables and figures. All references cited in the text must be on the reference list, and there can be no publications on the reference list that were not cited in the text. The author is responsible verifying this.

Because one of the purposes of the references is to allow others to retrieve them, information about each publication must be complete and accurate. Although there are numerous variations of reference formats, references to journals contain the following information:

- author(s) surname and initials
- year of publication
- title of article (and subtitle)
- name of journal
- volume number
- issue number if journal is paginated by issue, and
- inclusive page numbers.

For many reference styles, such as APA, the issue number is not included if pages are numbered consecutively across issues; however, other styles, such as AMA, require the issue number for all references to journals (AMA, 2007).

References to books contain the following information:

- author(s) surname and initials
- year of copyright
- book title (and subtitle)
- volume number and title if more than one volume
- edition number (other than first edition)
- place of publication
- name of publisher.

When referring to a chapter in a book, the reference also includes the:

- chapter author(s) surname and initials
- chapter title
- inclusive page numbers of the chapter.

There are specific formats for preparing references on articles in journals, books, book chapters, technical reports, proceedings of meetings and conferences, theses and doctoral dissertations, unpublished materials, online references, audiovisual media, and other sources of information. The author guidelines either provide examples of how to prepare each type of reference or indicate the reference style to be used for manuscript preparation. For instance, the author guidelines for *Western Journal of Nursing Research* direct authors to use the most recent edition of the APA *Publication Manual* and also to limit references for research reports to 40 citations, although review papers may include more. APA style is used by many nursing journals. Others use the citation-sequence system in which references are numbered consecutively in the order in which they appear in the text. For example, the *Journal of Nursing Administration, Journal of Nursing Care Quality,* and *Cancer Nursing,* among others, use the *AMA Manual of Style,* which is a citation-sequence system; text citations are numbered and the references are listed in numerical order.

Authors cannot assume that the reference style they used for writing papers in their nursing programs or with which they are familiar is the same one used by the journal for submission of the manuscript. It is critical for authors to prepare references according to the style specified by the journal (Oermann, 1999, 2010). If the manuscript is rejected and then sent to a different journal, the author is responsible for revising the citations and references to be consistent with that journal's style.

Name-Year System: Citations

In the name-year system, citations in the text include the surname of the author(s) and year of publication in parentheses. The author's name and publication date are placed next to the statement being referenced:

> Smith (2010) found a significant relationship between student stress in the clinical setting and performance.

> A significant relationship was found between student stress in the clinical setting and performance (Smith, 2010).

Once the reference is cited in a paragraph, subsequent references in that same paragraph do not have to include the date of publication. For example:

> Smith (2010) found a significant relationship between student stress in the clinical setting and performance. The higher the level of stress, the lower the performance ratings. Smith also found differences in student stress across clinical courses in the nursing program.

For publications by multiple authors, different principles are followed for citing author names in the text. When the publication has two authors, both names are included each time the reference is cited in the text:

> Smith and Jones (2010) found a significant relationship between student stress in the clinical setting and performance.

A significant relationship was found between student stress in the clinical setting and performance (Smith & Jones, 2010).

When there are three to five authors, the names of all the authors are included the first time the reference occurs in the text, but for subsequent citations only the name of the first author is included followed by "et al." and the year published (APA, 2009). For example:

Smith, Jones, Kaelig, Brown, and Dowd (2010) reported that…(first citation in text)

Smith et al. (2010) reported that…(subsequent citations).

For references with six or more authors, only the surname of the first author is cited followed by "et al." (APA, 2009). In using "et al" (which means "and others"), only the surname of the first author is included, without a comma after the name and with a period after "al."

If the citation refers to a specific part of the original work, such as a quotation or statement on a particular page, then the page number also is included in the citation. An example follows:

Patients described their conditions as living with a "time bomb with no possible way out" (Doe, 2010, p. 24).

Name-Year System: References

In the name-year system, the references are listed at the end of the manuscript in alphabetical order based on the surname of the first author. The year of publication, in parentheses, follows the last author name cited with the reference. When there is more than one reference by the same person(s), they are arranged by year of publication with the earliest listed first (APA, 2009). An example follows:

Basco, S., Gumbel, A. C., & Davies, R. (2007)

Jones, T. B. (2009)

Mathews, A. M. (2009)

Mathews, A. M., & Coleman, T. Z. (2010)

Smith, J. B. (2009)

Smith, J. B. (2010).

If there is more than one reference by an author, or by the same two or more authors in identical order, published in the same year, these would be arranged alphabetically by title (APA, 2009, p. 182). Lowercase letters are placed after the year of publication to differentiate the citations. For example:

Smith, J. B., & Thompson, M. (2010a). Behavioral…

Smith, J. B., & Thompson, M. (2010b). Stress…

The APA *Publication Manual* provides detailed information about preparing references using the name-year system. Some journals use a variation of this system by listing the references in alphabetical order and then numbering them. These numbers are used for the citations in the text rather than the name and year of publication. Exhibit 11.1 presents sample references prepared according to a few of the commonly used reference styles.

Citation-Sequence System: Citations

To improve uniformity across journals, the ICMJE developed the Uniform Requirements for Manuscripts Submitted to Biomedical Journals, which uses a citation-sequence style (ICMJE, 2008). The Uniform Requirements can be accessed from the ICMJE website at http://www.icmje.org/ and provide valuable guidelines for authors not only in citing references but also on ethical principles in the conduct and reporting of research and other aspects of writing. The Uniform Requirements are consistent with the National Library of Medicine's (NLM) recommendations for citing medical literature (Patrias, 2009). The AMA *Manual of Style* uses a citation-sequence system also based on the NLM's recommendations.

In the citation-sequence system, citations in the text, and in tables and figures, are placed in Arabic numerals and numbered consecutively. In the Uniform Requirements the numerals are placed in parentheses (ICMJE, 2008, p. 14). For example:

> Recently, these guidelines have been implemented in the emergency department and outpatient clinic.(1–4)

In the AMA *Manual of Style* superscripts are used instead of parentheses. For formats using superscripts, the superscript numeral is placed outside periods and commas and inside colons and semicolons (AMA, 2007, p. 43). When more than two references are cited, a hyphen is used to join the first and last number of the series. Two examples follow:

> Recently, these guidelines have been implemented in the emergency department and outpatient clinic.[1–4]

> The teacher can prepare different types of objective test items for the course[7]: true-false, multiple choice ....

One advantage of using the citation-sequence system is that the numbered citations do not interrupt the text and flow of ideas as sometimes occurs with the name-year system. A long list of references cited in a sentence may interfere with the ease of reading it and may affect remembering the preceding idea; at minimum it can be distracting.

Citation-Sequence System: References

In the citation-sequence system, references at the end of the manuscript are numbered consecutively in the order in which they are first cited in the text (AMA, 2007; ICMJE, 2008). Journal titles are abbreviated, and the year of publication follows the title, which differs from APA. Authors cannot shorten the titles themselves, and instead the titles of journals should be abbreviated according to the style used by the NLM (Lang, 2010). The list of journal title abbreviations can be accessed through PubMed by using the link to the Journals Database (http://www.ncbi.nlm.nih.gov/journals).

In preparing the draft, citations in the text should be indicated by the author's name and publication date rather than numbered. Otherwise, as revisions are made in the draft and references are reordered, these numbers will change. The citations should be numbered in the final version of the paper. Reference management software automatically renumbers the citations as changes are made in the paper.

EXHIBIT 11.1

Different References Styles With Examples of References to Journal Article and Book

American Psychological Association (APA) Style[1]

Patrician, P. A., & Brosch, L. (2009). Medication error reporting and the work environment in a military setting. *Journal of Nursing Care Quality, 24,* 277–286. doi:10.1097/NCQ.0b013e3181afa4cb

Oermann, M. H., & Gaberson, K. B. (2009). *Evaluation and testing in nursing education* (3rd ed.). New York: Springer.

American Medical Association (AMA) Style[2]

Patrician PA, Brosch L. Medication error reporting and the work environment in a military setting. *J Nurs Care Qual.* 2009;24(4):277–286.

Oermann MH, Gaberson KB. *Evaluation and testing in nursing education.* 3rd ed. New York: Springer; 2009.

Uniform Requirements for Manuscripts Submitted to Biomedical Journals Style[3]

Patrician PA, Brosch L. Medication error reporting and the work environment in a military setting. J Nurs Care Qual. 2009 Jan-Mar;24(4):277–86.

Oermann MH, Gaberson KB. Evaluation and testing in nursing education. 3rd ed. New York: Springer; 2009.

Chicago Style[4]

Patrician, Patricia A., and Laura R. Brosch. "Medication Error Reporting and the Work Environment in a Military Setting." *Journal of Nursing Care Quality* 24, no. 4 (2009): 277–86.

Oermann, Marilyn H., and Kathleen B. Gaberson. *Evaluation and Testing in Nursing Education.* 3rd ed. New York: Springer, 2009.

Modern Language Association (MLA) Style[5]

Patrician, Patricia A., and Laura R. Brosch. "Medication Error Reporting and the Work Environment in a Military Setting." *Journal of Nursing Care Quality* 24 (2009): 277-286.

Oermann, Marilyn H., and Kathleen B. Gaberson. *Evaluation and Testing in Nursing Education.* 3rd ed. New York: Springer, 2009.

---

[1]American Psychological Association (APA). (2009). *Publication manual of the American Psychological Association* (6th ed.). Washington, DC: APA.
[2]American Medical Association. (2007). *AMA manual of style: A guide for authors and editors* (10th ed.). New York: Oxford Press.
[3]Uniform Requirements format is based on NLM style. See: Patrias, K. (2009). *Citing medicine: The NLM style guide for authors, editors, and publishers* (2nd ed.). Bethesda, MD: National Library of Medicine. 2007 [updated 2009 Oct 21]. Retrieved from: http://www.nlm.nih.gov/citingmedicine
[4]*The Chicago Manual of Style* presents two documentation systems, the humanities style (using footnotes or endnotes and a bibliography that lists all of the works cited in the notes and others) and the author-date system. See: University of Chicago Press Staff. (Eds.). (2003). *The Chicago Manual of Style* (15th ed.). Chicago: The University of Chicago Press.
[5]Modern Language Association (MLA). (2009). *MLA Handbook for Writers of Research Papers* (7th ed.). New York: MLA.

The references for the following citation are prepared using the *AMA Manual of Style.* A few other examples are presented in Exhibit 11.1. Because there are many variations to the citation-sequence system, the author needs to follow the journal guidelines.

Citations

The decision-making process begins with identifying a clinical question to which the nurse needs more information, searching for evidence to answer that question, critiquing the evidence, and incorporating it into practice if warranted.[1,2] Clinical nurse specialists are well positioned to facilitate the use of evidence in practice.[3]

References

1. Oermann MH, Floyd JA, Galvin EA, Roop JC. Brief reports for disseminating systematic reviews to nurses. *Clin Nurse Spec*.2006;20(5):233–238.

2. Thompson C, Cullum N, McCaughan D, Sheldon T, Raynor P. Nurses, information use, and clinical decision making—the real world potential for evidence-based decisions in nursing. *Evid Based Nurs*.2004;7(3):68–72.

3. Hopp L. The role of systematic reviews in teaching evidence-based practice. *Clin Nurse Spec*.2009;23(6):321–322.

▓ ELECTRONIC REFERENCE FORMATS

The proliferation of electronic information resources continues, and authors need to follow the style manual for citing these references. Internet resources are prone to being moved and deleted, resulting in URLs in the reference lists that can no longer be accessed (APA, 2009). In a study of 573 Web citations in articles published in nursing journals, 414 (72.3%) were still available, but 159 (27.7%) of the references could not be found (Oermann, Nordstrom, Ineson, & Wilmes, 2008). Authors should be cautious about using Web sites as primary sources of information for manuscripts (Lang, 2010; Oermann et al., 2008).

Because of these problems with electronic information sources, publishers have starting assigning a digital object identifier (DOI) to journal articles and other bibliographic materials. A DOI is a unique alphanumeric string assigned to a digital object such as an electronic journal article or a book chapter (CrossRef, 2009). The DOI provides a persistent link to the digital content, allowing the material to be found no matter where it is on the Internet (Paskin, 2010). Once a DOI number is registered, it never changes. More information about the DOI system can be found at http://www.doi.org/. The DOI system is implemented through agencies such as CrossRef, which is a not-for-profit organization that provides citation linking services for publishers. The most recent edition of the APA *Publication Manual* includes the DOI with references to journal articles if one was assigned. For example:

Patrician, P. A., & Brosch, L. (2009). Medication error reporting and the work environment in a military setting. *Journal of Nursing Care Quality, 24*, 277–286. doi:10.1097/NCQ. 0b013e3181afa4cb

The DOI is generally located on the first page of the article, including papers published ahead of print and in the published version. The DOI is also listed on the article's database page (Exhibit 11.2).

EXHIBIT 11.2

Location of Digital Object Identifier for Article in MEDLINE Database

PMID — 19584755
OWN — NLM
STAT — In-Process
DA   — 20090916
IS   — 1550–5065 (Electronic)
VI   — 24
IP   — 4
DP   — 2009 Oct-Dec
TI   — Medication error reporting and the work environment in a military setting.
PG   — 277–86
AB   — This study examined nurses' reasons for medication errors, reasons for not reporting errors, and perceived unit-reporting practices. It compared nurses' anonymous reports of medication errors with those from institutional reporting mechanisms. Qualities of the work environment, staffing, and workload were evaluated to

determine associations with perceived error-reporting practices. The study findings have immediate applicability as a baseline for system improvements.

AD — School of Nursing, The University of Alabama at Birmingham, NB 324, 1530 Third Ave S, Birmingham, AL 35294, USA. ppatrici@ uab.edu
FAU — Patrician, Patricia A
AU — Patrician PA
FAU — Brosch, Laura R
AU — Brosch LR
LA — eng
PT — Journal Article
PT — Research Support, U.S. Gov't, Non-P.H.S.
PL — United States
TA — J Nurs Care Qual
JT — Journal of nursing care quality
JID — 9200672
SB — IM
SB — N
EDAT — 2009/07/09 09:00
MHDA — 2009/07/09 09:00
CRDT — 2009/07/09 09:00
AID — **10.1097/NCQ.0b013e3181afa4cb [doi]**
PST — ppublish
SO — J Nurs Care Qual. 2009 Oct-Dec;24(4):277–86.

Sayers, E. W., Barrett, T., Benson, D. A., Bolton, E., Bryant, S. H., et al. (2010). Database resources of the National Center for Biotechnology Information. *Nucleic Acids Research, 38*(Database issue), D5–16. Epub 2009 Nov 12.

In general, citations for Web documents and other electronic resources follow a format similar to that for print, with additional information about the location of the site (URL). For example, the citation for a document found at the Agency for Healthcare Research and Quality Web site using APA style is:

U.S. Department of Health and Human Services, Agency for Healthcare Research and Quality. (2008). *Treating Tobacco Use and Dependence: 2008 Update*. Retrieved from http://www. surgeongeneral.gov/tobacco/treating_tobacco_use08.pdf

In citing an entire Web site, rather than a specific document on it, it is usually sufficient to give the address of the site in the text without including a reference. For example, "The American Heart Association provides valuable information on how to maintain a healthy life style, cardiac diseases, early warning signs of heart attack and stroke, and children's health. This information can be found at http://www.americanheart.org." In this situation, the resource would not need to be included on the reference list.

The author should be aware of the type of information required for electronic references to ensure that information is recorded when the materials are accessed. In a search, the author can copy the URL and other information from the Web page that will be needed for the reference or can print the page. Because of the rapid changes on the Web, the author is cautioned to check the reference prior to submitting the paper to the journal and again when reviewing the page proofs to validate the URL and other information. To ensure that electronic resources, of which they are many types, are cited correctly, authors should follow the style manual used by the journal or the author guidelines.

▨ REFERENCE MANAGEMENT SOFTWARE

Reference management software, such as EndNote®, Reference Manager®, and ProCite®, allows authors to search online bibliographic databases, store records, organize references in a database, and create reference lists automatically. It also enables the author to format manuscripts complete with citations and references for hundreds of reference styles. If the author decides later to submit the manuscript to another publication, which uses a different reference style, the software automatically reformats the citations and references. This avoids retyping them. If using this software, the author needs to select the style that is required by the journal, making preparation easier of the citations and references.

▨ VERIFYING REFERENCES

Being careful to prepare accurate references cannot be overemphasized. Errors that can occur with reference lists are: (1) mistakes in the information provided in the reference, (2) errors in matching the citation with the correct reference, (3) not including all of the information needed with the reference, and (4) incorrect reference style. Authors can avoid these problems if they take time to review their references before submitting the manuscript (Oermann, 2010; Oermann, Mason, & Wilmes, 2002).

The author should verify the accuracy of each reference against the original document, paying particular attention to the spelling of authors' names, initials, order of names, title of the document and publication it is in, and publication data. Book titles should be taken from the title page rather than the cover.

In reviewing the paper, the author should check that each citation is placed properly in the text and that the name or number corresponds to the correct reference at the end of the manuscript. In the name-year system, the spelling of authors' names and the year of publication cited in the text should be identical to the reference list, and references should be alphabetized correctly. In the citation-sequence system, the author should check that the citation number in the text matches the correct reference on the list at the end of the paper. Once the information is verified, then the author can check that all of the data are included in the reference, depending on the style, and the reference format is correct. Exhibit 11.3 provides a checklist for verifying the references.

EXHIBIT 11.3

Checklist for Verifying References

Verify the Following Before Submitting a Manuscript:

Spelling of authors' names and year of publication in text with spelling and year in reference list, or

Number of citation in text with correct reference on reference list

Spelling of authors' names and accuracy of initials on reference list

Order of authors' names listed in reference and if all names included

Date of publication

Accuracy of title of document (e.g., title of article, chapter, report)

Accuracy of title of publication in which document appears (e.g., journal title, book title)

Abbreviation of journal title if relevant (using MEDLINE Journals Database)

Accuracy of volume number, issue number (if included with reference style), page numbers

Capitalization

Order of references

SUMMARY

Journals differ in the styles they use for citations and references. Citations are how the work is documented in the text. The citation informs the readers that the statement or idea in the text was developed by the author(s) cited. A reference list includes the resources actually used in preparing the manuscript whereas a bibliography provides additional readings about the topic not cited in the manuscript. Most journals require reference lists not bibliographies.

Two of the reference styles used widely in nursing and healthcare journals are the name-year system and citation-sequence system. In the name-year system, citations in the text include the author name and year of publication in parentheses. References are listed at the end of the manuscript in alphabetical order based on the surname of the first author.

In the citation-sequence system, citations in the text are placed in Arabic numerals (in parentheses or superscript) and numbered consecutively. References are listed and numbered at the end of the manuscript in the order they are first cited in the text. There are many adaptations of these systems by journals—authors need to follow carefully the journal guidelines or style manual adopted by the publication.

Authors make errors in their references that can be avoided by verifying the reference with the original document and matching the citations in the text with the reference list. In the name-year system the spelling of authors' names and the year of publication cited in the text should be identical to the reference list, and references should be alphabetized correctly. In the citation-sequence system, the author should check that the reference number cited in the text matches the correct reference at the end of the paper. Reference management software prevents some of these errors. With this software, authors can select the reference style required by the journal; the citations and references are then prepared according to this style.

▓ REFERENCES

American Medical Association. (2007). *AMA manual of style: A guide for authors and editors* (10th ed.). New York: Oxford Press.

American Psychological Association (APA). (2009). *Publication manual of the American Psychological Association* (6th ed.). Washington, DC: Author.

CrossRef.org. (2009). *FastFacts*. Retrieved from http://www.crossref. org/01company/16fastfacts.html

International Committee of Medical Journal Editors. (2008). *Uniform requirements for manuscripts submitted to biomedical journals: Writing and editing for biomedical publication*. Retrieved from http://www.icmje.org/urm_full.pdf

Lang, T. A. (2010). *How to write, publish, and present in the health sciences: A guide for clinicians and laboratory researchers*. Philadelphia: American College of Physicians.

Oermann, M. H. (1999). Writing for publication as an advanced practice nurse. *Nursing Connections, 12*(3), 5–13.

Oermann, M. H. (2010). Writing for publication in nursing: What every nurse educator needs to know. In L. Caputi (Ed.), *Teaching nursing: The art and science* (2nd ed., pp.). Glen Ellyn, IL: College of DuPage.

Oermann, M. H., Mason, N., Wilmes, N. A. (2002). Accuracy of references in general readership nursing journals. *Nurse Educator, 27,* 260–264.

Oermann, M. H., Nordstrom, C., Ineson, V., & Wilmes, N. A. (2008). Web citations in the nursing literature: How accurate are they? *Journal of Professional Nursing, 24,* 347–351. doi: 10.1016/j.profnurs.2007.12.004

Paskin, N. (2010). Digital Object Identifier (DOI®) System. In M. J. Bates & M. N. Maack (Eds.). *Encyclopedia of Library and Information Sciences* (3rd ed., pp. 1–7). London: Taylor & Francis. doi: 10.1081/E-ELIS3–120044418

Patrias, K. (2009). *Citing medicine: The NLM style guide for authors, editors, and publishers* (2nd ed.). Bethesda, MD: National Library of Medicine. 2007 [updated 2009 Oct 21]. Retrieved from: http://www.nlm.nih.gov/citingmedicine

12

TABLES AND FIGURES

Tables are essential when the author needs to report detailed information and numeric values. It is often clearer and more efficient to develop a table than to present the information in the text. Figures, such as graphs and charts, are valuable for demonstrating trends and patterns. For some manuscripts the author may even include an illustration of a new procedure or equipment, or a photograph of a patient. Not every manuscript, though, needs tables and figures, and whether to include them is a decision made during the drafting phase of writing the paper. This chapter provides guidelines for deciding when to prepare tables and figures and how to develop them.

■ NUMBER OF TABLES AND FIGURES

In writing the draft the author needs to know the maximum number of tables and figures allowed. With this information the author can avoid developing too many tables and figures for the length of the manuscript and specifications of the journal. It is helpful to prepare a draft of each table and figure as the manuscript is being written to confirm that the essential data are presented. The author can format these at a later point when the manuscript is revised.

Many journals limit the number, often to three, of tables and figures because of the space they require in the publication. Vintzileos and Ananth (2009) emphasized the need for authors to consider "editorial space" when planning tables and figures for a manuscript. If the author guidelines do not specify the limit for tables and figures, the author can review current issues of the journal for the typical number of tables and figures per article.

Tables and figures taken from journals and other copyrighted materials cannot be reproduced in a manuscript without written permission from the copyright holder, for example, the publisher of the journal or book where the original document was found. Permission to reuse published material can be obtained from the Copyright Clearance Center (http://www.copyright.com/), and many journal Web sites have links to facilitate this process. In addition to obtaining this permission, authors need to add a credit line at the bottom of the table or figure that indicates the original developer and copyright holder and that the material was "reprinted with permission." Authors need to consider if it is "worth the space" in the manuscript to reproduce tables and figures that readers can find elsewhere; instead, authors can refer readers to the original publication.

▨ TABLES

Tables are an effective way of presenting detailed and complex information succinctly and clearly. Tables should be used when the author wants to report exact values, present a large amount of information, display different quantitative values simultaneously, and show relationships among data. The table can be used to show patterns in the data, allowing the readers to compare findings side-by-side (Lang, 2010). For research articles tables are valuable for presenting the findings of the study with statistical results. In a table the author can compare groups and show how differences across the groups were analyzed with accompanying results.

The purpose of tables is to present detailed information that supplements the text and supports statements made in it but without duplicating it. In the text the author can discuss main findings from the table and highlight key points for readers to look for in the table. As an example, using the data from Exhibit 12.1, a statement in text might be:

Of the 150 registered nurses, the majority (122, 81.3%) were in classifications II and III (Table 1).

EXHIBIT 12.1

Presenting Information in Table and as Text: Text Preferred

As table:

Table 1
Classifications of Registered Nurses

Classification	*n* (%)
I	28 (18.7)
II	56 (37.3)
III	66 (44.0)

As text:

Of the 150 registered nurses, 28 (18.7%) were in classification I, 56 (37.3%) were in classification II, and the remaining nurses (*n*=66, 44.0%) were in classification III.

Additional information about the number of nurses in each classification is available in the table, which avoids duplicating the text.

While tables support the text, they should be clear enough to "stand alone." Sufficient information should be included in the table for readers to understand it without referring to the explanation in the text. The author should reread each table when the draft of the manuscript is completed to ensure that the tabled material is integrated into the text yet clear enough to be understood without reference to the text.

The data in tables should be accurate and consistent with the information reported in the text. To check this, the author can place each table next to the page(s) in the text where it is referenced and compare them for accuracy and consistency.

Types of Tables

There are two types of tables authors can include in a manuscript: a traditional table and tabulation. Boxes or textual tables can be developed for non-tabular material to supplement the text. These are discussed later in the chapter.

Table

A table contains information arranged in columns and rows. It is used to present quantitative data, statistical results, and detailed information. Most of the examples in this chapter are tables. Each table has a title, headings to explain the columns and rows, and lines that visually organize the data for the reader. Examples are provided in Exhibits 12.1 and 12.2.

EXHIBIT 12.2

Presenting Information in Table and as Text: Table Preferred

As table:

Table 1

Differences in Importance Ratings Between Men and Women

Importance Ratings	Men M (SD)	Women M (SD)	t
Able to ask nurse questions	4.13 (.83)	4.12 (.85)	0.07
Having nurse teach me about illness and treatments	4.58 (.81)	4.51 (.89)	0.61
Having nurse teach me self care after discharge	4.56 (.89)	3.91 (.98)	2.51*

*$p = .006$

As text:

There was no difference in the importance of being able to call a registered nurse (RN) with questions after the visit to the nurse-managed clinic between men ($M = 4.13$, $SD = .83$) and women ($M = 4.12$, $SD = .85$), $t(120) = 0.07$, $p = .47$. Teaching by the RN about the illness and treatments also was equally important to men ($M = 4.58$, $SD = .81$) and women ($M = 4.51, SD = .89$), $t(120) = 0.61$, $p = .27$. However, having an RN teach patients about self care at home was significantly more important to men ($M = 4.56$, $SD = .89$) than to women ($M = 3.91$, $SD = .98$, $t(120) = 2.51$, $p = .006$.

Tabulation

A tabulation is a short, informal table in the text that sets the content off from the text (American Medical Association [AMA], 2007). Tabulations usually contain only one or two columns that are not placed within a formal table structure and instead are developed as part of the text (Exhibit 12.3).

EXHIBIT 12.3

In-Text Tabulation

Nursing faculty reported the use of multiple strategies for assessing student performance in the clinical setting. As expected, the predominant method in all schools of nursing was observing students as they care for patients. The strategies used by educators in baccalaureate nursing programs were:

Observation of performance by faculty	114 (93%)
Written assignments	100 (82%)
Skills testing	79 (65%)
Contributions to clinical conferences	90 (74%)
Self-assessment	70 (57%)
Simulations	56 (46%)

In associate degree programs, some differences were found in assessment methods in clinical courses.

Use of Tables

In planning the manuscript, the author determines what information should be reported and then decides if this information is best communicated in a table or in the text. There are two general principles for using tables in a manuscript.

First, tables should not be used when the information can be reported in the text. Sometimes authors develop tables with information that could be presented easily in the text. When that is the case, tables should not be used. Readers may have difficulty following the data presented in a large number of tables and may lose track of the message (American Psychological Association [APA], 2009). Too many tables "break up" the text, and tables and figures are expensive to produce in a publication. For these reasons, tables should be used judiciously by authors.

An example of this principle can be seen in Exhibit 12.1. The information in the exhibit is presented in the form of a table and as text. As can be seen in this example, the information can be conveyed easily and concisely in the text, and for this reason, a table should not be developed.

Second, tables should be used when the author needs to report a large amount of data and exact numbers. Tables are an efficient way of presenting detailed information in a small amount of space and facilitating the comparison of information. In Exhibit 12.2 data are presented in two ways, as a table and in the text. In contrast to the previous example, these data are best reported in the form of a table. They

TABLE 12.1

Sample Correlations Table

Table 1

Correlations of Patient Satisfaction Scores With Health Status

SF-36	Medical Care	Patient Teaching	Provider Competence	Type of Provider	Nurse-Patient Interaction	Convenience of Appointments
Physical Functioning	.10	.42**	.23*	.11	-.24*	-.48**
Role Limitations (Physical)	-.22*	-.36**	-.04	.10	-.23*	-.24*
Pain	.08	-.09	-.03	.04	-.03	-.32**
Vitality	.12	-.06	-.04	.11	-.12	-.18*
Social Functioning	.09	-.06	-.03	-.02	-.14*	-.12
Role Limitations (Emotional)	.06	-.26*	.01	.04	.02	-.32**
Mental Health	.12	-.18*	.02	.01	-.26*	-.09
General Health	.25	-.47**	.23	.34**	-.12	-.46**

$*p < .05$ $**p < .01$

are too detailed for readers to follow in the text, limiting the ability to draw comparisons between the groups. Another example is Table 12.1. The correlations reported in this table are too extensive to include in the text, and the table provides a means for presenting all of the correlations, significant and not significant, in one place.

Guidelines for Constructing Tables

The content in tables should be arranged logically and presented clearly for readers to understand it and to locate specific data easily. In drafting the manuscript the author plans what information will be reported in the text and in tables. The next decision is how best to organize the information so it is clear to readers. The content is usually organized into columns (vertical) and rows (horizontal). Most tables are read first from left to right (horizontally), then from top to bottom (vertically) (AMA, 2007, p. 84). In deciding how to place data in a table, the author should keep this mind: the key information should be placed horizontally on the table. For example, if the table is intended to compare groups or make before and after comparisons, it should be constructed for readers to review the data horizontally across the table. In Exhibit 12.2 readers can compare scores for men and women on each of the three importance items by reading the scores horizontally across the table.

Tables contain five major parts: title, column headings, row headings, body of the table, and footnotes (Figure 12.1). This chapter provides general guidelines

FIGURE 12.1

Parts of Table

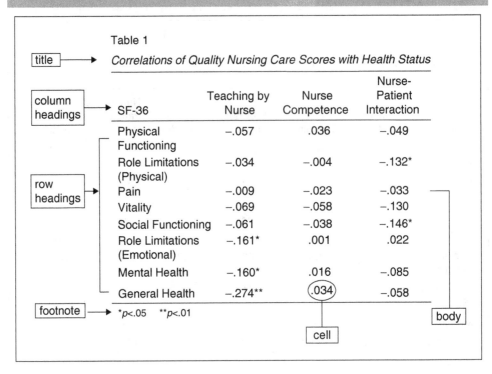

Table 1

Correlations of Quality Nursing Care Scores with Health Status

SF-36	Teaching by Nurse	Nurse Competence	Nurse-Patient Interaction
Physical Functioning	−.057	.036	−.049
Role Limitations (Physical)	−.034	−.004	−.132*
Pain	−.009	−.023	−.033
Vitality	−.069	−.058	−.130
Social Functioning	−.061	−.038	−.146*
Role Limitations (Emotional)	−.161*	.001	.022
Mental Health	−.160*	.016	−.085
General Health	−.274**	.034	−.058

*p<.05   **p<.01

Labels: title, column headings, row headings, footnote, body, cell

on how to construct tables, and the author is directed to a style manual such as APA *Publication Manual* (APA, 2009) and *AMA Manual of Style* (American Medical Association [AMA], 2007) for more details.

Title

Every table needs a title. The title should be short, descriptive of the content in the table, and written as a phrase rather than as a sentence. The word "table" and its number are part of the title. In some style manuals such as the *AMA Manual of Style*, the entire title is placed on one line (example 1), while in other styles such as APA *Publication Manual*, two lines are used and the title is italicized (example 2):

Example 1:   Table 1. Classifications of Registered Nurses
Example 2:   Table 1
              Classifications of Registered Nurses

The first letter of each major word should be capitalized but not articles, prepositions, nor conjunctions such as "and" and "but."

Column Headings

A table provides a means of organizing information and presenting it logically, and the headings inform the reader of how the information is organized. The main categories of information should be in a separate column (AMA, 2007). Each column should have a brief heading that identifies the type of information reported in it. This includes the left-hand column of the table, referred to as the stub column. For research papers, this column usually contains the independent variables. When numerical data are reported in a column, the heading should include the unit of measure, which should be consistent for all of the information in that column. Only one category of information should be reported in a column.

If groups of columns relate to one another, they can be labeled with a heading, and a line can be placed over the column headings included under it. For example:

	Education			
Measure	ADN	BSN	MSN	PhD

Row Headings

The left-most column of a table contains the row headings that describe the content included in the rows of the table. Similar to column headings, these should be brief statements that adequately label the row and all of the items in that row. If groups of rows are related, a heading can be included and subheadings used to clarify this in the table. This can be seen in Table 12.2 where race/ethnicity, highest education, and marital status are used as headings to group the information reported in the rows that follow.

Body of Table

The body of the table is also referred to as the field (AMA, 2007). The body is the content of the table – its numerical values or words and phrases—organized in columns (vertical) and rows (horizontal). The intersection of a column and row, a cell, is where the specific numbers and text are placed. If the cell is empty because the information is not applicable, the cell can be left blank. If the cell is empty because data are missing, however, the author should insert a dash and include a footnote if further explanation is necessary.

Numerical values are usually placed in the columns; this facilitates totaling the scores and percentages. The author should verify that totals and percentages reflect the numbers and percents given in the table. When a discrepancy exists, such as the percents not equaling 100 because of rounding, an explanation can be included in the footnote to the table if needed. Column data should aligned vertically, for example, by decimal points, so the numbers are not misinterpreted. This can be seen in the sample tables in this chapter.

Information in the rows of a table should be aligned horizontally to facilitate reading from left to right across the table. If the lines of text do not fit in the space allotted and run over into the next line, the numbers or words in the cells are

TABLE 12.2

Sample Table With Subheadings to Group Information in Rows

Table 1
Background of Patients Receiving Home Care

Variable	*n*	%
Race/ethnicity		
Caucasian	67	56.8
African-American	46	39.0
Hispanic	3	2.5
Asian	2	1.6
Highest education		
<12th grade	40	34.8
High school graduate	64	55.6
College graduate	11	9.6
Marital Status		
Married	72	61.0
Divorced/separated	19	16.1
Widowed	9	7.6
Single	18	15.3

placed on the first or top line. For example, in Table 12.1, because the text "Physical Functioning" and "Role Limitations (Physical)" runs over into the next line, the numeric values within the table cells are positioned on the first or top line.

When reporting the results of statistical analyses, the author should check in a style manual or statistics book the information that should be contained in the table. Statistical abbreviations, such as M (mean) and standard deviation (SD), may be used in tables without an explanation in a footnote. A list of statistical abbreviations is provided in Appendix 1. In the text and tables, the exact probability values should be reported to two or three decimal places rather than using $p < .05$ or $p < .01$ (AMA, 2007, p. 96; APA, 2009, p. 139). These values should be reported to two digits to the right of the decimal point; if those digits are zeros then the three digits should be used, e.g., $p = .003$. When the p values are less than .001, then $p < .001$ should be used in both the text and table (AMA, 2007; APA, 2009).

Footnotes

Footnotes provide additional details about the table in general or a specific column, row, or cell. They also are used to explain abbreviations in the table and define the symbols, for example, asterisks, to indicate the p values. Footnotes make the table understandable for readers.

Styles manuals differ in how footnotes are designated. APA *Publication Manual* (2009) refers to a footnote that pertains to the entire table as a general note. These are labeled as *Note* (in italics and followed by a period) and are placed at the bottom of the table. For example,

Note. S = student; RN = registered nurse.

Footnotes for columns, rows, and the specific entries in the cells are designated by superscript lowercase letters ([a,b,c]) placed after the item and then explained at the bottom of the table. These superscripts are ordered from left to right and top to bottom, beginning at the top left point in the table (APA, 2009, p. 138). An example is:

[a]n = 125. [b]n = 129. [c]Control variables were age, gender, and smoking history.

The third type of footnote, a probability note, explains the symbols used in the table to represent the p values. The exact probability values should be reported unless it makes the table difficult to prepare and read, such as with a correlation matrix. In those instances, p values are designated by asterisks, such as $*p < .05$ and $**p < .01$. Sample footnotes are seen in Table 12.3.

AMA style designates footnotes for both tables and figures with superscript lowercase letters (AMA, 2007). The style indicated in the author guidelines dictates how tables and their components parts are prepared in a manuscript.

TABLE 12.3

Table With Footnotes

Table 1

Differences in Role Stress Based on Highest Degree of New Graduate

	ADN[a]		BSN[b]		Master's[c]			
Role Stress Scores[d]	*M*	*SD*	*M*	*SD*	*M*	*SD*	*F*	*p*
Overload	2.89	.69	3.36	.72	3.93	.70	5.96	.004
Conflict with physicians	2.88	.96	3.36	.89	3.54	.78	3.28	.04
Lack of support from manager	2.65	.71	3.23	.78	3.34	.83	3.86	.05
Personal impact	2.57	.48	2.93	.61	3.14	.43	3.69	.02

Note. New graduates completed tool within first six months of practice.
[a]n = 46. [b]n =52. [c]n = 6. [d]New Graduates' Role Stress Assessment

Relationship of Table and Text

Every table must be referred to in the text, and the author should inform readers what to look for in the table. Tables are numbered consecutively, using Arabic numerals, in the order they are first mentioned in the text. This number is then used in the text to refer the reader to the table. Two examples follow:

> As seen in Table 1, there were differences in the importance of teaching by the nurse to men and women.
>
> Men and women differed in the importance they placed on teaching by the nurse (Table 1).

When the article is published, tables are placed close to where they are first referenced as determined by the publisher. As such, authors should not write "the table above/below" or the table on "page 7" because it may not be in that position or place when published.

Formatting Tables

Tables are double-spaced throughout including the title and headings. Because journals differ in how they format tables, the author should follow the style manual or use a standard format such as found in this book. Generally, horizontal lines (rules) are placed between the table title and column headings, used to separate the column headings from the body of the table, and placed at the bottom of the table to separate it from the footnotes. Lines also are used to group similar columns together as shown earlier in the chapter. If any additional formatting is needed for a particular journal, this will be done by the publisher.

Authors generally construct tables using the "Table" feature of their word processing program. Some word processing programs enclose tables in boxes and include additional lines between rows and columns; if so, authors will need to modify this to meet the style requirements, as discussed earlier. Tables should be saved as .doc files, making it easier for the editor to modify them if needed and the publisher to prepare them. In some situations authors may attempt to use scans of tables that were developed using other formats, but generally these will not be clear enough for publication. Smaller type should not be used because the submitted table will be reduced in size when published, making smaller type difficult to read. The author guidelines will specify requirements for producing tables and figures, and authors should adhere to them. If unfamiliar with developing tables, the author should practice how to develop them with the word processing program before beginning to type the manuscript to avoid being distracted during the writing phase.

Each table is placed on a separate page. When tables extend beyond one page, they are continued on the next page and labeled with the table number and title, followed by the word "continued" (AMA, 2007). For wide tables, the author might orient them horizontally (landscape) rather than vertically (portrait), consider preparing two tables, or shift the columns with their headings to the rows, and the rows and headings to the columns if appropriate. Exhibit 12.4 provides a checklist for authors to ensure their tables reflect principles for their development.

EXHIBIT 12.4

Checklist for Reviewing Tables

- Is the table essential to the paper, or can the information be conveyed in the text?
- Does the table stand alone—is the information in the table sufficient for readers to understand it without referring to the explanation in the text?
- Does the title communicate the content in the table and is it short?
- Does every column and row have a heading, and do the headings reflect the information in them?
- Is the content in the table arranged logically and presented clearly for readers to understand it?
- Is the table designed for readers to easily locate specific data?
- Are the data in the table accurate and consistent with the information reported in the text?
- If the table has totals and percentages, are they correct based on the numbers given in the table?
- Are abbreviations and symbols in the table explained in the footnotes?
- Are the notes listed in this order: general, specific, then probability (APA, 2009)?
- Are the lines in the table done correctly, e.g., horizontal lines between the title and column headings, to separate the column headings from the body of the table, and at the bottom?
- Are p values identified correctly?
- Are exact probability values reported and asterisks used only when needed?
- If part or all of a copyrighted table is reproduced, is there a note in the caption giving credit to the copyright owner?
- Was written permission obtained to reproduce the table in the manuscript, and was a copy of the permission sent to the journal editor?
- Is each table numbered (consecutively) and referenced in the text?
- If there are multiple tables in the paper, are they consistent in format, font type and size, and other aspects of the presentation?

Non-Tabular Material

Word or textual tables can be used to highlight key points, summarize information, and provide additional details to support the text. These are used to set the material off from the text, emphasizing it to readers. Word tables display words, phrases, and sentences, usually in lists. Similar to tables that present numerical data, word tables convey information that helps readers understand the content but is too detailed to be included in the text. For example, a word table may be developed for a paper on care of the burn patient that lists potential patient

TABLE 12.4

Sample Word Table

Table 1

Phases of Nursing Process

Phase	Definition
Assessment	Recognizing problems and collecting data
Diagnosis	Analyzing data and identifying nursing diagnoses
Plan	Setting priorities, developing goals, selecting interventions
Implementation	Carrying out nursing interventions
Evaluation	Evaluating outcomes of care

problems, data to collect in an assessment with related laboratory tests, and interventions for each problem. Boxes, sidebars and similar types of exhibits (that have one column only) may be used in place of a word table. Word tables, similar to ones that report quantitative data, should not be developed if the information can be presented clearly and concisely in the text. Table 12.4 is an example of a word table that could be included in a publication.

▨ FIGURES

Figures include graphs, charts, diagrams, photographs, and other illustrations. They can be used to illustrate the findings of a study, display trends in the data, make comparisons, and show equipment, procedures, and other objects described in the text. For research papers figures have the advantage of allowing readers to visualize trends and patterns in the data more easily than when written in the narrative.

Figures should be used only when essential to facilitate understanding of the content in the paper. They should add value to the paper, displaying the results and other information more clearly than can be done by the text alone. Figures are useful for illustrating trends in data over time and showing the relationships between variables. However, if those same outcomes can be described adequately in the text, figures should not be developed. Journal editors are allotted a certain number of pages for each issue of the journal, and tables and figures take space to produce.

Types of Figures

There are varied types of figures that can be prepared by the author. These include:

▨ *Graphs*: Graphs show the relationship of two variables, for example, hospital length of stay to number of days on a ventilator. Graphs displaying quantitative data are valuable to indicate changes and patterns in the data. These include line graphs, survival plots, scatterplots, histograms and frequency polygons, bar graphs, pie charts, and dot or point graphs (AMA, 2007).

■ *Diagrams*: Diagrams depict the sequence of a process, such as a flowchart to show the steps in a process or how subjects moved through a study. A flow diagram to report the progress of participants through a randomized control trial, from the CONSORT (Consolidated Standards of Reporting Trials) Statement, is included in Figure 12.2. Authors can download a template of this diagram from the CONSORT Web site to use in their own manuscripts (CONSORT, 2008). Diagrams also include charts such as an organizational chart and algorithms.

FIGURE 12.2

CONSORT Flow Diagram

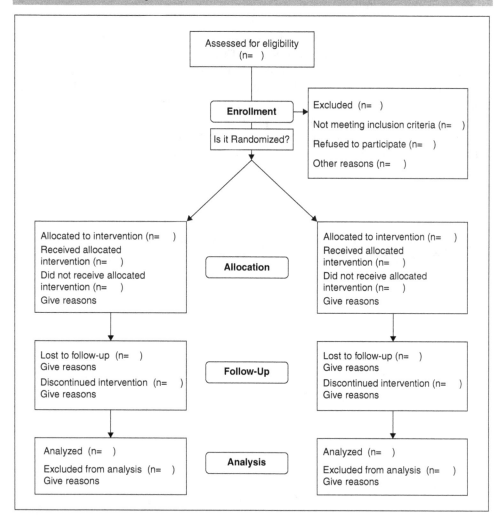

From: CONSORT. (2008). *CONSORT Flow Diagram*. Retrieved from http://www.consort-statement.org/consort-statement/flow-diagram/. The CONSORT Statement is distributed under the terms of the Creative Commons Attribution License, which permits unrestricted use, distribution, and reproduction in any medium, provided the original author and source are credited.

■ *Maps*: Maps show relationships and trends that involve locations and distance (AMA, 2007). For instance, they may be used to display the prevalence of health problems in particular communities.
■ *Photographs*: Photographic images of patients and objects are submitted usually as separate digital files and need to have the appropriate level of resolution (APA, 2009). Photographs of patients require their signed release. When copied from another source, in addition to obtaining permission for use of the photograph, the author should request an original version; copies of figures are often blurry.

Guidelines for Developing Figures

How to develop each of the figures described earlier is beyond the scope of this book, and the author can obtain this information in a style manual. A few general guidelines, though, follow.

■ Use large enough letters, symbols, numbers, lines, and other objects to allow them to be read once reduced in size to fit the journal page. Figures are usually smaller when published, and this should be taken into consideration when they are constructed. The final printed figures must be easy to read and clear.
■ Use standard symbols, such as open and closed circles, triangles, and squares, that are defined in the legend or caption of the figure.
■ If shadings are used, they should be sufficiently different and limited to two or three types in one bar graph. The ideal option is to use no shading and black bars (APA, 2009, p. 161).

FIGURE 12.3

Sample Figure

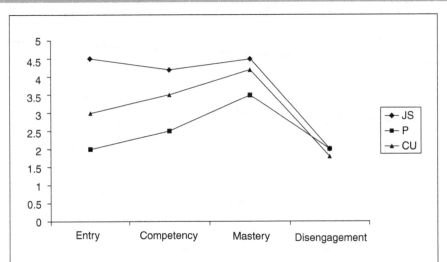

Figure 1. Scores are for new graduates' job satisfaction (JS), productivity (P), and commitment to the unit (CU) by stages.

- Label each axis as to what it is measuring and the units in which it is measured.
- Number figures consecutively, for example, Figure 1, Figure 2, and so forth, and include a title immediately following the number. This is not part of the figure.
- Prepare a legend or caption for each figure that is placed below the figure. The legend provides information for understanding the figure and all the symbols in it without referring to the text. This is illustrated in Figure 12.3.
- Submit the originals of all figures with the manuscript. Most figures will be reproduced as submitted, and for this reason it is important to be careful that the original is without flaws.
- Follow the author guidelines or style manual as to how to prepare the figures. Figures developed for presentations with PowerPoint, for example, are likely to need revision because the type will be too large for use in a manuscript. APA (2009) style indicates that lettering should be no larger than 14 points.

Exhibit 12.5 provides a checklist for authors to ensure their figures reflect principles for their development.

EXHIBIT 12.5

Checklist for Reviewing Figures

- Is the figure essential to the paper, or can the information be conveyed in the text?
- Does the figure stand alone—is the information in the figure sufficient for readers to understand it without referring to the explanation in the text?
- Does the title communicate the content in the figure and is it short?
- Is the information shown in the figure accurate and consistent with what is reported in the text?
- Is the figure easy-to-read and understand?
- Is it free of unnecessary details?
- Are standard symbols used, and all parts of the figure labeled clearly?
- Are letters, symbols, numbers, lines, and other objects large enough to be read once reduced in size to fit the journal page?
- Is there a caption with each figure, which is placed below it?
- Does the caption provide information for understanding the figure and all the symbols in it without referring to the text?
- If there is more than one figure, is the same scale used for their preparation? (APA, 2009)
- Are the figures in a file format consistent with the author guidelines and publisher specifications?
- Are the figures at a sufficiently high resolution to allow for accurate reproduction? (APA, 2009)
- If a copyrighted figure is reproduced, is there a note in the caption giving credit to the copyright owner?

Continued

Exhibit 12.5 *Continued*

■ Was written permission obtained to reproduce the figure in the manuscript, and was a copy of the permission sent to the journal editor?
■ Is each figure numbered (consecutively) and referenced in the text?

Relationship of Figure and Text

Similar to tables, figures are numbered consecutively, using Arabic numerals, in the order they are first mentioned in the text. Every figure is referred to in the text by its number, for example:

Changes in infant mortality over the time period of the evaluation project are shown in Figure 1.

When the article is published, figures are placed close to where they are first referenced in the text. Similar to tables, authors should not write "the figure above/below" because it may not be in that position when published.

As far as placement in the manuscript, tables and figures follow the references, with tables first, then figures. As one last reminder: tables and figures should only be used when essential, and it is the author's responsibility to know the maximum number allowed with a manuscript.

■ SUMMARY

Tables are an effective way of presenting detailed and complex information succinctly and clearly. Tables should be used when the author wants to report exact values, present a large amount of detailed information, display different quantitative values simultaneously, and show relationships among data. Tables should not be used, however, when the information can be reported instead in the text.

There are two types of tables authors can include in a manuscript: the traditional table with information arranged in columns and rows, and a tabulation, a short, informal table developed as part of the text. Boxes also can be developed; these are valuable for emphasizing important information from the text and highlighting key concepts.

Tables contain five major parts: title, column headings, row headings, body of the table, and footnotes. The title should be short, descriptive of the content in the table, and written as a phrase rather than as a sentence. The body or content of the table is usually organized into columns (vertical) and rows (horizontal). The intersection of a column and row, a cell, is where the specific numbers and text are placed.

A table provides a means of organizing information and presenting it logically, and the headings inform the reader of how the information is organized. Each column has a brief heading that identifies the type of information reported in it. Only one category of information is reported in a column. The leftmost column of a table contains the row headings that describe the content included in the rows of the table. Footnotes provide additional details about the table in general or a specific column, row, or cell in the table.

Every table is referred to in the text, and the author should inform readers what to look for in the table. Tables are numbered consecutively, using Arabic numerals, in the order they are first mentioned in the text. Each table is placed on a separate page following the references.

Figures include graphs, diagrams, maps, and photographs. They can be used to illustrate the findings of a study, display trends in the data, make comparisons, and show equipment, procedures, and other objects described in the text.

Figures are usually reduced when published, so the letters, symbols, numbers, lines, and other objects should be large enough so they can be seen once reduced to fit the journal page. The legend or caption for the figure is placed below it and includes details about the figure. Most figures will be reproduced as submitted, and the author should take care that the original is without flaws. Similar to tables, figures are numbered consecutively, using Arabic numerals, in the order they are first mentioned in the text. Every figure is referred to in the text by its number. Tables and figures should only be used when essential, and it is the author's responsibility to know the maximum number allowed with a manuscript.

▓ REFERENCES

American Medical Association (AMA). (2007). *AMA manual of style: A guide for authors and editors* (10th ed.). New York: Oxford University Press.

American Psychological Association (APA). (2009). *Publication Manual of the American Psychological Association* (6th ed.). Washington, DC: APA.

CONSORT. (2008). *CONSORT Flow Diagram*. Retrieved from http://www.consort- statement. org/consort-statement/flow-diagram/

Lang, T. A. (2010). *How to write, publish, & present in the health sciences: A guide for clinicians and laboratory researchers*. Philadelphia: American College of Physicians.

Vintzileos, A. M., & Ananth, C. V. (2009). How to write and publish an original research article. *American Journal of Obstetrics & Gynecology*. Advance online publication. http://dx.doi.org/10.1016/j.ajog.2009.06.038

FINAL PAPER THROUGH PUBLICATION

13

FINAL PAPER AND
SUBMISSION TO JOURNAL

At this point in the writing process, the author has completed the revisions of the content and format of the paper; has prepared the references, tables, and figures; and is ready to submit the paper to the journal. Prior to submission, there are some final responsibilities of the author to ensure that the manuscript is consistent with the journal requirements and contains all the required parts for submission. The manuscript is then ready to send to the journal for review.

Chapter 13 describes the steps in preparing all elements of the final paper to submit to the journal and details associated with this submission. Examples of these elements are provided in the chapter, and a checklist is included for authors to ensure that all items are sent with the manuscript to avoid delays in its review.

PREPARATION OF FINAL PAPER

Chapter 10 provided guidelines for revising the content and format of the paper so it is ready for submission. Because journals differ in their requirements, the author needs to complete one final check of the manuscript to ensure it is consistent with these requirements. This final check begins by reviewing the guidelines for preparing manuscripts described in the author information page. The author read these while preparing the manuscript, but this final review confirms that the paper has all essential parts and meets these requirements. Some journals provide a pre-submission checklist that summarizes the requirements. The author also notes whether the manuscript may be submitted electronically or in hard copy and how many copies are sent.

Most journals either require or permit electronic submissions (American Medical Association [AMA], 2007; American Psychological Association [APA], 2009). Electronic submissions include submissions by email, compact disc, or downloading onto a proprietary website supported by the journal. Manuscripts submitted by email, disc or hard copy are pre-assembled by authors prior to submission. Downloaded submissions are not pre-assembled. Instead, the digital software prompts the author to enter separate elements of information that the software assembles into the required format. Regardless of the submission method, authors must gather the same elements in preparation for submission.

This chapter begins by describing all of the required elements for submission of a scientific manuscript. Exhibit 13.1 provides a checklist for authors to use to ensure that all of the essential elements. The chapter concludes with considerations for using a website to submit a manuscript, followed by considerations for submitting pre-assembled manuscripts.

EXHIBIT 13.1

Checklist of Elements for All Submissions

- ☐ Manuscript title
- ☐ Contact information for all authors
- ☐ Designated corresponding author
- ☐ Running title
- ☐ Funding support
- ☐ Abstract
- ☐ Keywords
- ☐ Text with appropriate headings, subheadings, citations, table and figure placements
- ☐ Acknowledgements
- ☐ References
- ☐ Tables
- ☐ Figures
- ☐ Disclosures
- ☐ Manuscript Type
- ☐ Preferred and Non-preferred reviewers
- ☐ Permissions
- ☐ Cover Letter
- ☐ Copyright forms

■ ELEMENTS OF A FINAL SUBMISSION

Title Page

Every manuscript needs a title page, which is the first page of the paper. Journals differ in their requirements of elements on the title page. Journals that use APA formatting require five elements: title, running title, all authors, their organizational affiliations, and an author note (APA, 2009). Journals that use AMA style do not require a running title but rather compose running heads during the production process after acceptance (AMA, 2007).

For refereed journals, manuscripts are reviewed anonymously. Reviewers must receive title pages that include only the title(s) and omit elements that could identify the authors or their affiliations. If one or more title pages are required by the journal, authors should read the journal's author guidelines carefully to learn what elements are required on each version of the title page and to prepare them accordingly. For pre-assembled submissions with only a complete title page, the editor removes the title page prior to sending the paper to the reviewers.

When elements are entered separately into software fields online, each is coded and assembled into requisite versions of the title page, depending on the stage of the submission. For example, full and running titles are entered separately and placed automatically on title pages that will go to reviewers. Title pages that are sent to copy-editors after acceptance include some combination of the following elements: the title of the paper; authors' names, credentials, positions, and institutions in which employed or to which affiliated; corresponding author and contact information; grant support or other type of support; disclosure of financial or other benefits and non-duplication of material; keywords; and a running head. Prior to submission online or hardcopy submission, authors should gather the following material.

Title

As discussed in Chapter 10, the title may have undergone multiple changes as the manuscript emerged. In the pre-submission phase, the author has the opportunity to refine the title to capture the essence of the article. The author should craft a final draft of the title to capture the attention of the target audience.

Contact Information

The author should confirm with each of the coauthors all of their contact information. This includes the full name with middle initials, correct academic degrees and clinical certification, institutional affiliations, physical addresses including street and box number, telephone and fax numbers, and email address. For faculty who may not be available during certain times of the year and consultants who are away from the office, home addresses and numbers may be provided to facilitate contact with editor during these time periods. This also allows for a faster turnaround time for review of page proofs if the manuscript is accepted for publication.

The authors should decide before submission who will serve in various submission-related capacities. The first author and all coauthors should be listed in order in the appropriate fields. One of these should be designated as the 'corresponding author.' The corresponding author is the one who will have responsibility for being available to the editorial office during the review process. One or more authors should be identified to serve as corresponding author in case the primary corresponding author is unavailable during brief periods of time. Some journals also require information from the "submitting agent", who may or may not be an author on the manuscript. For example, a staff assistant may submit the manuscript but not be either the first author or a coauthor.

Running Title

Some journals include a running title, which is a short version of the title, usually 50 characters or fewer, to be used on each page of the published paper. In the final printed copy, this short title is printed at the top (running head) or bottom of the page (running foot) to assist the reader to find the desired article. Journals differ regarding their requirement for authors to compose a running title. This is typically specified in the journal's information for authors.

Funding Support

If the author received a grant or another type of support for the project reported in the paper, this should be noted. Some grant-making agencies and organizations require that authors use specific language when acknowledging their support. This information is usually available on award letters or on the website for the agency. If there is any doubt about the correct acknowledgement, authors should contact the agency directly for information.

If the journal does not provide a separate field to enter funding information, the authors should use the field for Acknowledgements to include this information. Acknowledgement sections are described below. Exhibit 13.2 provides a sample of a complete title page.

EXHIBIT 13.2

Sample Title Page

Evaluation of Educational Program for Patients with
Congestive Heart Failure

Mary Smith, MSN, RN
Clinical Nurse II

John Peterson, MSN, RN, C
Advanced Practice Nurse

Jane Doe, MSN, RN
Nurse Manager

Robert Jones, PhD
Statistician

Grace Memorial Hospital
Reading, PA

Correspondence to:
Mary Smith, MSN
[mailing address,
phone and fax numbers,
and email address]

Project supported by Staff Development Department,
Grace Memorial Hospital

Abstract Page

The next page of the paper is the abstract page. How to write the abstract was described earlier in the book. In reviewing the abstract page, the author should confirm that the information is consistent with the text. The author also should check again that the length of the abstract is within the limits of the journal. Most word processing programs have a function that allows the author to check the number of words in a document.

For online submissions, the abstract is usually uploaded into a separate field and not included with the text of the manuscript. For hard copy submissions, the abstract is placed on a separate page following the title page. The heading "Abstract" can be centered at the top of this page. The abstract should be double-spaced consistent with the rest of the paper.

Keywords

Some journals require authors to designate a short list of key words (usually 3–10) that represent the most important topics of their article and that readers will use to search online databases for articles of interest (AMA, 2007). Keywords are usually listed at the end of the abstract in published manuscripts.

Several of the major databases use their own controlled vocabulary indexing system to assign keywords to published articles. MEDLINE uses the MeSH vocabulary; CINAHL uses the Nursing and Allied Health Subject Headings (AMA, 2007). If authors are requested to submit their own keywords, they should consider using a major online database to select terms that conform to these external indexing services. When keywords are consistent between the printed article and the indexing service, readers can most easily find individual and related articles on the topic desired.

Text

The next part of the paper is the text. Although this should be in final form, and not require any further revisions of content nor writing style and format, the author should check the leveling of the headings and subheadings for consistency throughout the manuscript, the citations, and the consistency between the text and any tables and figures.

Headings and Subheadings

Guidelines for determining the level of headings and where to position them in the text are determined by style manuals, publishers, or journals. The *AMA Manual of Style* (2007) defers to publishers and journals with regard to headings. The *Publication Manual of the American Psychological Association* (2009) describes how to use five levels of headings in a paper, although for most manuscripts only two to three levels are needed. The format and placement of the heading depend on its level. For instance, when Levels 1 and 2 of headings are used, the first one is centered, bolded, and uses uppercase and lowercase; the second level heading is also bolded and uses uppercase and lowercase but is placed at the left margin. The text begins on the following line (APA, 2009).

At the final pre-submission check, there are two important issues regarding headings. The first issue is to have consistency in how the headings and sub-headings are typed throughout the manuscript regardless of what format is used. It may be helpful to write the headings and subheadings, and their leveling, on a separate sheet of paper and confirm that this is how the content should be organized and divided into sections.

The second issue is to use headings strategically to link all elements of the manuscript. The words used as headings in the text may also appear in the title, abstract, or tables and figures. Sometimes the same words and phrases are repeated as headings across two or more sections of the text, e.g., the introduction, measures, results, or discussion. Such strategic use of headings links the manuscript into a coherent whole and helps the reader to keep track of what the author is describing. Crist and colleagues (2009) used this strategy throughout their article, as seen in Exhibits 5.1–5.3, 5.7, 5.10–5.12 (pp. 96–123).

Citations

Although the need for accuracy in preparing citations and references has been discussed throughout the book, the author should check the citations in the text one final time. Citations should be consistent with the style used by the journal, all citations should be included, and they should match the reference on the reference list.

Consistency of Text With Tables and Figures

The need for consistency between the text and related tables and figures has been emphasized in prior chapters. The author should check that the data in the text are consistent with the tables and figures and that each one has been cited accurately in the text. The tables and figures also should be numbered correctly.

Acknowledgments

Online submissions will include a field for the acknowledgements. For hard copy submissions, the next page after the text is for the acknowledgments, which allows the author to give credit to people who made contributions to the manuscript. These contributions can be in many forms: consultation on the content of the paper, statistical assistance, editing of the paper, and financial support, as described in Chapter 3. Remember that written permission is needed to publish the names of people listed in the acknowledgments.

References

The reference list will follow any acknowledgements and is prepared according to either a citation-sequence system, in which references are listed in the order they are first cited in the text, or name-year system, in which they are alphabetized. The author should have verified already the accuracy of the references against the original documents, but if this was not done previously, it is an important step in preparing the final copy for submission. The author also checks that each reference on the list is cited at the correct place in the text, the reference format is consistent with the journal requirements and style manual, and each reference includes complete information.

For manuscripts cited in the text that are "in press", the author can include these on the reference list and insert in the appropriate space "In press." Papers under review should not be included as background information or listed in the reference list. Other unpublished papers should be noted according to the style manual required by the journal.

Tables

Each table should begin on a new page and numbered consecutively in the order to which they are referred in the text. The author checks that the tables are cited in the text at the correct place and the information in the table supports the text. The author also should review the titles of the tables and if they are formatted consistent with the style used by the journal or general principles provided in this book. The author should have identified earlier how many tables and figures are allowed with each manuscript, but if not done, this limit should be confirmed before submitting the manuscript. Tables follow the Reference List in pre-assembled manuscripts.

Figures

Figures follow the tables, with each figure beginning on a new page similar to the tables. Figures are numbered consecutively in the order they are cited in the text. Figure captions

For online submissions, figures are usually uploaded into a separate field from the manuscript text. These are added in the correct order in the version seen by the editor and reviewers. For hard copy submissions, remember not to staple or paper clip the originals of the figures to the manuscript when submitting it because they might be damaged from this.

Disclosures

Online submissions may have separate fields for disclosing pertinent information related to responsible author practices. Such checklists or statements may be related to having complied with author guidelines, blinded the manuscript, not previously published the article or simultaneously submitted it to another journal, removed track changes from the final version, or other concerns that will impede the prompt processing and review of the manuscript. It is imperative that the submitting author or agent pay special attention to these disclosures. Careless or incorrect information in these fields can come back to haunt the group of authors at best by delaying review or publication and at worst by requiring retraction of an article or being barred from future publications at the journal.

If there were any financial or contractual associations between the authors and others that might bias a study or how the findings are interpreted, this should be disclosed to the editor (AMA, 2007). A statement may be included in the cover letter, and the authors may be asked to sign a separate form to this effect. For example, the guidelines for journal of the Association of periOperative Registered Nurses (AORN, 2009) direct the author to disclose if there was a financial association between the author and the commercial company that makes the product featured in the manuscript.

In addition to financial interest, authors need to disclose any other type of involvement that might represent a potential conflict of interest such as being a paid consultant on a project evaluated highly in the manuscript, owning stock in the company that manufactures the product described in the paper, and receiving an honorarium for participating in the evaluation of the product, to name a few. For example, a statement such as this might be included in the cover letter:

> Ms. Smith is a consultant for Software Incorporated that produced the software evaluated in this paper.

The author also might include a statement in the cover letter that indicates no commercial, proprietary, or financial interest in the product or subject matter discussed in the paper (AMA, 2007).

■ OTHER ELEMENTS OF ONLINE SUBMISSIONS

Journals must often triage incoming submissions to the appropriate persons across multiple layers of editors and reviewers. In order to sort and track different types of manuscripts to the appropriate associate or review editor, online submission Web sites may request additional information from the authors about their manuscript at the time of submission. Types of information may include whether or not the manuscript reports original research, the type of data analysis (qualitative, quantitative, or mixed methods), or subject characteristics (diagnostic focus, setting, age group, or other.) The author will probably be familiar enough with the content in order to provide the requested information but should confer as needed with coauthors.

Some journals request submitting authors to provide the names of reviewers who would have the requisite expertise to serve as invited reviewers as well as any persons whom the authors prefer not be invited to reviewer their manuscript. Authors may suggest authors whose work has been important to the development of their ideas, but authors should not inquire directly of any suggested reviewers whether they would be willing to serve as a reviewer of the manuscript, as this information would compromise the blinded peer review process.

Authors might list as non-preferred reviewers any colleagues at other universities or organizations who have served in an advisory capacity on the material in the article but who were not coauthors. This information also supports the blinded peer review process. Authors may be tempted to list as non-preferred other researchers with known disagreements about the topic area or whom they would suspect to be skeptical of the findings. These should not be listed. The editors are free to disregard both preferred and non-preferred reviewers at the time of reviewer selection.

If relevant, the author should have available any permissions needed. These may include permissions to reprint information in the manuscript, letters granting permission to publish the acknowledgments and to cite the names of institutions in the manuscript, and permissions to publish photographs and other illustrations.

FORMATTING THE FINAL MANUSCRIPT

The manuscript must be formatted according to the journal specifications in the journal's information for authors. Papers are double-spaced throughout including the title page and abstract and continuing through the last page of the manuscript. This includes double-spacing the references, tables, and figure captions. The references themselves are double-spaced, not only the lines between each reference on the list.

There are some other important guidelines for keyboarding the paper of which the author should be aware. If the paper is too long, do not attempt to include more lines per page by using narrow margins. The journal guidelines may specify the size of the margins, but if unsure about them, refer to the style manual or use 1 to 1½ inch margins on all sides. Paragraphs should be indented, and spaces should not be left between each paragraph. Words should not be divided at the end of a line, and most word processing programs take care of this. Pages should be left-justified (aligning the text at the left margin), not double-justified (where the text is aligned at both the right and left margins). When double-justified, there may be large spaces between words and symbols in a line.

Pages are numbered consecutively, considering the title page as the first page. Some journals specify the placement of page numbers, but if not indicated in the author guidelines, pages can be numbered in the right-hand corner of each page either at the top or bottom. Remember that each section of the paper begins on a new page.

For hard copy submissions, the manuscript should be printed on a high quality white paper, using a high quality printer. After printing the necessary number of copies, the author should check each page of each copy to be sure that it printed correctly and pages are in the correct order. Some authors prefer to print an original and make copies to submit with it. This same principle holds true – each page of each copy should be checked as well as their order. Except for the originals of the figures, the paper may be stapled or paper clipped. Coauthors should have a final digital or hard copy of the paper for their files.

SUBMISSION OF MANUSCRIPT TO JOURNAL

The paper is now ready to submit to the journal. Submission to the journal requires writing a cover letter to accompany the manuscript, obtaining signatures on the transfer of copyright form if required for submission, and creating an author account on the journal website. If the journal permits hardcopy submissions, the authors must also prepare to pack the manuscript and related materials and mail them. These steps are described in this section of the chapter.

Cover Letter

The cover letter accompanies the manuscript and provides the editor with information about the paper and corresponding author (Exhibit 13.3). The cover letter should include the following elements, as relevant:

- title of the paper
- length of manuscript (pages or word count) and number of tables and figures
- statement that paper is original and has not published already
- information about previous presentations, e.g., at a scientific meeting
- information about closely related manuscript submitted to other journals, in press, or published
- explanation of financial interest in any aspect of the study
- notification of ethical treatment of subjects
- full name, affiliation, and complete contact information of the corresponding author
- confirmation that all authors have read and approved the final version
- copies of all permissions granted to reproduce copyrighted material
- recommendations for preferred and non-preferred reviewers, where requested
- type of review preferred, if blinded review is optional
- department of the journal for which it is submitted for consideration
- number of copies and other materials submitted in hardcopy (APA, 2009).

The cover letter does not need to be long but should contain the above information. Some of this information may be duplicated in other fields of an online submission process. However, having the following information in the cover letter insures that all of the information will be readily available to the editor upon receipt of the manuscript.

First, the complete title of the paper should be specified in the letter. If the title does not explain fully all of the content in the manuscript, or how the paper might fit in a department of the journal, the author might include a few sentences describing the focus of the paper. In the example in Exhibit 13.3, the title "Evaluation of Educational Program for Patients with Congestive Heart Failure" may not sufficiently explain that the program begins during the patient's hospitalization, continues through home care, and includes periodic teaching and follow-up via telephone contact with the patient. A sentence to this effect might be included in the cover letter.

Second, some journals have departments that publish different types of articles. For example, *Applied Nursing Research* accepts papers in six main categories: original research, clinical methods, research briefs, special features, international column, and as an expert (Elsevier, 2009). The *Journal of Obstetric, Gynecologic, and Neonatal Nursing* has a number of possible types of submissions: Research, Principles and Practice (innovations and trends), Thoughts and Opinions, Letters to the Editor, Case Reports, In Focus (current issues) and In Review (integrated literature reviews) (Wiley Interscience, 2009). The cover letter should indicate if the paper was written for a particular department.

EXHIBIT 13.3

Sample Cover Letter

[Date]

Dr. Ann Brown
Editor, *Nursing Journal*
1234 Main Street
Anytown, AnyState 56789

Dear Dr. Brown:

Attached please find our manuscript, "Evaluation of Educational Program for Patients with Congestive Heart Failure," for your review for possible publication in *Nursing Journal*. The manuscript includes 4978 words, two tables, and one figure. We respectfully request its double-blinded review. As noted in the Acknowledgements, Drs. Rebecca Markham and Michael Hayes at Second University in Calista, CA, have provided extensive comments on the manuscript and would not be appropriate as independent reviewers.

The manuscript is based on a symposium paper delivered on November 4, 2009, at the 9th National Council of Nurses Education Summit meeting in Indianapolis, IN. A companion paper describing the development of the educational program is "in press" in the *Education Evaluation Journal*. That manuscript describes the pilot data (n = 32) from one hospital that informed the content of the program described in the current paper; however, the current paper is based on follow-up data and describes the process and outcome evaluations of the program in three hospitals (n = 291). Please let me know if you would like us to forward to you a copy of the companion manuscript. Neither the enclosed manuscript nor any part of its content has been submitted to, accepted for, or published by another journal.

The undersigned have no financial interests in any element of the study, which was approved by the institutional review boards of Our Town University and each of the three hospitals.

The study is based on a conceptual model copyrighted to Wiley Interscience. We attach a copy of the permission granted by that publisher to reprint the model herein.

Mary Smith will serve as the first author and corresponding author on this paper. The four authors have read and approved the current version. Mary Smith undertakes responsibility to keep them informed in each stage of the review process.

Thank you for your consideration.

Sincerely,
Mary Smith
Mary Smith
Our Town University
1 River Road
Reading, PA 19709
313.888.8888 (voice)
313.444.4444 (fax)
mary.smith@otu.edu

John Peterson
John Peterson

Jane Doe
Jane Doe

Robert Jones
Robert Jones

Third, because of issues with duplicate publications, discussed in the beginning of this book, authors should include a statement in the cover letter indicating that the paper is original and has not published already, in its entirety or in part. A sample statement that can be used is: "Neither the entire paper nor any part of its content has been published or has been accepted by another journal. The manuscript is submitted only to this journal." Inclusion of this statement in the cover letter can be seen in Exhibit 13.3.

If the manuscript being submitted is based on the same data set or has similar content as previously published or submitted papers, the author should indicate exactly how the manuscript differs from these other publications. Journals also may ask the author to submit these articles with the manuscript. If the manuscript is based on a conference presentation, the author should indicate such to the editor. Other ethical considerations to verify in the cover letter include conflicts of interest and humane treatment of human or animal subjects.

Fourth, the author is responsible for informing the editor about any options afforded all authors. Options may include the naming of preferred or non-preferred reviewers as well as blinded versus open review. Chapter 14 discusses these options more fully.

Fifth, the cover letter should specify the full name and affiliation of the corresponding author. Contact information, including mailing address, telephone and fax numbers, and email address, should be included; this information should be consistent with that listed on the title page or elsewhere in the online submission website. For faculty who may not be available during certain terms of the year, or consultants who are away from the office, home addresses and numbers may be provided or an alternate individual may be listed for contact during these time periods. For papers written by more than one author, the *Uniform Requirements* specify that the cover letter must state that the submitted version of the manuscript has been read and approved by all authors and that they meet criteria for authorship as described in Chapter 3 (International Committee of Medical Journal Editors, 2008). A clear designation of the corresponding author is particularly important so the editor knows whom to contact.

Finally, for hardcopy submissions, the cover letter also includes the number of copies and other materials submitted with the manuscript. If copyrighted material was included in the manuscript, proof of permission to reprint should be forwarded to the editor.

Copyright Forms

For some journals the author submits the signed transfer of copyright form with the submission, while for others this is only completed when the paper is accepted for publication. If the copyright form is needed for submission, this will be noted on the author guidelines and will probably be available at the web site of the journal. If not, the author needs to obtain the copyright transfer form from the editorial office. This should have been done when the journal was selected so it is available when the manuscript is ready to be sent.

Creating an Author Account for Web-Based Submissions

The first time that authors log onto a journal website, they will be instructed how to initiate an account dedicated to their submission. If the author is already a reviewer of manuscripts for that journal, an account may already be available for manuscript submissions.

The same author account is used to process manuscripts being submitted, to track the progress of submitted manuscripts through the editorial process, and to respond to invitations to revise and resubmit an article. For a new manuscript being submitted, the author is prompted through sequential steps to provide each element needed and respond to specific queries relevant to the submission. Usually the final screen provides the opportunity to check all of the inputted elements and displays any missing elements, which can then be uploaded. Once the author is satisfied with all uploaded elements, the author clicks a link that 'submits' the manuscript to the editorial office. The author account may confirm the receipt of the manuscript, and the corresponding author may also receive an email confirmation. Chapter 14 describes the editorial processing of a manuscript.

Submission of Pre-Assembled Manuscripts

With the cover letter done, the author is ready to assemble all elements into a complete manuscript in preparation to upload to the journal website or to submit by mail, disk, or email. Most manuscripts are submitted online at the journal's website; however, some journals may still request manuscripts by mail, disk, or email, and authors generally submit hard copies of book manuscripts with the electronic files. If sending copies through the mail, the author must send the correct number of copies of the paper as specified in the author guidelines; remember to check each copy to ensure that it has all the pages, in the correct order.

If the manuscript includes original figures, they can be placed in a separate envelope that is labeled clearly. Copies of the figures may be included with each copy of the manuscript as long as the editor has the original illustrations. Be careful when packaging the manuscript to protect the originals from damage during mailing. Cardboard can be placed in the envelope to avoid bending them.

Other materials submitted are the permissions to reprint information in the manuscript, letters granting permission to publish the acknowledgments and to cite the names of institutions in the manuscript, and permissions to publish photographs and other illustrations. If requested by the journal, the author should include the transfer of copyright form. Documents such as these can be scanned and uploaded with the manuscript files during the submission.

If the journal requires hard copies of the manuscript and a copy on a compact disc (CD), the disk should be labeled clearly with the author's name, title of the manuscript, platform (PC or MAC), and software program (e.g., Word, Word Perfect, or others, including the version number). A new disk should be used, and it should be packaged in a mailing folder to avoid damage. Some of the materials such as permission letters would have to be mailed under separate cover. Manuscripts are not returned if rejected. If the author wants the original of the paper returned, a self-addressed and stamped envelope should be sent with the submission package.

For the first submission, when there is no deadline to meet, the materials can be mailed first class. When there are deadlines to be met, express mail might be worth the additional cost. Authors should have one complete copy of all the materials mailed, not only the manuscript itself.

SUMMARY

The author needs to complete one final check of the manuscript to ensure that it is consistent with the requirements of the journal specified in the information for authors page. This final review confirms that the paper has all essential parts and meets these requirements. The author also notes whether the manuscript may be submitted electronically or in hard copy only and how many copies are sent.

The author should check the title page, abstract page, and text. Although the manuscript should be in final form, and not require any further revisions of content nor writing style and format, the author should check the: (1) leveling of the headings and subheadings and if typed consistently throughout the manuscript, (2) citations, and (3) consistency between the text and any tables and figures. The author should complete one last check of the references.

Each table and figure is typed on a separate page and numbered consecutively in the order referred to in the text. The author checks that the tables and figures are numbered consistently with their placement in the text.

The manuscript should be typed according to the journal specifications. Most manuscripts are submitted online at the journal's website, but some journals still request manuscripts by mail, disk, or email. Authors generally submit hard copies of book manuscripts with the electronic files.

Submission to the journal requires writing a cover letter to accompany the manuscript, obtaining signatures on the transfer of copyright form if required for submission, and either uploading or emailing the file or packing the disk or manuscript and related materials for mailing. The author now awaits the results of the review of the paper.

REFERENCES

American Medical Association. (2007). *AMA manual of style: A guide for authors and editors* (10th ed.). NY: Oxford University.

American Psychological Association. (2009). Publication manual of the American Psychological Association (6th ed.). Washington DC: Author.

Crist, J. D., McEwen, M. M., Herrera, A. P., Kim, S-S., Pasvogel, A., & Hepworth, J. T. (2009). Caregiving burden, acculturation, familism, and Mexican American elders' use of home care services. *Research and Theory for Nursing Practice: An International Journal, 23*(3), 165–179. doi: 10.1891/1541-6577.23.3.165

Association of periOperative Registered Nurses. (2009). Author information. *Applied Nursing Research.* Retrieved from http://www.aornjournal.org/authorinfo

Elsevier. (2009). Author information. *AORN Journal Online.* Retrieved from http://www.appliednursingresearch.org/

International Committee of Medical Journal Editors. (2008). Uniform requirements for manuscripts submitted to biomedical journals: Writing and editing for biomedical publication. Retrieved from http://www.icmje.org/urm_main.html

Wiley Interscience. (2009). Guidelines for authors. Journal of Obstetric, Gynecologic, & Neonatal Nursing. Retrieved from http://www3.interscience.wiley.com/journal/118495258/home

14

EDITORIAL REVIEW PROCESS

The last chapter presented the final steps in preparing a paper for submission to a journal. This same process is used in writing a grant, a report for an organization, and other types of papers. When the paper is completed, another person or group will more than likely read and critique it whether for publication, funding, or some other purpose. The process of writing drafts and revising them for content and format was emphasized in earlier chapters so the final paper contains the essential content, is organized clearly, and is well written. The cycle of writing a draft and revising it, combined with attention to other details described earlier, results in a paper that should be competitive with others that are also being reviewed.

Chapter 14 presents the editorial review process from the point at which the paper is received in the journal office through the final editorial decision. The roles and responsibilities of the editor, editorial board, and peer reviewers are discussed, and examples are provided of criteria used by reviewers when asked to critique a manuscript for publication. Peer review is not without issues, and some of these are examined in the chapter.

Manuscripts submitted to a journal may be accepted without revision or accepted provisionally pending revision, may be returned to the author for a major revision and resubmission, or may be rejected. Each of these editorial decisions has implications for the author and how the author responds to the editor.

■ WHO IS INVOLVED?

When the manuscript is completed, and all materials assembled, the manuscript and supplementary document are forwarded to the editorial office of the journal to begin the review process. The editorial office might include a large number of staff in a dedicated office for journals widely circulated and published frequently or an editor and limited if any support staff working online from their home offices. Journals differ in the resources needed to process manuscripts and, once accepted, to prepare them for production. For example, health-related newspapers and journals published monthly will need more editorial staff to handle the number of manuscripts to be processed in comparison with a specialty nursing journal published quarterly which receives and processes fewer manuscripts. The number of people involved in the editorial process and their roles, therefore, will differ based on the needs of the journal.

Editor

The editor of a nursing journal is an expert in the nursing specialty or content area covered by the journal. Depending on the focus of the journal, editors may have expertise in clinical practice, administration, management, education, research, and other areas. Few nursing editors are prepared as such, and most are selected for the position because of their knowledge of the topics covered by the journal.

In addition to content expertise, editors usually have additional knowledge and skills related to the types of articles published in the journal. For example, editors of journals that publish research have an understanding of statistics and research methods and have often conducted research themselves. Clinical journals that focus on a particular nursing role, such as publications for nurse practitioners, are generally edited by someone functioning in that role or with an understanding of it.

To maintain their expertise, editors spend much of their time keeping current by reading the professional literature; by attending professional meetings; through their own research, writing, and work; and by maintaining contact with experts in the field. This also serves as a way of soliciting manuscripts for the journal.

Some editors of journals began initially as assistant or associate editors, then moved into the editor's position. Most, however, served on editorial or advisory boards of journals, were manuscript reviewers, and have experience themselves writing articles, books, and other types of publications.

One or more editors are appointed by the owners of a journal. While the owner is responsible for all important business decisions about the journal, the editor is accorded full authority over journal content (International Committee of Medical Journal Editors [ICMJE], 2008). Editors work with their owner-publishers under contractual arrangements that state the duties, responsibilities and terms of both parties.

Functions of the Editor

Editors may work full time in their role or function as part-time editors who hold other positions in nursing. Part-time editors receive an honorarium by the publisher for serving in that role. The publisher of the journal is the individual or group that produces, distributes, and markets the journal. Editors report to the publisher of the journal through different types of organizational arrangements.

The editor is accountable to the readers for quality manuscripts that promote the development of the field. The editor also is accountable to the editorial board and reviewers for carrying out the editorial process and arriving at decisions consistent with their recommendations and advice. Since editors report to the publisher, they are responsible for meeting the publisher's expectations associated with editing the journal.

Responsibilities of the Editor

The editor's first responsibility is to readers: to inform and educate them by providing high quality scholarly papers that were fairly selected (American Medical

Association [AMA], 2007). In service of this first responsibility, the editor's overall responsibilities are for the editorial content and quality of the journal; direction of staff and consultation with board members; development and maintenance of procedures; and creation and enforcement policies that focus efforts to achieve the journal's mission effectively, efficiently, expeditiously, and ethically (AMA, 2007, p. 260).

To fulfill these responsibilities, the editor functions to:

- solicit high quality manuscripts
- work with authors to develop their ideas into manuscripts that are suitable for publication
- assess honestly and impartially the quality of manuscripts submitted to the journal
- select reviewers to critique papers
- decide on manuscripts to publish based on recommendations from the reviewers
- address appeals of decisions and conflicts of interest
- maintain confidentiality concerning all submitted manuscripts
- edit manuscripts
- decide on the papers to include in each issue
- complete other tasks to prepare the manuscripts for publication
- exhibit courtesy, tact, and empathy with authors and reviewers (AMA, 2007).

With most journals, the editor is responsible for deciding whether to accept or reject a manuscript. With refereed journals, peer reviewers critique the submitted manuscript and advise the editor on the acceptance decision, but the editor makes the final decision. For tenure and promotion considerations, refereed publications carry more weight because they include this peer review process, thereby providing an external review of the quality of the work and its contribution to nursing. There are other journals though that are not peer reviewed, and the editors read and critique the manuscripts in-house and make the acceptance decisions. These are considered non-refereed journals.

Editors work with authors, editorial board members, peer reviewers, the production editor, and other personnel associated with publishing the journal. Because the editor interfaces with the production editor, there is an opportunity to maintain the quality of the content of the manuscript as it moves through production.

The editor also establishes the editorial policies for the journal and develops the author guidelines for submitting manuscripts. These policies and guidelines are generally prepared with input from the editorial board and peer reviewers. If the journal is an official publication of a professional organization, the editor works closely with the officers and board of the organization so there is consistency between the goals of the journal and those of the organization.

In some journals the editor writes an editorial or solicits other people to write it. When associated with a nursing organization, the editorials often reflect the positions of that organization.

For journals with columns and departments, the editor has a role in soliciting manuscripts for them or working with the assistant or associate editor who has this responsibility. The editor and assistant or associate editor review these papers and suggest revisions to the authors rather than sending them to peer reviewers for critique.

Managing Editor

In addition to the editor, some journals also have a managing editor. The managing editor is the staff member responsible for the administrative details associated with processing the manuscripts from submission through publication. The managing editor sends the manuscripts to reviewers, tracks the status of reviews, and oversees the processing of the manuscripts once accepted for publication.

Editorial Board

Editors do not make decisions in isolation about the journals they edit. They consult with an editorial board, which is a group of individuals with expertise in the content covered by the journal and who contribute that expertise in advising the editor about strategic plans for the journal as well as in reviewing the quality, accuracy, and currency of manuscripts submitted to the journal. The editor makes the decisions as to who will serve on the editorial or advisory board to the journal.

The editorial board members may represent the board in community outreach; give the editor advice on policies, content and direction of the journal; provide feedback from journal constituencies; review and write manuscripts; and assist with editorial decisions (AMA, 2007). Board members are listed on the journal website and in the masthead. Editorial boards meet at least annually and confer by conference call as needed.

Peer Reviewers

Peer reviewers are experts in the topic of the manuscript; they are considered "peers" of the author because they have similar expertise allowing them to critique the paper. Depending on the journal and type of manuscript, peer reviewers may have published on the topic, may be practicing in the same specialization as the focus of the manuscript, or may have research or statistical expertise needed for the review. The principle is that peer reviewers have expertise to critique the manuscript and make recommendations to the editor. Peer reviewers are sometimes called external reviewers or referees.

The panel of peer reviewers of a journal is usually larger than the editorial board because expertise is needed for a wide range of topics. The editor chooses peer reviewers based on their expertise. The editor also may ask ad hoc reviewers, people who do not serve on the review panel but have specialized knowledge, to read a particular manuscript. With some journals, the editorial board also serves as the review panel, with the board members reviewing manuscripts in their areas of specialization.

Peer review is a privilege. Peer reviewers have an obligation both to conduct their review within the domain dictated by the particular journal and also to adopt a professional approach to the review (Happell, 2008). The domain of a review includes whether the manuscript topic will be of interest to the journal's usual readers and whether its quality will contribute to their scholarly endeavors. It is not within the purview of the reviewer to agree or disagree with the findings or conclusions. A professional approach to reviewing a manuscript includes identifying positive features of the work, treating the process as a learning experience rather than a test, providing as much detail as possible about literature that should be but was not considered, and to acknowledge one's own limitations of expertise when evaluating the work of others (Happell).

PEER REVIEW

Peer review is an extension of the scientific process whereby a journal submits the manuscripts it receives to outside review (ICMJE, 2008). The review policies and procedures used by these journals to review manuscripts differ widely across journals. For this reason general principles of peer review are described, recognizing that each journal will have its own way of conducting peer reviews and its own criteria and format. Some journals publish statements in the information for authors page on their peer review process and policies.

Peer review began in the eighteenth century when committees were set up by medical societies to evaluate papers sent to them for publication in their journals (Benos et al., 2006). As medicine became more specialized and more journals developed, editors found they lacked the knowledge to review manuscripts out of their specialization and sought experts to give them opinions about the submitted papers. Specialization became a driving force in the acceptance of peer review (AMA, 2007). As more manuscripts became available, peer review also was seen as a way of accepting the best papers for the journal.

Blind Review Process

Many peer reviewed journals use a process of blind review in which submitted manuscripts are sent to reviewers with the identity of the author and institution concealed. The editor removes the title page or otherwise conceals identifying information that might suggest the author and institutional affiliation. The principle behind sending a "blinded" copy, free of identifying information, is that there is less chance of bias when the reviewer does not know who wrote the article or the author's credentials. When the author also does not know the name of a reviewer, the process is called "double-blinded."

Blinding of authorship does not always work because in specialized areas often the reviewers know the research and projects of others. Baggs and colleagues (Baggs, Broome, Dougherty, Freda, & Kearney, 2008) reported that, even when a blinded copy was sent, reviewers thought they could identify the authors about 38% of the time, often by self-referencing. Even so, double-blind review was favored by 93.6% of the reviewers in the study because they believed it eliminated bias. The advantages of open review cited by the reviewers were that it imposes transparency on the process and allows comparisons across reviewers and across revisions of the manuscript (Baggs et al.).

Authors are usually blinded as to the identity of the reviewers. When reviews are returned to the author, the identities of the reviewers are masked so the author does not know who evaluated the paper. With this anonymity, reviewers are free to evaluate a paper honestly and without fear of repercussions from the author if they give a negative review. It is believed that these reviews are fairer. Unblinded reviews could deplete the ranks of reviewers significantly (Baggs et al., 2008).

Unfortunately, some authors have had experience in receiving highly critical reviews without feedback that could be used to modify the manuscript. Unless the editorial decision is to accept the manuscript, reviews can be considered negative. Some novice authors, upon receiving a negative review, may abandon all future attempts to write for publication. However, research shows that even the most experienced and highly cited authors (including Nobel laureates) receive negative reviews and rejection of their manuscripts (Campanario & Acedo, 2005). We discuss later in the chapter how authors can prepare proactively for the results of the review process by developing strategies to address negative reviews.

Whether certain kinds of peer review procedures actually improve the quality of scientific publications is debatable. A recent Cochrane review evaluated evidence for the impact of seven types of procedures on quality of a published paper: ways of screening, assigning, and blinding of manuscripts; use of reviewers who were internal and external to the journal; group versus single-person editorial decision-making; and types of feedback (Jefferson, Rudin, Brodney Folse, & Davidoff, 2007). The authors found little evidence that either the blinding or training of reviewers or the manner of feedback improved quality. Checklists and standardized media used for reviews were found to have a positive effect on overall quality. Editorial comments on grammar and style made articles more readable, based on a small sample of studies. Despite the complexity of such research, more studies are needed on the effects of editorial peer review on biomedical publications, including on the quality of nursing journals.

Purposes of Peer Review

The review process assists the editor in establishing the importance of the manuscript, its relevance to the journal, the value of its content to readers, the timeliness of the manuscript, and its overall quality, thereby providing a sound basis for the editor's decision. Peer reviewers give the editor and author their judgment and expert opinions about the manuscript. The editor uses the review as a basis for making the acceptance decision, and authors use the review for revising the paper.

With some journals, reviewers do not state their judgments on whether the paper should be published. For others reviewers recommend to the editor if the manuscript should be accepted, revised, or rejected; the editor then makes the acceptance decision considering these recommendations.

Journals differ in the focus of the manuscript reviews by the nature of the articles they publish. Journals that publish clinical articles emphasize more of the practical implications of the paper and how readers might use the ideas. Reviewers for journals that publish research focus more on the adequacy of the research design, how the research was carried out, appropriateness of the statistical methods, and conclusions drawn from the evidence.

Although there are differences across journals, reviewers commonly evaluate if the:

- ideas and information in the paper are new and innovative
- paper contributes to nursing and to the knowledge and skills of readers
- content is important and warrants publication
- content is relevant to readers of the journal
- content is at the appropriate level for readers
- content is applicable for the reader's practice
- paper is well organized
- ideas are expressed clearly and developed logically
- research methods are adequate
- evidence is sufficient to support conclusions drawn from the research
- point of view that is advanced is balanced
- references are current (within the last five years) and relevant (Penrose & Katz, 2004; AMA, 2007; American Psychological Association [APA], 2009).

Review Forms and Guidelines

Although some journals mail hardcopy or send email attachments of a manuscript and review forms to each reviewer, journals increasingly conduct peer reviews online. Reviewers establish online accounts for reviewing in the same way that authors establish online accounts for submitting manuscripts, as described in Chapter 13. Once the reviewer accepts an invitation to review, the journal administrator makes available digital links to the manuscript, instructions, and the review forms.

Online reviewing entails some general responsibilities for reviewers. Reviewers should familiarize themselves with the journal's web page and review-related links, addressing any questions to the journal administrator or managing editor. Spam filters may interrupt the flow of some crucial information or communication and should be disabled. It is important for reviewers to monitor whatever email inbox they designated for journal communication so that no messages are missed. Reviewers should not hesitate to alert the journal staff or editors about any special needs or considerations related to their participation. If professional or personal circumstances will prevent them from accepting any invitations to review for a significant period of time, the software program can automatically be set to alert the editor not to interrupt the reviewer with unwanted messages during that time. The setting also avoids delaying the completed review process. If a reviewer recognizes an assigned manuscript as having been authored by a close colleague or student or otherwise suspects a conflict of interest, the reviewer should contact the journal immediately so that the manuscript can be reassigned.

Most journals use review forms or checklists that specify the criteria for judging the manuscript and provide space for reviewers to support their ratings with comments about the paper. An example of a checklist and rating form is shown in Exhibit 14.1.

Review forms vary in the format and wording. Most forms give the reviewer an opportunity to rate features of the paper as present or absent. For example,

EXHIBIT 14.1

Sample Manuscript Review Form

The Journal of Nursing Administration
Manuscript Review Form

_____Are edited manuscript pages being faxed (###-###-####) to the office?

_____Are edited manuscript pages being scanned and emailed to the editor?

YES   NO

Is the content:

_____	_____	timely/relevant?
_____	_____	logically and clearly developed?
_____	_____	sophisticated enough for our readers?
_____	_____	innovative?
_____	_____	on cutting edge of knowledge on topic?
_____	_____	Introduction: Is the purpose of the paper clear?
_____	_____	Are most references from the last 3 years?
_____	_____	Are the references relevant?
_____	_____	Is the content's application/utility made explicit to the reader's
_____	_____	If there is no cost-benefit analysis, does the content warrant its addition?

Methods (if applicable):

_____	_____	IRB approval obtained (This is a research manuscript as evidenced by intervention to evaluate new or existing practices, adds subject risks beyond standard care, generates new knowledge, and/or findings have implications beyond the unit or institution).
_____	_____	This is a quality improvement manuscript but meets criteria (see above item) for a research paper. Ask authors to provide justification as to why IRB approval was not obtained.

———— ———— This is a quality improvement manuscript (reports internal process improvement, results are specific only to author's institution and are not intended for use in other organizations, describes standard of care, and is informational in nature/lessons learned). No IRB approval needed.

———— ———— Are the sample and sampling method adequate?

———— ———— Are the instruments reliable and valid?

———— ———— Are statistical tests appropriate?

———— ———— Are data adequately and appropriately presented?

———— ———— Do conclusions/generalizations/implications go beyond what findings/data/theory support?

General:

———— ———— Does the paper present new findings or ideas?

———— ———— If no, does it present old material better?

———— ———— Was the paper interesting to read?

———— ———— Publish ahead of print (PAP), when revised, on website (Critical, time-dated information that needs immediate publication)

————Please rate the overall quality of this manuscript on a scale of 1–5 (1=excellent; 2=good; 3=acceptable; 4=uncertain of acceptability; 5= unacceptable)

Comments:

Reprinted by permission of Suzanne P. Smith, EdD, RN, FAAN, Editor-in-Chief, *The Journal of Nursing Administration.*

(yes or no) "does the abstract accurately reflect the text, are the references current, etc."? Some forms ask the reviewer to compare the features of the submitted manuscript to other published papers in the field. For example, "compared to published articles of similar content or methods, is the quality of the data presented (or the mechanics of the writing, etc.) in the top 10%, top 25%, top 50%, lower 50%, or lower 25%?" Following the specific ratings, the review form may ask for an overall assessment of the manuscript and a recommendation to the editor concerning the editorial decision. The editor takes such comments under consideration, but the final decision rests with the editor. Examples of overall assessment and recommendation schema are shown in Exhibit 14.2.

Following the forced-choice ratings, the reviewer is invited to expand on the ratings in a narrative format. The additional comments are not required but are useful both to the editor as well as the author. The narrative customarily begins with a sentence or two that summarize the topic of the manuscript and one or more strengths or contributions. This is followed by an evaluation of each part of the manuscript that could be improved; the most helpful reviews are specific in these comments, suggestions, and questions. They encourage

EXHIBIT 14.2

Example of Scales for Reviewer's Overall Rating and Recommendation to Editor

- **Rating of the manuscript overall as:**
  - Excellent—Presents an important new approach, new ideas, or new information
  - Good—Improves significantly on previous work of its type or contains new interesting information
  - Average—Good work, but contains little novelty and may be of limited interest to most readers
  - Routine—No errors, but likely to have narrow or little interest to journal's main readership
  - Flawed—contains serious flaws in project design, data analysis, or presentation
- **Recommendation of action to Editor:**
  - Accept subject to minor revision. No need for re-evaluation by reviewer.
  - Possibly accept with moderate revision. May need re-evaluation by reviewer.
  - Do not accept. Major revision required, with re-evaluation by reviewers.
  - Possibly reject. May be more suitable for publication in another journal.
  - Reject. Not acceptable for publication by this journal.

the authors to refine and focus their manuscript for their intended readership. Exhibit 14.3 presents questions that a reviewer may consider appropriate to discuss in a narrative evaluation when reviewing research and other types of manuscripts.

These reviews and narrative comments are given to the author for use in revising the paper. They also provide documentation for the editorial decision. With some journals reviewers comment directly on the manuscript pages, which also are returned to the author for feedback, or indicate the page and line of the manuscript in question or needing revision, such as with online reviews.

Peer reviewers should be provided with guidelines for an appropriate review, so that it is fair and unbiased. Journals take care that reviews are solicited consistently for each manuscript submitted, using the same process, criteria, and format. Reviewers are required to disclose to the editor any conflict of interest that would bias their judgment of the manuscript and disqualify them from the review process (ICMJE, 2008).

Editors, editorial board members, and peer reviewers treat manuscripts and reviews as privileged communication. The manuscript is not publicly discussed

EXHIBIT 14.3

Topics Appropriate to Reviewer's Narrative Evaluation of Manuscript Sections

- Title
  - Does the title contain key words that interested readers would logically use in an index search?
  - Was the title too long, too general, inaccurate, non-professional, or boring?

- Abstract
  - Was the abstract complete, i.e., did it contain the objectives or research questions; study design, sample, and measures (if appropriate); key findings; and conclusion?
  - Were there discrepancies between the abstract and the full manuscript?

- Keywords
  - Did the keywords accurately reflect the content of the manuscript?

- Rationale, Background, and Objective(s)
  - Rationale
    - Did the introduction identify a significant problem?
    - Was the chief aim of the article stated clearly and concisely?
  - Background
    - Were there gaps in the background literature described? Did the reviewer need more or different information about prior research?
    - Was unnecessary background literature described?
    - Was the background literature described logically, e.g., from the more general to the more specific problem?
    - Was the reviewer ultimately convinced of a significant gap in knowledge and the importance of filling it?
  - Objective(s)
    - Do the authors propose specific and concrete objectives or research hypotheses or questions?

- Substantive *original* contribution
  - For a data-based study:
    - Was the design of the study appropriate to the rationale?
    - Were subjects chosen with clear inclusion and exclusion criteria and any groups clearly distinguished? Was the sample size large enough to draw useful conclusions? Were human or animal subjects protected?

Continued

Exhibit 14.3 *Continued*

- Were the assessment measures appropriate to the problem described in the Introduction?
- Was the data analysis strategy fully explained and did it fit the research questions?
- Was there enough information provided to support replication in another setting?
- Were results described completely and logically, in accordance with the tables?
- For non-data-based manuscripts:
  - Did the newly proposed material follow logically from the background literature?
  - Were all elements and dimensions of the new material identified, defined, and explained?
  - Did you have enough information to apply the new material in another setting, if appropriate?

- Conclusions and Implications
  - Were the conclusions justified or were they 'over-interpreted', i.e., did they claim more than flowed logically from the background and original material?
  - Did the authors discuss similarities and differences between their work and the work of others, and possible reasons for differences?
  - Did the authors discuss implications of their findings for patients, students, communities, human subjects, faculty, clinicians, and/or researchers?
  - Did the authors discuss potential limitations to their conclusions and how future work might improve or extend their work?

- References
  - Were the references more than 5 years, or were classic articles on the topic missing?

- Tables and Figures
  - Were the tables and figures clear, complete, and effectively designed?
  - Could tables and figures be improved to reduce bias when displaying results?

- Style
  - Did the authors use standard English prose style?
  - Was the prose style direct and clear? If not, what are specific examples of difficult sections?
  - Did the authors avoid jargon, typographical and grammatical errors?
  - Was the manuscript compliant with required style guidelines, e.g., headings, citations, references, tables, etc.

prior to publication, and reviewers are not allowed to copy the manuscript they receive, use the ideas in a paper for their own work, nor share the ideas with others (ICMJE, 2008).

Manuscript Review Process

When the manuscript is submitted to the journal, it is given a number that is used throughout the review process to track the manuscript. This number is recorded in the author account on the journal website or on the email to the author acknowledging receipt of the manuscript and should be used by the author in all subsequent correspondence with the editor.

The editor or managing editor establishes careful records so the manuscript can be tracked through the review process beginning from its receipt in the editorial office, through the review and revision stages, and into production. Records are increasingly digitalized into audit trails, based on the software used by the journal and including email correspondence. For larger journals the managing editor usually assumes responsibility for this function. It is important that this record system be followed carefully so the whereabouts of each copy of the manuscript are known at all times and triggers are built in the system to signal delays in reviews (AMA, 2007).

Reasons Manuscripts Returned to Author

Not all manuscripts are sent out for review. If the manuscript is not relevant for the journal, the editor will likely return it to the author without its being reviewed. The editor usually will specify in the letter to the author why the manuscript is not suitable for the journal and its readers or other reasons for its return. The editor may suggest an alternative target journal for the topic. The author, however, can avoid this situation by carefully selecting journals for submission as discussed earlier in the book.

The second reason a manuscript may be returned to the author rather than its being reviewed is when it is incomplete or does not conform to the journal requirements. The manuscript may not be properly formatted, may not be written using standard English grammar and syntax, or the reference format may not be consistent with the journal guidelines. The importance of carefully preparing the manuscript and checking it before submission was described earlier. If authors do not follow these principles, the review of the manuscript may be delayed.

Steps in Review Process

After the editor determines the suitability of the manuscript for the journal, then the review process begins. How many peer reviews are done depends on the journal, but generally at least two reviews are completed of each manuscript. For some papers an additional review might be included to assess a specific aspect of the paper such as the statistical analysis used for a research study.

The editor decides who should review the manuscript. This decision is based on who has the expertise to evaluate the manuscript and make a judgment of its relevance for readers, importance, timeliness, and quality, among other criteria. For papers with highly specialized content, the editor may seek ad hoc reviewers, i.e., people not on the review panel and who do not normally review for the journal. They may have the expertise, however, to judge a particular manuscript.

The results of the peer review are then sent to the author with the editorial decision on whether the paper is accepted, should be revised and resubmitted, or is rejected. The editor also sends questions about the content, issues to be resolved, and suggestions for revision that were identified during the review process. The reviews provide data for the editor to use in making an acceptance decision and feedback for authors in revising the paper to strengthen it. In some instances the manuscript may be accepted without further revision, but usually authors revise their papers using the comments and suggestions from reviewers.

After revising the manuscript, the author returns it to the editor who in turn may review the changes and make a final acceptance decision without another external review. If substantial changes were made in the manuscript or the author was directed to revise and resubmit it, the reviewers will critique the revised version and make recommendations to the editor. This revision process continues until the paper is accepted for publication.

■ EDITORIAL DECISIONS

Not every paper sent to a journal will be accepted nor should it be, to maintain the quality of the journal and meet reader needs. Rejection rates vary across journals. Some journals receive a large number of manuscripts, significantly more than could be published within a reasonable time frame, and therefore reject many of these papers. Other journals have fewer submissions and work with authors in revising their papers until acceptable for publication. Authors may inquire about rejection rates to the Editor, as this information is proprietary and calculated by publishers.

Editors monitor the number of papers accepted for publication to avoid a backlog of papers accepted but not published. Journals are allotted by the publisher a predetermined number of pages for each issue. This is known as a "page budget." Because of the cost, only this contracted number of pages is allowed. As such, the editor plans which manuscripts to include in each issue, estimating the number to accept so the time between acceptance and publication is not unreasonable. A delay in publishing accepted papers hinders disseminating new knowledge to readers, and when too much time elapses, papers may need to be updated. Some backlog though is needed to insure that a sufficient number of papers is available for each issue and to allow for fluctuations in submissions without creating a delay in publication.

Criteria for Acceptance of Manuscripts

The criteria used by editors to decide whether or not to accept a manuscript vary by journal, but the AMA (2007) identified nine criteria for importance and quality that most editors use in making this decision:

Importance

1. Represents a non-trivial scientific advance
2. Has clinical relevance (for clinical specialty journals)
3. Presents original information
4. Will be interesting to reader

Quality

1. Design and methods are appropriate to the research questions or hypotheses
2. Research questions and methods are adequately described and rigorously conducted
3. Data analysis is appropriate
4. Conclusions are supported by the findings
5. Subjects are treated ethically (pp. 303–304)

The editor also considers the number of papers on the same or similar topics that have already been accepted. It is unlikely that the editor will accept too many articles on similar topics because of the need to publish new content for readers. If the author is notified that the paper is rejected, the backlog of papers may have been an influencing factor, and the rejection may have less to do with the paper's quality and relevance for readers than the backlog of manuscripts.

Types of Editorial Decisions

Editors generally make one of three decisions, based on their own review and suggestions from reviewers: (1) accept for publication, (2) revise and resubmit, and (3) reject.

Accept for Publication

Accept for publication decisions may involve an acceptance with no revisions or limited ones, or a tentative acceptance pending revision. An acceptance without revisions is rare. Even if the paper is accepted for publication because of its important and timely content, it is likely that the author will need to make some changes to strengthen it. The author should make these revisions, or provide a rationale for not making them, and return the paper as soon as possible to the editor. It may be that the editor has space to include the paper in an upcoming issue or, if not, the paper will have a better chance of earlier than later publication.

Other acceptances are provisional, with the final decision resting on whether the author revises the manuscript to reflect the changes suggested by the editor and reviewers. Changes might be needed in the content, for example, adding or deleting content, preparing or omitting a table, including a new section of content, and so forth, or the changes might be in the writing style and format. As with acceptance decisions, the author should revise the paper without delay.

Revise and Resubmit

A second type of editorial decision is to revise and resubmit the manuscript for another review. When authors are asked to revise and resubmit the manuscript, it suggests that the paper has merit and would be strengthened by a revision. Although a revision does not guarantee acceptance, there is interest by the editor and reviewers in the paper and its message. For this reason, the author should take the time to revise the paper as recommended. Once again the author should not delay in resubmitting it.

Reject

The third editorial decision is a rejection. Perhaps the content was not new, and the author missed this in the literature review. The journal might have recently published a series of articles on the same or a similar topic or accepted a paper with the same theme. The content may be too specialized or not specialized enough for readers of the journal, or may be of limited interest to readers. The organization of the paper and writing style may be unclear. These are only a few of many reasons for a rejection.

Editors intend no personal offence when they reject a manuscript (AMA, 2007), and authors should not take a rejection personally. There are many reasons a manuscript may not be suitable for a publication, and the feedback from the editor and reviewers gives the author information about why the paper was rejected. Many well-written papers are rejected because the content and focus do not reflect the needs of the readers, and the paper would be better suited for a different journal and audience. When the reasons for rejection relate to the quality of the writing and development of the content, the author should get editorial assistance in revising the paper and should ask colleagues to critique the content. An example of a rejection letter is shown in Exhibit 14.4.

Except for unqualified acceptances, all other editorial decisions following peer review are returned to the authors with feedback in the form of comments or suggestions. Murray and Moore (2006) provided a taxonomy of six types of negative reviews that accompany non-accepted manuscripts: non-specific but scathing, scathing but useful, damning with faint praise (rejection), redirecting (to another journal), editorial (grammar and style), and inviting revision and resubmission. When an author receives any of the above, Murray and Moore (2006) strongly recommend digesting a negative review within a trusted group setting including coauthors or other colleagues in the process of writing for publication. This strategy serves several functions. First, the group can debate how to interpret reviewer responses, what may have prompted them, and how to revise the manuscript in response to the comments in a way that preserves the essence of the manuscript and the voice of its authors. Second, the group can brainstorm to generate ideas for how to frame the current and future manuscript in such a way as to avoid a harsh response, if one was received. Third, group members can

EXHIBIT 14.4

Sample of a Rejection Letter

Ref: JRN-D-09–00452
Manuscript Title: Clergy-laity support and patients' mood during serious illness
Journal of Research Nurses

Dear Dr. Turnbull,

Thank you for submitting your manuscript to the Journal of Research Nurses. We have now completed the review of your manuscript. Based on the comments and concerns of the external reviewers, we cannot accept your manuscript for publication. As you will see, our reviewers felt that, while the paper addressed an issue that is clearly of importance, the manuscript topic will not likely meet the needs of our readership. Taken together, the reviewers' comments resulted in a priority score for your manuscript that did not reach the bar for acceptance. The manuscript may be a better fit with a palliative care or religion and health journal. We hope that you find the three reviews to be helpful in improving this paper, should you decide to send the paper elsewhere.

We hope this decision will not discourage you from submitting other work to us in the future. Thank you for letting us consider your work.

With best wishes,
Dr. Mary Jones
Dr. Frank Barton
Senior Editors of *Journal of Research Nurses*

share stories of their own experiences with negative reviews, how they reacted and responded, and to what end, in order to provide mutual support.

Campanario and Acedo (2005) found that the most common arguments given by reviewers against papers were that the findings did not advance science or understanding enough to warrant publication, they lacked practical implications, or they posed the wrong research question or were based on the wrong conceptual model. Despite these complaints, the authors who received them acknowledged the positive effect of receiving constructive feedback. The strategies used by highly regarded scientists in the face of criticism were to resist distraction and discouragement, to persevere, to communicate directly with the editor, and to seek support from colleagues.

The author should evaluate the comments made by the editor and reviewers, for these may provide a basis for revising the paper and submitting it to another journal. It may be that the second or third journal is a better fit for the content and writing style, or these journals may have fewer submissions and accept more papers than did the first journal to which the paper was sent. In revising the paper and submitting it to a different journal, remember to reformat it to fit the journal requirements, including the reference format, writing style, page limits, and so forth, so it appears to be written for that journal.

This revision and resubmission process can be continued until the manuscript is accepted or the author determines that no further revisions are possible. The author might even try a non-refereed journal or newsletter as an option for publication.

▦ MANUSCRIPT REVISION

Authors should understand the review process. Few papers are accepted without some revision. Generally manuscripts need to be revised whether they are accepted for publication, tentatively accepted pending revision, or need a major revision prior to resubmission. If the paper is not rejected, the author should revise it using the feedback from the editor and reviewers and resubmit it to the journal within the deadline specified by the editor.

Authors should adhere to this deadline because some editors may accept the manuscript when returned. If the modifications were substantial, the editor may elect to send it back to one or more of the previous reviewers. If the criticisms made by the reviewers were resolved, an acceptance decision is more likely.

An invitation to revise and resubmit is accompanied by suggested changes that the author should consider. The comments from reviewers are intended as constructive criticism, and usually their questions point out areas needing revision. The author can respond by revising the paper as suggested or can provide a rationale as to why those changes are not appropriate.

Not all revisions have to be made in the paper, but the author should justify why changes were not made rather than sending the paper back without the suggested revisions. The author should indicate which revisions would not strengthen the paper and provide a rationale. "Slavish compliance with all recommendations of all reviewers may result in a manuscript that is difficult to comprehend, which is not the intent of the review process" (APA, 2009, p. 228). Sometimes the proposed revisions would not strengthen the paper, but they also might give the author a clue as to areas of the paper that are not clearly written or have missing information. It may be that the writing is unclear or there is another flaw in the presentation that created the problem for the reviewer.

Letter to Send With Revision

In revising the paper, the author should prepare a letter to accompany the revised version of the paper that explains each revision suggested and made in the paper as well as changes not made and why. The letter should indicate:

- each change proposed by the editor and reviewers;
- the specific revisions made in response to each of these proposed changes;
- the location of the revisions, for example, the exact page number, paragraph, and sentence (or line) where the revision is located; and
- changes proposed and not made in the manuscript with a rationale.

Exhibit 14.5 provides an example of a cover letter to submit with a revised manuscript; Exhibit 14.6 presents two alternatives for summarizing the changes suggested by the editor and reviewers and those made in response by the author.

EXHIBIT 14.5

Example of a Cover Letter Sent in Response to Reviewer Comments

Dear Dr. Smith,

Thank you for your invitation to revise and resubmit Manuscript #2010–0074 Medication Safety Initiative in Intensive Care. We found the comments and suggestions from you and the reviews helpful to us in strengthening and focusing the paper. Please see below the changes made to the manuscript in response to each comment.

We appreciate your time and attention and hope you will find the manuscript improved and appropriate for publication. Please do not hesitate to contact us with any other concerns or questions. We look forward to hearing from you at your earliest convenience.

Sincerely,
Jane Doe, MSN, RN

EXHIBIT 14.6

Examples of Alternative Formats for Displaying Revisions Made by the Authors in Response to Comments and Suggestions by Editors and Reviewers

Example #1

Outcomes of Using Admission and Discharge Nurses in Acute Care Settings

Revisions Proposed (page numbers refer to original manuscript)	Revisions Made (page numbers refer to revised manuscript)
Editor: Change first heading of abstract to Issues and Purpose and include statement of issue that prompted research	Heading revised and statement added (p. 2, paragraph 1)
Discuss rationale for factor analysis considering sample size of 75	Factor analysis was done in the original study with 120 admission and discharge nurses throughout the healthcare system. Paragraph on factor analysis revised to clarify this (p. 10, paragraph 2, sentence 1)

Continued

Exhibit 14.6 *Continued*

Reviewer #1: Add "qualitative portion" to description of questionnaire in abstract (p. 2)	Sentence revised (p. 2): "Nurses ($n = 75$) completed a modified satisfaction questionnaire *that collected both quantitative and qualitative data.*"
On pp. 3–4, include edits on text	Included as suggested
On p. 5, include statement as to why nurses were concerned about initiative	Sentence included on p. 5, paragraph 1, sentence 2
On p. 7, line 4, add "as compared to nurses on other units"	Added (see p. 7, line 11)
On p. 8 (and on p. 9, paragraph 3, line 1; p. 11, paragraph 1, line 1), were stress and challenge measured as separate variables? How did instrument collect qualitative data (also questioned on p. 10, paragraph 3, line 1, and on p. 15, line 3)?	Stress and challenge measured by individual Likert scales; 6 open-ended questions collected qualitative data. Description of instrument revised (p. 8, paragraph 2)
P. 8, Procedure: Were instruments anonymous?	Instruments were anonymous; no identifying information was collected. Added on p. 8, paragraph 1, line 3. Also added to text as recommended (p. 9, paragraph 2, line 3)
Add table with data	Table 1 added (p. 19)
On p. 10, paragraph 2, last sentence: How did these findings compare with other groups in the study?	Consistent with original study of new role for nurses; added (p. 10, last sentence)
P. 12, paragraph 2, line 2: Move M and SD to follow "staff"	Moved (p. 12, paragraph 2, line 4)
Reviewer #2: In abstract and on p. 11, only report p (not r)	Prefer to include the actual correlations with the p values. Rationale from *AMA Manual of Style* (10th ed.): Correlations should be reported with coefficient followed by significance, e.g., $r=0.61$, $p<.001$ (p. 541)
On p. 3, paragraph 2, line 7: Change patient to patients	Done
On p. 4, line 5: Add n	$n = 75$; added (p. 4, paragraph 1, line 3)
P. 4, paragraph 1, delete last sentence	Deleted
On pp. 4–5: Move paragraph 2 to p. 5 and sentences on Klehamer et al. study (p. 5, lines 4–6) to p. 4	Revisions made as suggested, with minor editing
On p. 5, paragraph 2, lines 4 and 5: Were the goals the same as patterns found in ethnographic data analysis?	Author of article uses "goals"

On p. 6, paragraph 1: Change "area" to "theme"	"Area" changed to "theme"
On p. 6, paragraph 2 and 3: Consider moving these two paragraph to earlier section of literature with other quantitative studies	The first set of studies reported in literature review (pp. 4–5) relate to experiences of nurses with other new models of care. Research on p. 6 is on studies about admission and discharge. For this reason, literature review was not reorganized
P. 7, line 1, change "Several studies" to "The studies noted here"	Done
Results: Add table	Table 1 added (p. 19)
On p. 13, delete last 2 sentences	Sentences deleted
P. 15, add sentence written on text	Sentence added and all other editing done as recommended (p. 15, last paragraph)

Example #2

Parents' Views of Quality Healthcare

Editorial Suggestions:

1. Add a table on demographic data, comparing the two groups: Table added (see p. 16, Table 1).
2. Include a list of pertinent Web sites: Added (see pp. 18–19).

Reviewer 1 Comments/Suggestions:

1. Weakness of study is lack of information about consumers: Findings added in text (see pp. 6–7, lines 12–16). Table added that presents demographic data (see p. 16, Table 1).
2. Add information on consumers such as age, educational level, marital status, views of nursing care of children, etc.: Ages of consumers (see p.7, lines 2–7); educational level (see pp. 6–7, lines 12–13 and p. 16, Table 1); marital status (see p. 7, lines 8–10 and p. 16, Table 1). Other demographic data presented on p. 7, lines 10–12. Views of nursing care of children are part of the Results.
3. Indicators not specific to care of children but, nevertheless, are general enough to provide information on perception of quality; investigator should have completed a pilot study: Paragraph on this limitation was rewritten (see p. 11, lines 3–4). Pilot study was completed but did not reveal this limitation (see p. 6, paragraph 1).

Reviewer 2 Questions/Suggestions:

1. How were subjects identified and accessed? Sentence added on p. 5, paragraph 2, sentence 3.
2. Did the study go through IRB? Yes, sentence added on p. 5 (line 8).

Continued

Exhibit 14.6 *Continued*

3. In terms of the Quality Health Care Questionnaire (QHCQ), is most of the literature used to identify indicators (for instrument) included in reference list of manuscript? Is so, add statement to this effect: No, the literature used to identify indicators for the QHCQ is much more extensive than that reported in manuscript. For this reason, statement was not added.
4. Indicators and factors used interchangeably in this section: Differences between the indicators and factors are explained on pp. 5–6 (lines 9–11). No revisions were made in this section.

Both formats include an example of how to respond to a reviewer's suggestion that was not made in the revised version of the paper. Authors should refer to each change suggested by reviewers using the reviewer's number, for instance, Reviewer #1, so it is clear to the editor who had suggested the revision.

Conflicting Reviewer Comments

There are times when reviewers might give conflicting advice to authors. One reviewer may suggest expanding a content area while another recommends eliminating it. As a result, the author is unsure how to revise the paper to improve it. The first step is to reread the comments to confirm that they are conflicting. It may be that both reviewers identified the same problem in the text or graphics, even though their suggestions for revision are quite different. If the author is asked to expand a content area by one reviewer and to delete it by the other, it may be that the paper is not clearly written in that section; the conflicting comments suggest some problem with that area of content. If neither of the reviewers suggested a change that would solve a specific concern, the author should develop another approach that could be used.

Decision Not to Revise

There are times, however, in which authors cannot modify the paper sufficiently to reflect the concerns of the editor and reviewers. In these situations, the author might send it to another journal or rewrite the paper for a different type of publication, for example, modifying a research report for submission to a clinical journal with more of an emphasis on patient care rather than the research itself, describing how the instrument was developed and validated, and preparing an integrated literature review for a publication. At some point the author may need to abandon the attempt to publish the work.

In other situations the author may decide not to take the time to revise the manuscript substantially in order to address the editor's and reviewers' concerns. This decision should be made carefully by weighing the alternatives of revising the paper for a journal with some interest in it versus sending it to another journal where there may be minimal interest in its content. If the author decides not to revise and return the manuscript, the editor should be notified so records can be kept up-to-date.

Time Frame for Decision

If the editor decides not to review the manuscript, the author will be notified of this decision within a few weeks. If the manuscript is sent to peer reviewers, the length of time varies widely for the reviewers to critique a manuscript, for the editor to compile and summarize the reviews, and for an editorial decision to be made. Many journals ask peer reviewers to complete their critiques within three weeks, but not everyone is able to meet this deadline. Reviewers have competing demands, and it sometimes takes longer than anticipated.

The earliest the author would be notified about the decision on whether to publish the manuscript is approximately eight weeks after it is submitted to the journal. Some editors make their editorial decisions more quickly than others, but generally it takes at least eight weeks to complete the review process and notify the author of the publication decision. If the author has not heard by twelve weeks, the author should contact to editor to inquire about the status of the review.

Length of Time to Publication

Journals vary in their backlogs of accepted manuscripts waiting to be published. Some journals have a backlog of a year or two while others may publish the manuscript six months after the final version is accepted. Journals are increasingly publishing papers electronically before print, either the final version of the manuscript as it will appear in print or prior versions so readers can follow the revisions of the paper. These papers are identified in MEDLINE as [Epub ahead of print], and journal subscribers can often access them at the journal website at no cost. Other readers can obtain these electronic versions similarly to print publications.

Honorarium

Most scientific journals do not reimburse the author when a manuscript is accepted for publication. Unlike consumer magazines that generally pay authors for an accepted paper, most nursing and healthcare journals do not give an honorarium. When they do, though, this is often specified in the author guidelines. For example, *AORN Journal* indicates that an honorarium will be sent to the author after publication as well as a copy of the issue and reprints of it (Elsevier, 2009). *Nursing 2009* pays authors approximately $50 per printed page. When the article is published, the editor sends an honorarium to the primary author plus complimentary copies of the issue in which the article appears (Lippincott Williams & Wilkins, 2009).

Some journals provide complimentary copies of the issue in which the article appears as well as a specified number of hardcopy reprints. Reprints can usually be downloaded from the journal's website to members of subscriber organizations such as libraries. Reprints can also be purchased following publication through the publisher website.

SUMMARY

The primary responsibilities of the editor are to solicit manuscripts, work with authors to develop their ideas into manuscripts that are suitable for publication, assess the quality of manuscripts submitted to the journal, decide on manuscripts to publish based on recommendations from the reviewers, edit manuscripts, and complete other tasks to prepare them for publication. Editors work with authors, editorial board members, manuscript reviewers, the production editor, and other personnel associated with publishing the journal. In addition to these roles, some journals also have a managing editor who is a paid professional responsible for the administrative details associated with processing the manuscripts from submission through publication.

Journals rely on external or peer reviewers, sometimes called referees, to read and critically judge the manuscripts submitted to the journal. Peer reviewers are experts in the topic of the manuscript; they are considered "peers" of the author because they have similar expertise allowing them to critique the paper. Peer reviewers give expert opinions about the manuscript and make recommendations to the editor concerning its acceptance.

Many peer reviewed journals use a process of blind review in which submitted manuscripts are sent to reviewers with the identity of the author and institution concealed. The editor conceals identifying information that might identify the author and institution with which affiliated. The principle behind sending a "blinded" copy, free of identifying information, is that there is less chance of bias.

Reviewers also are unknown to the author. When reviews are returned to the author, the identities of the reviewers are masked so the author does not know who read the paper. With this anonymity, reviewers are free to evaluate a paper honestly and without fear of repercussions from the author if they give a negative review. It is believed that these reviews are fairer.

When the manuscript is submitted to the journal, it is given a number that is used throughout the review process to track the manuscript. Not all manuscripts are sent out for review. If the manuscript is not relevant for the journal, the editor will likely return the manuscript to the author without its being reviewed. The second reason a manuscript may be returned to the author rather than its being reviewed is when it is incomplete or does not conform to the journal requirements.

After the editor determines the suitability of the manuscript for the journal, then the review process begins. The editor decides who should review the manuscript based on who has the expertise to evaluate the manuscript. There are usually at least two reviews completed of each paper. The results of the peer review are then sent to the author with the editorial decision on whether the paper is accepted, should be revised and resubmitted, or is rejected. The reviews provide data for the editor to use in making an acceptance decision and feedback for authors in revising the paper to strengthen it.

The criteria used by editors to decide whether to accept a manuscript vary by journal, but there are some general criteria most editors use in making this decision: (1) relevance of the paper for the journal, (2) importance of the content, (3) if the content is new and innovative, (4) validity of evidence to support the conclusions of the paper, (5) usefulness to the journal considering other topics published in it, and (6) the number of papers on the same or similar topics that have already been accepted.

There are three main types of decisions that can be made by the editor based on own review and suggestions from reviewers: (1) accept for publication, (2) revise and resubmit, and (3) reject. Accept for publication decisions may involve an acceptance with no revisions or limited ones, or a tentative acceptance pending revision. An acceptance without revisions is rare; even if the paper is accepted for publication, because of its important and timely content, it is likely that the author will need to make some changes to strengthen it. Other acceptances are provisional, with the final decision resting on whether the author revises the manuscript to reflect the changes suggested by the editor and reviewers.

The second type of decision is to revise and resubmit for another review. When authors are asked to revise and resubmit the manuscript, it suggests that the paper has merit and would be strengthened by a revision. The third editorial decision is a rejection.

A good review suggests changes that the author should consider. The author can respond by revising the paper as suggested or can provide a rationale as to why those changes are not appropriate. Not all suggestions have to be made in the paper, but the author should justify why changes were not made rather than sending back the paper without the suggested revisions. The author should prepare a letter to accompany the revised version of the paper that explains each revision suggested and made in the paper as well as changes not made and why.

When the manuscript is accepted for publication, the paper moves into the next phase. The author has some responsibilities here, such as answering queries and correcting page proofs, but the publisher completes most of the work performed at this stage

▦ REFERENCES

American Medical Association. (2007). *AMA manual of style: A guide for authors and editors* (10th ed.). New York: Oxford University Press.

American Psychological Association. (2009). *Publication manual of the American Psychological Association* (6th ed.). Washington, D.C.: Author

Baggs, J.G., Broome, M.E., Dougherty, M.C., Freda, M.C. & Kearney, M.H. Blinding in peer review: The preferences of reviewers for nursing journals. *Journal of Advanced Nursing, 64*(2), 131–138. Doi: 10.1111/j.1365–2648.2008.04816.x

Benos, D.J., Bashari, E., Chaves, J.M., Gaggar, A., Kapoor, N., LaFrance, M.,...Zotov, A. (2007). The ups and downs of peer review. *Advances in Physiology Education, 31,* 145–152. doi:10.1152/advan.00104.2006

Campanario, J.M. & Acedo, E. (2005). Rejecting highly cited papers: The views of scientists who encounter resistance to their discoveries from other scientists. *Journal of the American Society for Information Science and Technology, 58*(5), 734–743. doi: 10.1002/asi.20556

Elsevier. (2009). Author guidelines. *AORN Journal.* Retrieved from http://www.aorn.org/AORNJournal/

Happell, B. (2008). The responsibility of review: Guidelines to promote professional courtesy and commitment through the peer review process. *International Journal of Psychiatric Nursing Research, 13*(3), 1–9.

International Committee of Medical Journal Editors. (2008). Uniform requirements for manuscripts submitted to biomedical journals: Writing and editing for biomedical publication. Retrieved from http://www.icmje.org/urm_main.html

Jefferson, T., Rudin, M., Brodney Folse, S. & & Davidoff, F. (2007). Editorial peer review for improving the quality of reports of biomedical studies. *Cochrane Database of Systematic Reviews*, Issue 2, Art. No. MR000016. doi: 10.1002/14651858.MR000016.pub3

Lippincott Williams & Wilkins. (2009). Author guidelines. *Nursing 2009.* Retrieved from http://edmgr.ovid.com/nursing2009/accounts/ifauth.htm

Murray, R. & Moore, S. (2006). The handbook of academic writing: A fresh approach. NY: McGraw-Hill.

15

PUBLISHING PROCESS

When the manuscript is accepted for publication, the paper moves into the publishing phase. The author has some responsibilities here, such as answering queries and correcting page proofs, but most of the work is done by the publisher of the journal or by the group or individual responsible for the publication. The manuscript is edited for clarity and consistency with the journal style and format; the copyeditor more than likely will have questions about the manuscript for the author to answer. These questions, or queries, must be answered and the proofs must be reviewed, to confirm the accuracy of the content after editing and to check other details, in the time frame allowed.

Chapter 15 describes the publishing process that begins with the acceptance of the paper through its publication. Publishers have different ways of handling the manuscript editing phase and forms of the manuscript that they return to the author for proofing. The publishing process is described in the chapter, but the author should recognize that may differ across journals. When the paper is published by an organization or individual, the process may vary from what is described in the chapter.

WHAT HAPPENS NEXT?

The time from acceptance of the paper to its publication varies with the journal depending on its backlog and other factors such as the relationship of the topic to others waiting to be published, the focus of a particular issue, and other editorial priorities. It could take a few months to a year or longer before the paper is published. When the editor decides on the issue in which the paper will appear, the author is notified of this and when to expect the proofs to review. The manuscript is edited first by a copyeditor who formats the manuscript to be consistent with the journal style, corrects grammatical errors, and edits the paper. The copyeditor works for the publisher, not the author, and will not rewrite the manuscript; authors who need help with writing should get editorial assistance before they submit the paper to the journal (Lang, 2010). The author receives proofs of the edited manuscript, which are in portable document format (PDF): these proofs appear like the pages in the journal but will have queries for the author to check (Figure 15.1).

In this stage of publication, the author reviews the proofs, answers questions raised by the copyeditor, corrects any errors in the paper as a result of the

FIGURE 15.1

Sample Proof of Journal Page

4   JOURNAL OF NURSING CARE QUALITY/JANUARY–MARCH 2010

The systematic review included information collected from 6 well-executed RCTs. The review showed significant benefits with aspirin [AQ6] use for total coronary heart disease, nonfatal MI, and total CVD events ($P < .001$ in each case).

One cohort study conducted by Goldstein [AQ7] et al was appraised using the Scottish Intercollegiate Guidelines Network checklist.[13,15] This was a multicenter study to assess the role of aspirin in the progression of coronary heart disease in patients currently receiving therapy. The results of the study concluded significant outcomes related to long-term aspirin use in cardiac death, all-cause mortality, and nonfatal infarction ($P = .005, .009,$ and $.029,$ respectively). This study was not an RCT.

SYNTHESIS

The evidence collected through the evaluation of the 10 documents supports the use of aspirin for prevention of cardiovascular events. On the basis of the combined results of these studies, aspirin decreases total CVD events. Heterogeneity was present across some studies for outcomes including stroke and mortality. This was mainly attributed to the results of 3 different RCTs that concluded there was insufficient evidence for or against recommending aspirin for the prevention of CVD events. Possible reasons for the heterogeneity include patient selection, randomization, and the presence of baseline disease patterns.

The remainder of the studies all possessed consistent and strong evidence that supports the use of aspirin for prevention of CVD events. Furthermore, Sanmuganathan et al[12] and Hayden et al[10] presented supplemental information regarding the benefits and risks of using aspirin for preventative therapy. Gaps in the evidence remain about the efficacy of aspirin use for prevention of CVD in women and dose-specific outcomes related to CVD. Further research is warranted in these areas to provide strong evidence to guide practice. Nine of the 10 data sources reviewed, though,

provide evidence that is strong enough to support the use of aspirin therapy for the prevention of CVD events. The literature demonstrated an obvious benefit associated with aspirin as the studies were compounded.

NURSING IMPLICATIONS

The findings from this review provide important evidence-based implications to consider when planning nursing care. Documentation of a thorough patient history is imperative to the delivery of care at all levels of nursing practice. Cardiovascular risk factors, including family history, nicotine use, physical activity, obesity, hypertension, diabetes, and elevated cholesterol levels, should be discussed in detail with patients.[2] Every attempt should be made to modify risk factors as indicated; however, the evidence shows that patients with cardiovascular risk factors benefit from aspirin therapy.[4] Furthermore, patients who have a history of cardiovascular events including MI should be treated with daily aspirin therapy indefinitely.[1] Likewise, patients with a coronary artery intervention including stent placement should receive daily aspirin indefinitely.[16] Absolute contraindications to aspirin therapy include true aspirin allergy.[1]

Careful consideration should be given in discontinuing therapy once it has been initiated, and the risks and benefits of doing so must be considered. Patients should be monitored for GI tract and bleeding complications. In addition, a complete blood cell count, platelet count, prothrombin time, liver function studies, serum urea nitrogen, and serum [AQ8] creatinine should be obtained periodically.[17] Patients should be educated to monitor for bleeding complications and consult their cardiovascular provider before discontinuing antiplatelet therapy.

CONCLUSION

On the basis of the information gathered for this review, regular aspirin use is positively correlated with the reduction in editing or formatting, and checks other details such as word divisions, accuracy of tables, and accuracy of author information. Even though the author reviewed the manuscript thoroughly prior to sending the final version, the paper has since been edited, and the author needs to verify that the changes made during editing did not alter the intended meaning. This is the last chance for the author to find errors in the paper prior to its publication.

Authors need to read the proofs carefully because copyeditors are not nurses, and they do not have expertise in the topic; the copyeditor may have altered the meaning of a sentence when grammatical errors were corrected or the paper was formatted for consistency with the journal style. In this process of editing the paper, some of the meaning may have been changed and errors in the content may have resulted. The author is responsible for identifying these when reviewing the proofs. Authors should check carefully their tables and figures because they will be modified to conform to the journal style and formatting, and errors may have occurred as a result of this process.

There is generally a limited period of time, for some journals only 48 hours, for the author to read and correct the proofs of the manuscript. The author should adhere to this time frame. Otherwise, the article may be printed as is with any errors present. Generally, authors are emailed a link for them to access the proofs of their paper or the PDF is emailed to them. Authors should notify the editor if there is a change in email address or if an alternate one should be used for emailing the proofs. When registering at the journal website, it is a good idea to include a backup email address; then the proofs and other correspondence will be sent to both email addresses.

Formats for Author Review

With chapters and books, authors will be emailed the edited version of the manuscript that shows the corrections made in the paper. The edited manuscript displays the original text and each revision using track changes such as in Microsoft Word or a similar program. The author should read the edited version carefully, noting any errors or revisions that are needed because few changes can be made in the proof stage. With some edited books, the copyedited chapters are emailed to the editor rather than the individual author(s) of the chapter, and only the editor reviews the manuscript and proofs. Alternately, the copyedited chapters will be reviewed by the authors themselves and then sent to the editor to return to the production manager. With journals, however, as mentioned earlier, the author receives the edited paper in the form of proofs that incorporate the copyeditor's revisions. The proofs are in PDF format.

Proofing the Manuscript

Authors are emailed an edited version of their chapter or book, or proofs of their journal article for two purposes: to check for errors and answer queries about it. For chapters and books, authors can use the track changes function to indicate additional revisions or modify ones made by the copyeditor, and can insert notes in the edited version of the text. This will be the final chance to make revisions in the text. Authors should alter the color used in track changes to a different one from the edited version; that way the author's revisions of the edited manuscript will be apparent to the copyeditor.

For proofs of articles, however, the author cannot rewrite the text except for what is necessary to correct an error. The paper was accepted as submitted in the final version, following peer review, and the author cannot rewrite it at this stage. If the content has changed since the paper was accepted, this should be discussed with the editor rather than modifying the proofs. Changes at this point in the publishing process are expensive and therefore should focus only on the accuracy of the content (Chambers, Wakley, Nineham, Moxon, & Topham, 2006). Authors can print the proofs and can answer queries and note revisions in the margins and on the PDF pages; the marked up proofs can then be faxed to the production editor. Another way is to indicate the revisions and answer the queries on the PDF pages using the Comments function, which allows authors to insert and delete text and answer queries in notes to the editor.

Answering Queries

The author must answer each query raised by the copyeditor. Often this is done easily by checking a revision, inserting text, modifying a reference, and revising the table or text so they are consistent. Some queries require an explanation, which the author can add in the margin or as a note to the editor in the PDF file. If unable to answer a question, this should be noted.

Areas to Proof

What should the author check when reviewing the edited version of chapters and books, and the proofs of articles? First, the main goal is to ensure that there are no errors in the content. There are times when a minor editorial revision changes the meaning of the sentence, and this is the author's only chance to correct the paper prior to publication. The author should confirm that the content is accurate, the changes made by the editor did not alter the meaning, nothing was omitted from the paper that is essential, and the correct numbers are in the text, tables, and illustrations. In proofreading the paper, the author should compare the original copy sent to the editor against the proofs.

Second, the author should check for spelling and grammatical errors. Even though this was a done in preparing the final version, a misspelled word might not have been noticed, and words correctly spelled might have been used incorrectly, such as rational for rationale. The spelling of authors' names, their credentials, their positions, and the contact information of the corresponding author should be verified. The author should check the title of the article and spelling of words in it.

The author also should pay attention to how words are divided. In aligning the right margin of the text, some words may need to be divided. The author should check that these divisions of words are correct and make sense. If not, authors can add a note for the editor to check a "bad break" in a term.

Third, the author should review the abbreviations, numerical values in the text and tables, statistical results, references, tables, and figures. Errors may have occurred when these were formatted for the style of the journal. For research articles, the author should verify that the numbers used to report the findings are the same in the abstract, text, tables, and figures, and that no data are missing. The author should check carefully numbers with decimals, p values, and statistics. The copyeditor may have made changes in how the statistics are presented to conform to the journal's style, and the author needs to review these for any errors.

The names of authors cited in the text should be compared with the reference list. If numbers are used for the citations, these should match the correct reference.

For some journals tables require substantial reformatting; for this reason tables in the proofs should be checked carefully. Each column and row should be examined, paying attention to whether the numbers are accurate and are lined up properly. Footnotes from the original copy may be changed to the symbols used by the journal; the author should verify that footnotes are included and are correct. The proofs of figures such as flowcharts, guidelines, and other illustrations should be examined carefully to ensure that they are clear and can be read when published in the journal. Titles of the tables and figures also should be reviewed.

Exhibit 15.1 is a checklist authors can use when reading proofs. Authors should not take this step lightly because the author is responsible for identifying and correcting errors before the paper is printed (Lang, 2010).

EXHIBIT 15.1

Proofing Checklist

Use this checklist to review your manuscript before submitting it for publication and again to check the proofs.

Check:

- that the author information is accurate and all coauthor names are spelled correctly
- that all content is accurate, including any numbers, medication names and dosages, names of instruments and measures, statistical symbols and results, information in the tables and figures, and other content
- line by line for grammatical, punctuation, and other errors
- that acronyms are spelled out the first time cited in the paper and that only the acronym is used from that point on

Continued

Exhibit 15.1 *Continued*

- that all author names cited in the paper have a reference to the source
- that citations and references are accurate and formatted per journal style
- that the level of headings is correct based on how the content is organized and journal style
- that names of commercially developed products have the appropriate™ or ®marks
- that each table, figure, and other illustration is correct
- that individuals and hospitals cited in the acknowledgment, text, or elsewhere in the paper have given written permission, which was sent to the editor
- that written permission for using or adapting copyrighted material was received and the appropriate credit line was added

Citing in Press Papers

Manuscripts accepted for publication by the journal can be cited as "in press" (American Medical Association [AMA], 2007; American Psychological Association [APA], 2009). Some publications require authors to verify the paper has been accepted (AMA, 2007). Manuscripts that have been submitted to journals and are in review cannot be listed with the references. Instead, the author should cite the work in the text as "unpublished data" or an "unpublished paper." For example:

> Similar findings have been reported in a rural health clinic (J. A. Smith, DNP, unpublished data, June 2010).

If the "in press" paper is published by the time the author receive the proofs in which it was cited, the proofs can be updated; similarly, if a submitted manuscript is accepted, the proofs can be changed to "in press."

Ordering Reprints

After reviewing and correcting the proofs, the author has some assurance that the manuscript will be printed without errors and in the issue indicated by the editor. Generally the proofs are reviewed a few months prior to publication. Many journals email forms for ordering reprints with the proofs. If the author is interested in having reprints to distribute to colleagues, students, and others, they should be ordered when the proofs are reviewed or whenever the author receives the information about reprints. After the journal is published, reprints may be more expensive or may not be available. Thus, authors should decide early if they want reprints. The author decides how many reprints to order, but it is best to over-order them. Generally, the more reprints that are ordered, the less expensive they are for the author.

Some authors may want to distribute copies of their paper before it is published or post it on the Web. However, the copyright was transferred to the publisher, and any pre-publication of the paper would need to be consistent with the conditions in the copyright transfer.

After the article is published, the author will receive a limited number of complimentary copies of the journal or a final PDF of the paper, depending on the publisher. Complimentary copies are not mailed to coauthors: the corresponding author is responsible for distributing copies to them.

CORRECTIONS AND RETRACTIONS

If the author discovers after an article is published that there were errors in the data reported or the conclusions reached, the author should contact the editor and email a letter correcting the information. A correction or erratum of part of the work will be published in a later issue of the journal. The corrections will appear on a numbered page, be listed in the Table of Contents, and include the original citation (International Committee of Medical Journal Editors [ICMJE], 2008).

If there is scientific fraud, however, the paper should be retracted (ICMJE, 2008). The author should submit a letter, signed by coauthors, to the editor requesting a retraction and indicating the reasons. The retraction will be published in a subsequent issue of the journal. If the paper is not yet published, the editor more than likely will allow the author to withdraw it. Along the same line, if the author determines later that a coauthor published the same data in another paper, without indicating this in the current article, a letter is sent to the editor who will note this as a repetitive publication.

COPYRIGHT

Copyright is a form of legal protection to the authors of "original works of authorship," including literary, dramatic, musical, artistic, and other intellectual works, preventing others from copying them (U.S. Copyright Office, 2008). U.S. copyright law is defined by the Copyright Act of 1976. Copyright provides protection for any original material created by the author, including both published and unpublished works. Coauthors of papers written collaboratively have equal rights to the copyright.

The copyright law gives authors, or whomever holds the copyright, six exclusive rights: (1) to reproduce the work, (2) to prepare derivative works, (3) to publish or distribute copies of the work to the public, (4) to perform the work publicly, (5) to display it, and (6) for sound recordings to perform the work by means of digital audio transmission (U.S. Copyright Office, 2008, p. 1). The owner of the copyright is the only person allowed to exercise these rights; anyone else who wants to reproduce, modify, publish, perform, or display the work must get permission from the copyright owner.

Protected Works

Copyright protects original works "that are fixed in a tangible form of expression" (U.S. Copyright Office, 2008, p. 2). These protected works include:

1. literary works (e.g., articles, books, journals, software, and digital formats)
2. musical works including the accompanying words
3. dramatic works including the accompanying music
4. pantomimes and choreographic works
5. pictorial, graphic, and sculptural works
6. motion pictures and other audiovisual works
7. sound recordings, and
8. architectural works. (U.S. Copyright Office, p. 3)

For works created from 1978 to the present, the term of protection for copyright is the life of the author plus 70 years. For works created between 1964 to 1977, the protection for copyright is 28 years for the original term plus an automatic 67 year renewal; for materials created between 1923 and 1963, the protection extends for the original 28 year term with an additional 67 years if the copyright was renewed. Works created before 1923 are in the public domain.

Unprotected Works

Several categories of materials, though, are not protected by copyright. These include among others:

- works that have not been fixed in a tangible form of expression such as speeches or performances that have not been written or recorded
- titles, names, short phrases, and slogans; familiar symbols or designs; variations of typographic ornamentation, lettering, or coloring; and listings of ingredients or contents
- ideas, procedures, methods, systems, processes, concepts, principles, discoveries, or devices, as distinguished from a description, explanation, or illustration. Although the ideas may not be protected by copyright law, the written description of the ideas may be.
- works consisting entirely of information that is common property and has no original authorship, for instance, calendars and lists or tables taken from public documents or other common sources (U.S. Copyright Office, 2008, p. 3).

U.S. Copyright Office

Information about copyright is available to authors through the U.S Copyright Office at the following address:

Library of Congress
U.S. Copyright Office-COPUBS
101 Independence Avenue, SE
Washington, DC 20559–6304

Information about U.S. copyright, frequently requested circulars, copyright application forms, and related materials are available at http://www.copyright. gov/.

Transfer of Copyright

The copyright is held initially by the author, or coauthors, of the manuscript. When a manuscript is being considered for publication by a journal, each author contributing to the paper typically transfers the copyright to the publisher either at the time the manuscript is submitted or when it is accepted. Publishers usually require assignment of the copyright to them so they in turn may publish the article and distribute it in different forms. If the copyright transfer form is submitted with the manuscript, prior to its acceptance by the journal, the copyright reverts to the author, or coauthors, if the manuscript is not published.

Publishers have their own copyright transfer forms that are signed by each author. When the copyright is transferred, the publisher becomes the legal owner of the published paper. Neither the author nor others may reproduce the paper without written approval of the copyright holder—the publisher. Authors who want to reproduce any figure, table, or text from the copyrighted material must receive permission from the copyright holder. This is true even for the author's own article because the copyright was transferred to and is then held by the publisher.

This is an important principle for all manuscripts but especially for papers that include forms, tools, and other materials from clinical agencies, schools of nursing, and other institutions. The institution needs to grant permission for authors to include the material with their manuscripts; the credit line should indicate that the materials were reprinted by permission of that institution; and there should be a statement added that the institution retains the copyright to them. Otherwise the form, tool, guideline, or other document in the manuscript will be included in the transfer of the copyright to the publisher, and the institution will no longer be able to use it without the publisher's permission. Authors should check with the journal editor about how best to handle materials such as these in a manuscript.

Copying and Reproducing Copyrighted Material

The fair use provisions of the copyright law, contained in Title 17 of the United States Code, Section 107, allow the author to quote, copy, or reproduce a small amount of text from a copyrighted work without permission of the publisher or other holder of the copyright (U.S. Copyright Office, 2008). Fair use of copyrighted materials for purposes such as teaching, scholarship, and research, among others, is not considered an infringement of copyright. If it is more than a small section of copyrighted work, though, the author needs to get written permission from the copyright holder to use the material. Fair use does not give authors permission to reproduce complete articles nor to republish an article they wrote in a different journal.

In determining fair use, four factors are considered:

1. purpose of the use, including whether it is for commercial purposes or for nonprofit educational purposes
2. the nature of the copyrighted work
3. the amount of the material copied and how substantial it is in relation to the copyrighted work as a whole, and
4. the effect of the use on the potential market for or value of the copyrighted work (U.S. Copyright Office, 2009).

The amount of text subject to fair use is based on the proportion to the whole, but this proportion is not determined by number of words (AMA, 2007). There is no specific word length in the copyright law that is acceptable. For this reason the author needs to consider the above four factors when questioning whether permission should be obtained from the copyright holder. Some publishers may specify the number of words that are allowed to be reproduced without written permission. For example, the American Psychological Association (APA) provides guidelines for authors as to the extent of text and number of tables and figures published in an APA journal that may be reproduced without written permission from them (APA, 2009).

The author should be careful to include the reference to the original source. Any direct quotes should be placed in quotation marks, or indented to set off the quoted material, again with a reference to the original source.

Permission should be obtained for quotes that extend for a few paragraphs. The length quoted should not diminish the "value of the original work" (AMA, 2007, p. 198). Entire tables, figures, and illustrations may not be reproduced without permission. This includes use of a table, figure, or other type of graphic in a paper prepared for a course. Using one or two sentences from a table is acceptable if the original source is referenced, but reprinting the entire table is not. As discussed earlier, authors should obtain permission to adapt and reproduce tables, figures, and illustrations for a manuscript and for other types of writing projects.

The decision to reproduce text, tables, figures, and other illustrations in a paper is made early in the writing process, which is why permissions were discussed in chapter 4 on reviewing the literature. Authors need to allow sufficient time to receive these permissions to avoid delays in the submission and later publication of the manuscript. While a paper can be submitted for review pending the permissions to reprint, it cannot be published without them. How to obtain permissions was described in chapter 4 that also included sample letters and credit lines. It is best for authors to have these permissions in hand prior to submitting the manuscript because if permission is denied or not received in time for publication, the paper will need to be rewritten to avoid use of the quoted material, table, figure, and other illustration. For some manuscripts, this might require a significant amount of revision. Editors will likely ask authors for a letter from the copyright holder indicating approval to reproduce the material, but regardless of whether the permission letter is submitted to the editor, the author needs it to publish the copyrighted material.

Materials on the Internet and in Electronic Format

These same principles apply for materials published on the Internet and in electronic format. Works published on the Internet are not automatically in the public domain, and it cannot be assumed that they can be used in a manuscript. The fair use considerations identified earlier apply to Web sites, electronic documents, and digital works such as photographs, slides, and audio and video files. These materials are protected under copyright law and cannot be used in a publication without permission from the copyright holder (AMA, 2007). Copyright status varies widely across journals (International Committee of Medical Journal Editors, 2008). If there is any question about whether permission is needed, authors should seek permission to reproduce materials they did not develop themselves.

OPEN-ACCESS JOURNALS

Open-access is free and unrestricted online access to journals and their content. Journals that are open-access do not require transfer of copyright. Instead, they allow readers to freely download, copy, distribute, print, and link to the full text of articles (AMA, 2007, p. 184). These journals were discussed in Chapter 2. Open-access includes self-archiving and open-access publishing. With self-archiving, content is placed in an open archive prior to its publication, such as with preprints and advance online publishing of a paper, or in PubMed Central, which is the National Institutes of Health's free digital archive of biomedical and life sciences journals (PubMed Central, 2009).

Open-access publishing is when journals are freely open to use by consumers. These publications require authors, institutions, or another funding source to pay the costs of publishing the work (APA, 2007; Shieber, 2009). BioMed Central is an example of an open-access publisher (BioMed Central, 2009). Original research and other types of articles available at the BioMed Central Website are free to all users and accessible online immediately after their publication. The goal of BioMed Central is to provide open access to research findings to speed up dissemination.

SUMMARY

The publication stage provides an opportunity for the author to review the edited manuscript of chapters and books and the proofs of all types of publications, answer questions raised by the copyeditor, correct any errors in the proofs as a result of the editing or formatting, and check other details such as accuracy of tables and author information. Even though the author reviewed the manuscript thoroughly before sending the final copy, the paper has since been edited, and the author needs to verify that the changes made during editing did not alter the intended meaning. This is the last chance for the author to find errors in the paper prior to its publication. There also may be questions or queries about the text, references, or tables and figures that the author needs to answer.

There is generally a limited period of time for the author to read and correct the proofs of the manuscript, and the author should adhere to this time frame.

Otherwise the article may be printed as is with errors present. Authors should notify the editor if there is a change in email address for receiving the proofs or make this change at the journal website.

With chapters and books, the author or book editor is sent electronically the edited version of the manuscript that shows the corrections. The edited manuscript displays the original text and each change. With journals, the author receives a PDF of the proofs, which are the journal pages incorporating the copy-editor's revisions.

The proofs are sent to the author to identify errors, not for rewriting. After correcting them, the author has some assurance that the manuscript will be printed without errors and in the issue indicated by the editor. Generally the proofs are reviewed a few months prior to publication. Most journals send forms for ordering reprints at the same time as the proofs. When the article is published, the author receives either complimentary copies of the journal or PDFs of their paper.

Copyright is a form of legal protection to the authors of "original works of authorship." Authors own their manuscripts until they sign a copyright transfer form which then transfers the ownership to the publisher. This then gives the publisher the right to reproduce, modify, publish, perform, and publicly display the work. Authors who want to reproduce any figure, table or text from the copyrighted material must receive permission from the copyright holder. This is true even for the author's own article because the copyright was transferred to and is then held by the publisher.

REFERENCES

American Medical Association (AMA). (2007). *AMA manual of style: A guide for authors and editors* (10th ed.). New York: Oxford University Press.

American Psychological Association (APA). (2009). *Publication Manual of the American Psychological Association* (6th ed.). Washington, DC: APA.

BioMed Central. (2009). *What is BioMed Central?* Retrieved from http://www.biomedcentral.com/info/about/STM

Chambers, R., Wakley, G., Nineham, G., Moxon, & Topham, M. (2006). *How to succeed in writing a book*. Oxford: Radcliffe Publishing.

Copyright Clearance Center. (2009). *Copyright.com. Business.* http://www.copyright.com/viewPage.do?pageCode=bu1-n

International Committee of Medical Journal Editors. (2008). *Uniform requirements for manuscripts submitted to biomedical journals: Writing and editing for biomedical publication.* Retrieved from http://www.icmje.org/urm_main.html

Lang, T. A. (2010). *How to write, publish, & present in the health sciences: A guide for clinicians and laboratory researchers*. Philadelphia: American College of Physicians.

PubMed Central. (2009). *A Free Archive of Life Sciences Journals*. Retrieved from http://www.ncbi.nlm.nih.gov/pmc/

Shieber, S. M. (2009). Equity for open-access journal publishing. *PLoS Biol, 7*(8), e1000165. doi:10.1371/journal.pbio.1000165

U.S. Copyright Office. (2008). *Copyright Basics*. Retrieved from http://www.copyright.gov/circs/circ1.pdf.

U.S. Copyright Office. (2009). *Fair Use*. Retrieved from http://www.copyright.gov/fls/fl102.html

APPENDICES

APPENDIX 1

Selected Statistical Symbols and Abbreviations

Symbol or Abbreviation	Definition
$>$	Greater than
$\geq$	Greater than or equal to
$<$	Less than
$\leq$	Less than or equal to
α	Greek alpha, probability of Type I error; also reliability coefficient
ANCOVA	Analysis of covariance
ANOVA	Analysis of variance
β	Greek beta, probability of Type II error; also standardized regression coefficient (beta weight)
b	Regression coefficient
x^2	Chi-square test
CI	Confidence interval
d	Cohen's measure of effect size for comparing two sample means
df	Degrees of freedom
ES	Effect size
f	Frequency
F	F distribution, Fisher's F ratio
$F(v_1, v_2)$	F with v_1 and v_2 degrees of freedom
H_0	Null hypothesis
H_1	Alternate hypothesis
HSD	Tukey's (honestly significantly different) test
k	Kappa statistic
$KR20$	Kuder-Richardson reliability index
LR	Likelihood ratio
LSD	Least significant difference
$M\,(X)$	Mean of sample (arithmetic average)

Continued

347

Selected Statistical Symbols and Abbreviations   *Continued*

MANCOVA	Multivariate analysis of covariance
MANOVA	Multivariate analysis of variance
Mdn	Median
MS	Mean square
MSE	Mean square error
n	Number of cases (size of subsample)
N	Total number of cases (total sample size)
ns	Not statistically significant
OR	Odds ratio
p	Probability
r	Pearson product-moment correlation coefficient
r^2	Coefficient of determination; estimate of Pearson product-moment correlation squared
R	Multiple correlation
SD	Standard deviation of sample
SE	Standard error
SEM	Standard error of measurement
Σ	Sum
SS	Sum of squares
t	Student *t* (include *p* value, 1- vs. 2-tailed)
U	Mann-Whitney test
z	Z score; value of a statistic divided by its standard error

APPENDIX 2

Unnecessary Words in Writing

Unnecessary Words	More Concise
a decreased amount (number) of	less (fewer)
a number of	many, several
accounted for by the fact	because
along the lines of	similar, like
an adequate amount of	enough
as a consequence of	because of
as of this date	today
at a period of time when	when
at this point in time	now
by means of	with, by
consensus of opinion	consensus
due to the fact that	because
during the course of	during, while
fewer in number	fewer
for the purpose of	for, to
for the reason that	since, because
give an account of	describe
has been engaged in the study of	has studied
has the capability of	can
in a position to	can
in an effort to	to
in all cases	all, always
in close proximity to	near
in excess of	more than
in my opinion, I think	I think
in order to	to
in regard to	about

Continued

Unnecessary Words in Writing   Continued

in the event that	if
in view of, in view of the fact that	because
it has been reported by Smith	Smith reported
it would appear that	apparently
make reference to	refer to
many in number	many
of great benefit	beneficial
on account of	because
on the basis of	because, from
prior to (in time)	before
regardless of the fact that	even though
subsequent to	after
take into consideration	consider
the majority of, the vast majority of	most
with reference to	about
X-year period of time	X years

Adapted from Day, R.A. (1998). *How to write and publish a scientific paper* (5th ed.). Phoenix, AZ: Oryx Press, pp. 238–243; & Huth, E.J. (1999). *Writing and publishing in medicine* (3rd ed.). Baltimore: Williams & Wilkins, pp. 189–190.

APPENDIX 3

CONSORT (Consolidated Standards of Reporting Trials)	CONSORT Statement is intended for use in reporting a randomized controlled trial (RCT). It includes checklist and flow diagram available at http://www.consort-statement.org/consort-statement/ CONSORT Explanation and Elaboration Document enhances use and understanding of CONSORT Statement. It includes examples and explanations for each item in checklist. Available at http://www.consort-statement.org/extensions/extensions/
COPE (Committee on Publication Ethics)	COPE is concerned with integrity of peer-reviewed publications in biomedicine. Its Code of Conduct has defined best practice in ethics of scientific publishing to assist authors, editors, and others. Available at http://publicationethics.org/files/u2/Best_Practice.pdf. COPE has developed flowcharts that provide algorithms for editors if they suspect publication misconduct. Flowcharts and many other useful materials are available at http://publicationethics.org/
GPP (Good Publication Practice) Guidelines	GPP guidelines are intended to ensure that clinical trials sponsored by pharmaceutical companies are published in ethical manner. Available at http://www.gpp-guidelines.org/
ICMJE (International Committee of Medical Journal Editors) Uniform Requirements	ICMJE is group of medical journal editors who developed and update Uniform Requirements for Manuscripts Submitted to Biomedical Journals. Uniform Requirements document includes guidelines on ethical considerations, publishing and editorial issues, manuscript preparation, references, and other information relevant to writing for publication. Available at http://www.icmje.org/urm_main.html
PRISMA (Preferred Reporting Items for Systematic reviews and Meta-Analyses)	PRISMA Statement guides authors in reporting systematic reviews and meta-analyses; was referred to earlier as QUOROM (QUality Of Reporting Of Meta-analyses). PRISMA Statement is a 27-item checklist for reporting these reviews and flow diagram for identifying process used for the review and studies included at different phases. Provides Word templates that can be downloaded for authors' use, including a flow diagram, and other resources that can be accessed at PRISMA Website. Available at http://www.prisma-statement.org/

Continued

351

Guidelines and Resources for Preparing Manuscripts   *Continued*

SQUIRE (Standards for QUality Improvement Reporting Excellence)	SQUIRE guidelines should be used when preparing manuscripts on QI projects to adequately report: problem that led to QI project, intervention or initiative developed to solve it, setting, outcomes, and local conditions. Available at http://www.squire-statement.org/
STROBE (STrengthening the Reporting of OBservational studies in Epidemiology)	STROBE is a checklist for reporting items that should be included in articles describing observational research (case-control, cohort, and cross-sectional studies). Available at http://www.strobe-statement.org/index.php?id=strobe-home
WAME (World Association of Medical Editors) Policy Statements	Nonprofit voluntary, international association of editors of peer-reviewed medical journals. Developed resources for medical editors, which also are useful for authors. Available at http://www.wame.org/resources

INDEX

The letter *e* following a page number denotes an exhibit. The letter *f* following a page number denotes a figure. The letter *t* following a page number denotes a table.

DATE DUE			

Cressman Library
Cedar Crest College
Allentown, PA 18104